Neurorehabilitation
A MULTISENSORY APPROACH

SHEREEN D. FARBER, M.S., OTR, FAOTA

Associate Professor of Occupational Therapy
Division of Allied Health Sciences
Indiana University School of Medicine
Indianapolis

W. B. SAUNDERS COMPANY
Philadelphia/London/Toronto/Mexico City/Rio de Janeiro/Sydney/Tokyo

W. B. Saunders Company: West Washington Square
                           Philadelphia, Pa. 19105

                           1 St. Anne's Road
                           Eastbourne, East Sussex BN21 3UN, England

                           1 Goldthorne Avenue
                           Toronto, Ontario M8Z 5T9, Canada

                           Apartado 26370 – Cedro 512
                           Mexico 4, D.F., Mexico

                           Rua Coronel Cabrita, 8
                           Sao Cristovao Caixa Postal 21176
                           Rio de Janeiro, Brazil

                           9 Waltham Street
                           Artarmon, N.S.W. 2064, Australia

                           Ichibancho, Central Bldg., 22-1 Ichibancho
                           Chiyoda-Ku, Tokyo 102, Japan

Library of Congress Cataloging in Publication Data

Farber, Shereen D.

Neurorehabilitation: a multisensory approach.

1. Physically handicapped – Rehabilitation.   2. Nervous
   system – Diseases.   I. Title. [DNLM: 1. Central nervous
   system diseases – Therapy. WL 300 F221n]

RD798.F37   616.8'046   81–50835

ISBN 0–7216–3571–7   AACR2

Neurorehabilitation: A Multisensory Approach   ISBN   0-7216-3571-7

Last digit is the print number: 9   8

To Stephan Patrick Hagan
who will always be a miracle

and

To Mark Orrin Farber, M.D.
who will always be an inspiration.

CONTRIBUTORS

CATHERINE ERICKSON BARRETT, M.S., OTR

Adjunct Assistant Professor of Occupational Therapy, Division of Allied Health Sciences, Indiana University School of Medicine; Doctoral Candidate in Adult Education, Indiana University and Clinician, Activity Therapy, St. Francis Hospital, Beechgrove, Indiana

DAVID L. FELTEN, M.D., Ph.D.

Associate Professor of Anatomy and Neurobiology, Departments of Anatomy and Psychiatry (Joint Appointment), Indiana University School of Medicine

SUZANNE Y. FELTEN, Ph.D.

Post-Doctoral Fellow, Department of Pharmacology, Indiana University School of Medicine

SHEREEN D. FARBER, M.S., OTR, FAOTA

Associate Professor of Occupational Therapy, Division of Allied Health Sciences, Indiana University School of Medicine; Doctoral Student in Anatomy, Department of Anatomy, Indiana University School of Medicine

JUDITH HUNT KIEL, M.S., OTR

Assistant Professor of Occupational Therapy, Division of Allied Health Sciences, Indiana University School of Medicine

ZONA R. WEEKS, M.S., OTR

Associate Professor of Occupational Therapy, Division of Allied Health Sciences, Indiana University School of Medicine; Doctoral Candidate in Educational Psychology, Indiana University

SAMMY WILLIAMS, M.S., RPT

Formerly Instructor in Physical Therapy, Division of Allied Health Sciences, Indiana University School of Medicine; Consultant in Private Practice

FOREWORD

For many years various proponents of sensorimotor treatment approaches have, through their written and spoken word, challenged us to develop a better understanding of how the nervous system functions and how we may influence that function through therapy. At times, because each proponent was coming from a slightly different knowledge or clinical base or both, it seemed that the theories were in conflict or that suggested treatments were diametrically opposed. Yet empirical evidence indicated that the concepts worked. Perhaps some worked better than others or different approaches worked better for individual professionals or clients than others did. As a result, some professionals became convinced that one approach was better and consequently closed their minds to investigation of the alternatives. Some took bits and pieces from several approaches and did not take the time to thoroughly understand the total frame of reference for any of them. Others tried to meld the approaches, sometimes with success, but perhaps more often meeting with frustration. Yet no one approach has all of the answers for every patient.

Now at last, after many years of clinical practice involving patients with a wide variety of ages and disabilities, plus intensive study in the neurosciences and the various treatment approaches, Shereen Farber and her colleagues have bridged that gap for us. This book has been in process for seven years. It is thorough and well documented, logical in its approach and highly readable. Readers will be challenged to look at their current practice and to fill in whatever gaps there may be in knowledge and/or practice.

We are indeed indebted to Mrs. Farber for her major effort on our behalf. Many years ago she accepted the challenge of her teacher/mentor to pursue this area of study. She has now far surpassed that teacher, which is the greatest reward any mentor can receive. May we accept the challenge she offers to us and continue to develop our expertise.

A. Joy Huss, M.S., OTR, RPT, FAOTA
Associate Professor of Occupational Therapy
University of Minnesota

PREFACE

The purpose of this text is to synthesize current neurophysiological principles, sensorimotor integrative treatment rationales and techniques into a generic model of neurorehabilitation. The treatment approach presented in the text will be continually modified as research and practice elucidate new, effective methods of normalizing central nervous system function. All chapters are dovetailed in content design, and relevant research is cited whenever possible to increase the accountability.

It is hoped that this text will not be used as an end in and of itself but instead will serve to motivate the reader to further study, research and development of treatment principles. The book is intended for use by health professionals on many levels, and the author actively encourages their input to enhance its appeal.

SHEREEN D. FARBER

ACKNOWLEDGMENTS

In the writing of any manuscripts, many debts are incurred. My thanks go to:

The pioneers in sensorimotor and sensory integration treatment upon whose work we have built our current concepts.

A. Joy Huss, M.S., OTR, RPT, FAOTA, who opened the door to a whole new world of treatment concepts and gently pushed me through it.

Josephine C. Moore, Ph.D., OTR, FAOTA, whose encouragement over the years has helped me grow.

My students and patients, who have continually raised questions for which I had to seek answers.

The many therapists and scientists who read sections of the manuscript and provided helpful input.

Rebecca E. Porter, M.S., RPT, my partner and friend, for her content contributions and critique.

My former Program Director, Carol Nathan, A.M., OTR, FAOTA, whose encouragement and flexibility made an all too busy schedule liveable.

Anita Slominski, OTR, FAOTA, my first supervisor, who taught me to swim against the current.

Catherine Erickson Barrett, M.S., OTR, who, in addition to being a superb illustrator, is an innovator.

All my collaborators in this text for their great efforts.

The editorial staff at W. B. Saunders Co., especially Wendy Phillips.

My 9-year-old twin daughters, Aimee and Alison, whose forbearance during the writing of this manuscript belies their age.

Last but certainly not least, my husband Mark, who in addition to making significant editorial contributions to this text, provided me with essential emotional support and backrubs.

CONTENTS

CHAPTER 1

A REGIONAL AND SYSTEMIC OVERVIEW OF FUNCTIONAL NEUROANATOMY

David L. Felten, M.D., Ph.D.
and
Suzanne Y. Felten, Ph.D.

This chapter provides a functional overview of the nervous system. It is intended as a framework or as a foundation in neuroanatomy from both a regional and a systemic perspective. Illustrations are designed to provide a three-dimensional picture of the nervous system. An atlas at the end of the chapter includes cross-sections and a few sections of other orientations, labeled with structures mentioned in the discussion. The reader can refer to the atlas for structures not drawn in the illustrations.

We consider the basic neurosciences, particularly functional neuroanatomy, to be necessary for an understanding of the treatment of neurologically damaged patients. It is our belief that therapists lacking an understanding of the nervous system will be unable to synthesize a neurorehabilitation approach and will instead be dealing with scattered fragments of data. The basic neurosciences must provide the rationale for neurorehabilitative therapy as new research findings come to light.

THE THREE-NEURON NERVOUS SYSTEM

The human nervous system is extremely complex; it receives and interprets all outside stimuli, it integrates information from the outside world with that from inside the body, and it initiates appropriate responses to the environment, including all movements and all behavioral acts. The human central nervous system (CNS) contains close to a trillion (10^{12}) neurons, and connections between these neurons approach ten thousand trillion (10^{16}). The connections are not random but are highly organized and precise. These connections can be considered as specific systems performing specific functions and processing specific information. The organization of neural tissue into systems becomes clearer if we examine the nervous system of a primitive animal, the sponge. This will permit a brief look at steps in the evolution of the human nervous system.

The nervous system appears in sponges as a derivative of the ectoderm in contact

External environment

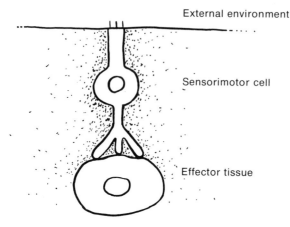

Sensorimotor cell

Figure 1–1. One-neuron nervous system.

Effector tissue

with the external environment. This modified ectoderm responds to noxious stimuli and causes the animal to withdraw from them. This primitive nervous system is a *one-neuron nervous system* in which a single type of nerve cell both receives external stimuli and initiates a withdrawal response by causing the contraction of muscles (effector tissue) (Fig. 1–1). Direct contact of nervous tissue with the external environment has persisted throughout evolution and is still present in the human (e.g., cutaneous receptors). However, to permit a diversity of response, the same neuron in humans that responds to external stimuli does not directly contact effector tissue. As the nervous system developed phylogenetically, specialization of neural tissue into sensory neurons in contact with the environment, and motor neurons in contact with effector tissue, occurred. This specialization produced a *two-neuron nervous system* found in coelenterates (Fig. 1–2). The sensory neuron in this system no longer interacts directly with the effector tissue. Rather, the sensory neuron conveys the stimulus to a second neuron, the motor neuron, which then communicates with the effector tissue, initiating a motor action in response to the sensory input. The motor neuron is no longer in contact with the external environment but is totally within the organism.

The direct communication between sensory input neurons and motor output neurons has persisted throughout evolution and can be clearly seen in humans in the form of *muscle stretch reflexes* (sometimes called *deep tendon reflexes*). This reflex is initiated by applying a sensory stimulus to a muscle tendon (a tap or stretch of the tendon with the reflex hammer). The stretching of the muscle activates the receptor of a sensory neuron. The sensory neuron communicates directly with a motor neuron in the spinal cord. The motor neuron communicates directly with the muscle being stretched and causes that muscle to contract. The same organization of neurons that originally evolved to allow

External environment

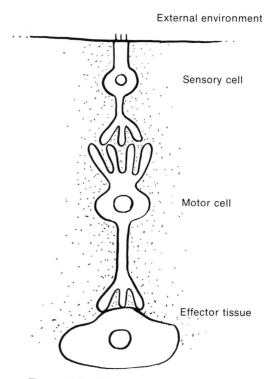

Sensory cell

Motor cell

Effector tissue

Figure 1–2. Two-neuron nervous system.

quick response to noxious stimuli has persisted in the human as a system that permits the unconscious regulation and maintenance of a particular state of muscle activity.

Such a reflex mechanism through just two types of neurons, *sensory* and *motor*, allows little flexibility in the behavior of the organism. Direct contact between sensory and motor neurons permits only a contraction or noncontraction of the effector tissue, an all-or-none response. It does not allow for a partial, or graded, response, nor does it allow the response to be integrated with other stimuli being received by the organism. Advanced behavior and adaptive responses require more complex processing between the sensory input and the motor output. This intermediate system of information processing is made possible by the addition of a third kind of neuron to the two-neuron nervous system, the *interneuron*. This final neuronal addition to nervous system evolution is present in worms and all other more advanced animals, including humans. It is designated the *three-neuron nervous system* and represents the most advanced and flexible of nervous system patterns (Fig. 1–3). The interneuron provides more processing of incoming information and allows more flexibility in the response.

This three-neuron nervous system has reached its highest level of development in the human brain. Specialization and complex communication networks have expanded the role of interneurons to the point to which the entire human brain, with the exception of a few million motor neurons supplying muscles of the head and neck, consists entirely of interneurons. Our ability to think, write, speak, and perform any complex action is based upon the functioning of interneurons. These interneurons are not in direct contact with either the external environment or the effector tissue but are clustered together into a complex central network — the CNS.

As complex as the human nervous system is, it can be broken down into basic components for study. The human nervous system can be thought of as having two basic parts: (1) a *peripheral nervous system* (PNS) that is in contact with the environment; and (2) a *central nervous system* (CNS) that is responsible for processing information and providing an appropriate

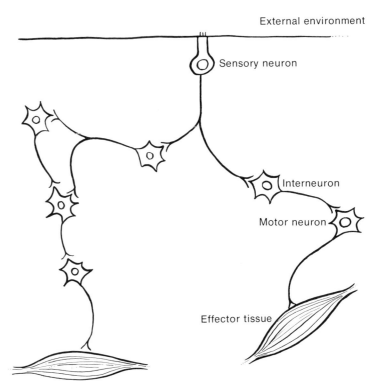

Figure 1–3. Three-neuron nervous system.

External environment

Sensory neuron

Interneuron

Motor neuron

Effector tissue

response to the environment. The PNS has a somatic component consisting of sensory input (sensory receptors and neurons) and motor output (axons and the neuromuscular junction of motor neurons) that controls the contraction of skeletal muscles. The PNS also has an autonomic component that controls smooth muscles, cardiac muscle, and glands, allowing for the continuous regulation of both basal homeostatic and stress-related functions of the body. This *autonomic nervous system* (ANS) is further subdivided into two components, the *sympathetic nervous system* (SNS) and the *parasympathetic nervous system* (PsNS). The sympathetic component is a widespread system that responds to stress by causing a general arousal and readiness of the body to cope with the perceived situation, often called a "fight or flight" response. The parasympathetic component is responsible for the control of homeostatic functions necessary for the well-being, basic maintenance, and repair of the body. An example of PsNS function is normal digestion.

The CNS is composed of a brain and a spinal cord. The spinal cord receives axons of sensory neurons bringing information into the CNS from the body. It also contains the cell bodies of the motor neurons and central autonomic neurons whose axons leave the spinal cord to exert control over effector tissue. The bulk of the spinal cord is made up of interneurons that mediate incoming sensory information and outgoing motor and autonomic information, and fiber tracts that represent communication channels with higher structures in the brain. The brain can be divided into a *brain stem* and a *forebrain*. The brain stem has four basic anatomical subdivisions continuing upward (rostrally) from the spinal cord. These are the *medulla*, the *pons*, the *midbrain*, and the *cerebellum*, which is associated with all three of the other subdivisions. The brain stem receives sensory input from general and special sensory systems of the head and neck and contains motor and central autonomic neurons supplying the head and neck and portions of the viscera. In this manner, the organization of the brain is similar to that of the spinal cord. In addition, the brain stem contains mechanisms and structures for more sophisticated sensory, motor, and

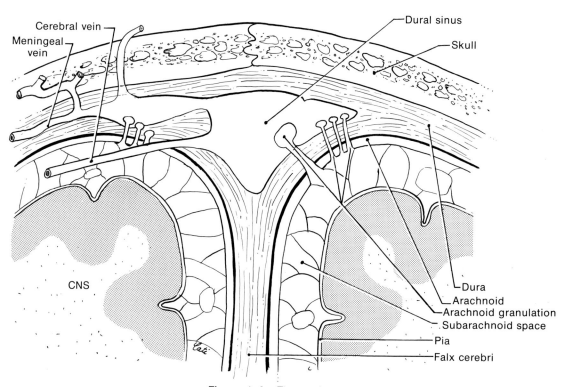

Figure 1–4. The meninges.

autonomic processing that are capable of integrating and coordinating this processing (e.g., respiratory rhythm, control of body tone, and eye movement responses to head position). The forebrain can be divided into a *diencephalon*, including mainly the thalamus and the hypothalamus, and a *telencephalon*, including the olfactory system, the limbic system, the basal ganglia (corpus striatum), and the neocortex. The functional role of these higher centers of the brain will be discussed later in this chapter.

In addition to the organization of neuronal structures of the brain, the study of the nervous system must also include its coverings, the meninges, and two fluid systems, the blood supply and the cerebrospinal fluid. The *meninges* comprise three layers of membranes covering the brain. The innermost layer, the *pia*, adheres very closely to the surface of the brain. The second layer, the *arachnoid*, encloses both the subarachnoid space, which contains the CSF, and the arteries and veins supplying the cortex. The third

or outer layer, the *dura*, is a tough protective membrane itself composed of two layers (Fig. 1–4). Major venous sinuses that drain blood from the brain lie between its two layers. The outermost layer is tightly adherent to the bones of the skull.

The blood supply to the brain comes from two sources: (1) two vertebral arteries that unite to form the basilar artery on the ventral midline surface of the pons, supply most of the brain stem; and (2) the internal carotid arteries supply most of the forebrain. The two arterial systems are connected at the base of the brain by communicating branches, forming the *circle of Willis* (Fig. 1–5). The venous blood drains into the major venous sinuses through superficial and deep veins. The sinuses then drain into the internal jugular veins. The *cerebrospinal fluid* (CSF), found in both the subarachnoid space and the ventricles within the brain, is an ultrafiltrate of blood. It is produced by the choroid plexus from arterial blood and by leakage of the extracellular fluid into the ventricular cavities

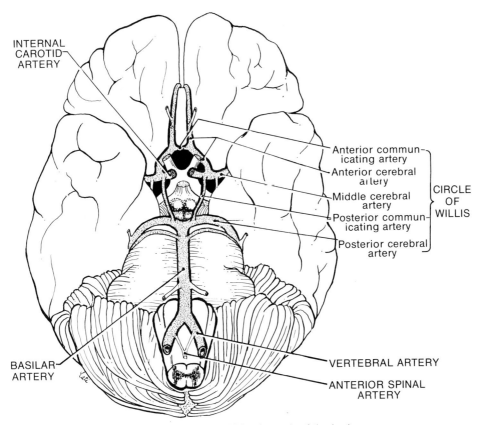

INTERNAL CAROTID ARTERY

Anterior communicating artery
Anterior cerebral artery
Middle cerebral artery
Posterior communicating artery
Posterior cerebral artery

CIRCLE OF WILLIS

BASILAR ARTERY

VERTEBRAL ARTERY

ANTERIOR SPINAL ARTERY

Figure 1–5. Arterial blood supply of the brain.

of the brain. The CSF circulates through the ventricular system, escapes into the subarachnoid space through foramina (the foramen of Magendie and the foramina of Luschka) at the caudal end of the fourth ventricle in the medulla, circulates around the external surface of the brain and spinal cord, and is absorbed into the venous blood through specialized one-way valve structures of the arachnoid, the *arachnoid villi*. The CSF provides a hydraulic cushion to protect the brain from contact with the hard bone of the skull and may provide a communication channel for CSF-borne substances to influence neurons.

The foregoing discussion provides a very general basic plan of the nervous system. Understanding the nervous system requires a knowledge of how the neuron functions and how groups of neurons function together as systems. The characteristics and properties of the neuron will be discussed next. The nervous system itself can be organized and studied in two different but complementary ways, regionally and systemically. Both of these organizations will be used to provide a framework for study. The PNS, including both somatic and autonomic components, will be discussed first, followed by a regional overview of the central nervous system. Finally, the nervous system will be studied longitudinally, according to functional systems.

NEURONS AND SUPPORTING CELLS

The Neuron

Morphological Characteristics of Neurons

The *neuron* is the fundamental unit of the nervous system. Its function is to communicate coded information over a distance. That distance may be very short, as with a local interneuron, or very long, as with a motor neuron whose cell body is in the spinal cord and whose axon terminates on a muscle of the foot. The neuron achieves this conduction of information by carrying an electrical potential down its axon. The shape of the neuron is particularly conducive to this function of information transport. Typically, the cell body

(soma) has two kinds of processes, called *neurites*, extending from it. *Dendrites* are usually relatively short and local. It is generally accepted that they receive information from other neurons and pass that information toward the cell body (Fig. 1–6). The branching patterns of dendrites may be very distinctive, reflecting the type and amount of information that a specific neuron is collecting. The other type of process is the *axon*. It usually originates at the cell body and is the long process through which the neuron communicates with other neurons or effector structures. Each neuron has one axon leaving the cell body, but that axon may branch to form several processes called *axon collaterals*. These collaterals may each communicate with different parts of the nervous system. Very near its end, the axon gives off a spray of fibers called *terminal arborizations*. Each of these arborizations has at its end specialized structures called *axon terminals* (or boutons). The terminal is in close proximity either to another neuron or to the effector tissue in the case of the PNS outflow. This gap between one neuron and another, or between neuron and effector tissue, is called a *synapse*. The flow of electrical information in a neuron is generally from the dendrites to the cell body, through the axon to the terminals, carrying the message toward the next neuron in that chain of communication or toward the effector tissue. Figure 1–6 shows a schematic representation of the basic neuron and a few examples of neurons with specific shapes.

The form and structure of each neuron reflects the role of that neuron. Very specific connections exist between neurons, establishing communication channels that may extend over long distances and may be composed of a chain of many neurons. The anatomy of these communication channels, called *neuronal connections* or *projections*, determines the hierarchical relationships and influences that one neuron population exerts over other neurons. A knowledge of these connection patterns is essential for the adequate evaluation of neurological disorders and their therapy. For example, a spinal cord injury removes motor neurons from the control of higher centers in the brain by severing or damaging descending pathways. Removal of this control, which normally holds these

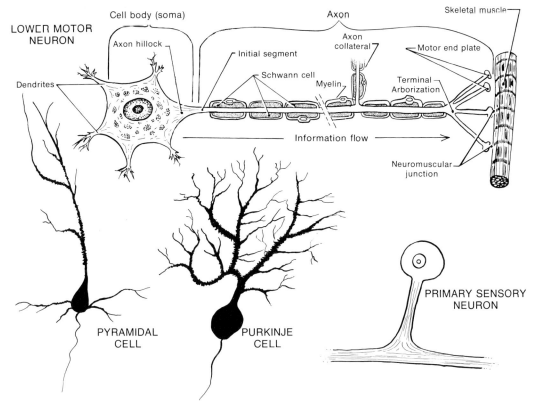

Figure 1–6. Cytologic features of neurons at the light microscopic level.

neurons in check and regulates their response to incoming sensory stimuli, results in hyperexcitability and over-responsiveness of spinal cord lower motor neurons (LMNs), manifested in the patient as spasticity. A knowledge of which connections were destroyed and which connections remain intact provides a rational basis for the therapy of such a patient.

Electrical Properties of Neurons

Understanding how neurons transfer information and how that information can be altered by outside influences can help to explain the mechanisms by which groups of neurons act together as integrated systems. The neuron has two properties that allow it to transfer information, *conductivity* and *neurotransmission*. The neuronal cell membrane is an excitable membrane; it is capable of conducting an electrical impulse over a distance. Because of the ionic balance that exists between the cytoplasm of a neuron and the extracellular fluid, an electrical potential, called the *resting po-*

tential, exists across the cell membrane. The resting potential is produced by the properties of the neuronal membrane itself, particularly the differential permeability of the membrane to sodium (Na^+) and potassium (K^+) ions. The resting potential is normally a voltage of approximately -70 mV. Excitation of the membrane causes that potential to change. If the stimulus is strong enough to allow the membrane potential to reach a higher specific voltage, called the *threshold*, the neuron fires an action potential. The *action potential* represents a special way of conducting an electrical impulse over a long distance, the whole length of the axon, without it dying out. That is to say, the action potential is nondecremental (does not decrease in size) over the whole length of the axon, even a meter or more. This is in contrast to the graded potential caused by the original stimulation. The *graded potential*, a small change of the membrane voltage away from the resting potential, will decay or die out after a short distance if it does not reach threshold. In general, graded potentials are carried by dendrites and cell bodies, while action potentials are carried by axons. The graded potential allows a great deal of flexibility in processing in the nervous system because it can be summed. In contrast to the action potential that, if it fires, is always a constant size and speed for a given neuron, under constant ionic conditions the graded potential may be increased owing to several inputs arriving at the neuron at the same time (*spatial summation*) or to individual inputs repetitively arriving so rapidly that the graded potential has not had a chance to die out (*temporal summation*). This means that increasing the input to a given neuron can cause it to fire an action potential. It also means that if one form of input is lost due to injury or disease, resulting in a failure of a given population of neurons to function, those neurons may then be caused to fire by increasing the input from another source. This principle is the basis for therapy of some disorders.

Neurotransmission

When an action potential reaches the axon terminal, it causes the membrane potential of that terminal to increase (i.e., to go from −70 mV toward 0). This change reduces the negativity of the potential across the membrane and is called *depolarization*. Depolarization of the nerve terminal results in the release of a chemical substance called a *neurotransmitter*. The release of neurotransmitter depends on the presence of calcium ion (Ca^{++}), which enters the cell during depolarization and permits the release of the neurotransmitter from the cytoplasm or from the prepackaged subcellular compartment, the *synaptic vesicle*. The vesicles in most terminals are approximately 50 nm in diameter, contain the neurotransmitter, will combine with the nerve terminal membrane in the presence of Ca^{++}, and will release the transmitter into the synaptic cleft. The vesicle membrane is later recycled (Fig. 1–7) by a process of *pinocytosis* (pinching off a membrane). The membrane of the axonal terminal pinches off fuzzy-coated vesicles inside the terminal, which then merge to form a cisternal apparatus. This apparatus then pinches off recycled synaptic vesicles, ready for use again in the process of *neurotransmission*. The neurotransmitter diffuses across the synapse between the neuron and the target cell, where it combines with receptors on the target cell surface. The combination of a neurotransmitter with a receptor (a surface protein) causes a change in the membrane of the target cell. The change can cause (1) a decrease in the potential difference or voltage across the cell membrane (making it more positive), called a *depolarization*, or (2) an increase in the potential difference across the cell membrane (making it more negative), called a *hyperpolarization*. Both these potentials are graded potentials and can be summed. A depolarization raises the potential toward the threshold, making it easier for the cell to fire an action potential. If a single depolarization is strong enough or if enough depolarizations occur, threshold may be reached and the neuron will fire an action potential. A hyperpolari-

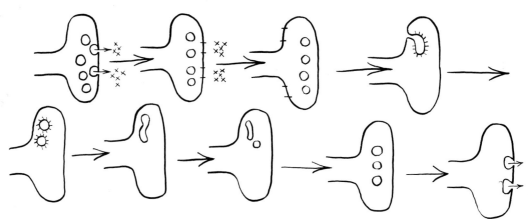

Figure 1–7. Recycling of vesicle membrane at a nerve terminal.

zation, on the other hand, lowers the potential away from the threshold, making it harder to fire an action potential. If a receptor response causes the depolarization of the cell membrane, it is excitatory, and the neurotransmitter stimulating it is called an *excitatory neurotransmitter.* Since it is generally accepted that only one neurotransmitter is released at a given synapse, this is an excitatory synapse. If a receptor response causes a hyperpolarization of the target cell membrane, it is inhibitory, and the neurotransmitter stimulating it is called an *inhibitory neurotransmitter.* This synapse is an inhibitory synapse. Recent evidence has shown that a single terminal may contain more than one neurotransmitter (for example, a catecholamine and a peptide), so this simplistic scheme of excitatory and inhibitory neurons may soon require extensive modification.

A nomenclature problem has developed as neurotransmitter research has demonstrated that a neurotransmitter can be excitatory at one kind of synapse and inhibitory at another. This seeming paradox is easily explained if it is realized that the single factor which determines whether the transmitter is excitatory or inhibitory is the receptor on the target cell, not the transmitter itself. The receptor on the target cell determines how that cell responds to the transmitter. The target cell membrane may contain receptors for many transmitters, but in general, a given neuron releases only one transmitter. A possible exception to this general rule is the peptide systems, which may synthesize and release more than one transmitter.

The evolution of chemical transmitters interacting with specific receptors provides the nervous system with additional flexibility in the processing of information. The neuron can sum information received from different sources, received at different rates, and received from both excitatory and inhibitory sources, and can integrate it to provide a single response based on the processing of a large amount of diverse information. It should be noted that other chemicals besides neurotransmitters may interact with receptors. Various drugs exploit an interaction with receptors in order to restore function when there is a lack of transmitter released, when the releasing neuron has been damaged, or when it is necessary to block the release or activity of a transmitter present in too high a quantity. These receptor interactions, whether excitatory or inhibitory, can be used to treat numerous disease states, such as Parkinson's disease, depression, and spasticity.

Patterns of Neuronal Connections and Interactions

Additional flexibility in information processing is brought about by diverse patterns of connections between neurons. The axon of one neuron may synapse with the dendrites of another neuron. This type of synapse is called an *axo-dendritic synapse.* Other types of synapses can occur, such as axons synapsing on cell bodies, called *axo-somatic synapses;* axons synapsing on axons, called *axo-axonic synapses,* dendrites synapsing on dendrites, called *dendro-dendritic synapses,* and so forth. Figure 1–8 illustrates the synaptic patterns just described. Because dendrites and cell bodies usually carry only graded potentials that may die out, synapses on these structures, especially if they are far from the axon, are less likely to cause an action potential to fire than a synapse near the origin of the axon. Synapses closest to the point at which the axon leaves the cell body, called the *axon hillock* (Fig. 1–6), are most likely to cause the firing of an action potential because the action potential originates at this point. A similar situation exists with inhibitory synapses.

Of particular interest is the axo-axonic inhibitory synapse on the axon terminal. It is the most effective way of preventing the axon action potential from releasing neurotransmitter at the axon terminal. If the terminal does not release a neurotransmitter, no message is communicated farther down the neuronal chain, even though an action potential did fire. This phenomenon, called *presynaptic inhibition,* depends upon an axo-axonic synapse.

Using a combination of excitatory and inhibitory synapses, sophisticated neuronal chains of control can be established. For example, Figure 1–9 illustrates a chain of three neurons. Each of the three neurons is excitatory, as indicated by the open cell body (closed cell bodies indicate inhibitory neurons). If A receives a stimulus, it

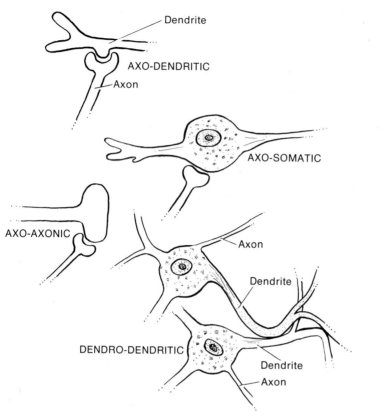

Figure 1–8. Types of synapses.

should be clear that it will excite B, which will excite C, which will excite the target tissue, T. In Figure 1–10, an inhibitory neuron has been introduced at B. A stimulus exciting A causes A to excite B. B, however, inhibits C and prevents it from firing. The target tissue is therefore not excited. Figure 1–11 adds a further complication. Both A and B are inhibitory. A will inhibit B and prevent it from inhibiting C. If C can receive an excitatory input from another source, or if it can fire spontaneously, the target tissue will be excited. This process of removing an inhibition is called *disinhibition* (or a release phenom-

enon). Disinhibition can occur when a previously inhibitory neuron is damaged, or when another inhibitory neuron inhibits the firing of the original inhibitory neuron. This happens in many motor disorders, such as spasticity, athetosis, and other involuntary movement disorders.

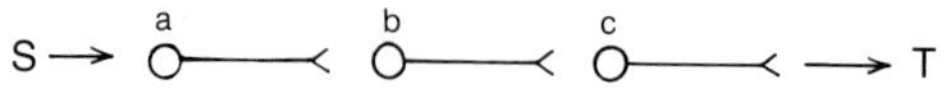

One more example of the possibilities of neuronal control mechanisms illustrates the process of feedback inhibition. Figure 1–12 shows neuron A exciting neuron B, which in turn excites the target tissue. However, an axon collateral from neuron B excites an inhibitory interneuron, C, which inhibits the firing of neuron A, causing the system to be shut off. As you can see from the foregoing discussion, neuronal control mechanisms can become very complicated and can involve chains of doz-

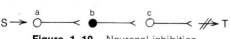

Figure 1–9. Neuron chain with excitatory influences.

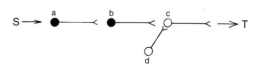

Figure 1–11. Disinhibition.

Figure 1–10. Neuronal inhibition.

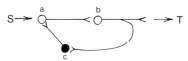

Figure 1–12. Collateral inhibition.

tonic mechanism

ens, or perhaps even hundreds of neurons. There are other examples of neuronal control that will be discussed with the systems in which they are active.

Neuronal Response to Injury and Manipulation

The foregoing discussion can aid in understanding of the manipulations that can be performed on a damaged or defective nervous system. Generally, neurons are not capable of replication in the adult brain, and only certain kinds of small neurons are still able to replicate during neonatal development. A dead neuron cannot be replaced or regenerated by cell division, in contrast to other organs such as liver or skin that can heal with new, functional cells. When a neuron is destroyed, its specific functions are permanently lost. When a neuron is damaged, it may cease to function altogether for a period of time, it may undergo a period of suboptimal or diminished function, it may totally recover its function and perform normally, or it may function in a hyperexcitable and excessive manner (producing seizure activity). If an axon is damaged in the PNS, regeneration of the distal portion of the axon may occur, accompanied by readjustments of metabolism by the cell body, a process called *central chromatolysis*. If an axon is damaged in the CNS, it is highly unlikely that appropriate regeneration of that axon or restoration of that function will occur. In the CNS, neuronal damage or cell loss can result in an anatomical and functional reorganization of remaining, intact neurons but not the destroyed neurons. When a specific input to a particular neuron, such as a motor neuron, is lost, as occurs in spinal cord injury, remaining neurons in the spinal cord or the dorsal root ganglia that are not damaged can sprout additional axonal terminals to reinnervate the partially denervated neuron. Neurons may be therapeutically facilitated to assume wider functional

(plasticity)

roles, such as when vestibular neurons are manipulated to influence motor tone in a cortically damaged patient. Perhaps neurons may also be therapeutically manipulated to assume new functional roles.

The limitations of therapy in neurological dyfunction must be clearly understood. The available therapeutic approaches, some occurring naturally and some aided by a therapist, include the following: (1) reinnervation and restoration of function in the PNS due to regeneration, generally achieved by nature, or aided by microsurgical reanastomoses of severed nerve fascicles; (2) recovery of function of neurons that have been temporarily but reversibly damaged, such as may occur in a stroke; (3) manipulation or stimulation of an intact system to overcome an imbalance produced by damage to another system (for example, use of vestibular manipulation to alter postural tone in a cortically damaged child, or administration of an anticholinergic drug to counterbalance the loss of a dopaminergic system in Parkinson's disease); (4) manipulation, stimulation or inhibition of a reorganized or reorganizing system following neurological damage (for example, training or eliciting reflex responses for bladder emptying or for sexual function following a spinal cord injury); (5) drug manipulation of intact neurons through alterations in neuronal metabolism, neuronal communication, or neuronal excitability; (6) surgical intervention to remove a mass, to restore a balance of functions, to temporarily alleviate pain, or to alter the hormonal milieu of the nervous system; and (7) transplantation of fetal neurons into a damaged adult brain.

Transplantation of fetal neurons into adult brain has only recently been achieved in experimental animals and has not been attempted in humans. However, the possibility exists that a fetal neuronal system, synthesizing and releasing a specific transmitter, could be transplanted to a damaged brain structure, where it could sprout axon terminals and reinnervate potentially functional but denervated structures. This has recently been achieved in a damaged (denervated) striatum of the rat, suggesting that fetal transplantation of dopaminergic cells to the striatum of a Parkinsonian patient may alleviate this disease. The future role for such therapy in the treatment of human neurological deficits still requires careful evaluation because of scientific, ethical, and sociological hurdles that must be overcome.

An additional approach to therapy involves altering neuronal functioning by environmental and other intangible influences not often viewed as part of current therapy for neurological disorders. Significant improvement of a patient's condition due to emotional and motivational factors is a real phenomenon and may exert a powerful influence on the progress of a neurologically damaged patient, through changes in neurotransmitter interactions. While the neurosciences cannot yet answer how these mechanisms work, or how emotional and cognitive factors interact in recovery from neurological disease, the empirical recognition and utilization of these phenomena is not to be overlooked. In some neurological conditions, the concern, determination, friendship, or empathy of the therapist may be equally as important as the actual physical benefits of therapy. It is admittedly difficult to teach a therapist how to persist in the face of overwhelming odds, how to truly care for the emotional well-being of a debilitated elderly patient, or how to emphathize with the hurt, the uncooperative, or the unlovely, but those who possess such capabilities should be given encouragement.

Supporting Cells

Neurons are supported by nonexcitable cells, called *glia* in the CNS and *Schwann cells* in the PNS. These cells help to insulate, separate, and protect neurons and may assist the neurons metabolically. These cells respond to injury by forming scar tissue and by phagocytizing debris. In the CNS the glia are of three types: astrocytes, oligodendroglia, and microglia. In addition, supporting ependymal cells line the ventricles of the brain and separate the cerebrospinal fluid (CSF) from the substance of the brain.

Astrocytes are responsible for forming scar tissue in response to injury. Within a week of the initial injury, astrocytes begin laying down fibrous processes that fill in spaces left open by the injury and add strength to the areas of necrosis and damage. Unfortunately, the astrocytic scar tissue can also form an irritative focus that can initiate seizure activity. Astrocytes also send *endfeet* (processes with bulbous endings) to contact the basement membranes of capillaries in the brain. Although tight junctions between adjacent cells linking the blood vessels exclude certain substances from the brain and form the cellular basis for a blood-brain barrier, the astrocytic endfeet may play a secondary role in the barrier by sequestering products, guarding the extracellular space, or inducing enzymes in the endothelial cells. Astrocytes also separate nerve cell bodies and processes by physically sending astrocytic processes between them.

Oligodendroglia are responsible for myelinating the axons of central neurons. *Myelin* is formed by the concentric wrapping around an axon of an oligodendroglial process that was formed from its cell membrane. The cytoplasm in the oligodendroglial processes is squeezed out during the wrapping, causing the membranes to abut each other, and forming a lamellar arrangement of wrapping around the axon. Myelin, which forms from fetal development through adolescence, is essential for normal nerve function. Its main purpose is to permit an increased speed of electrical conduction of the action potential down the axon. Proper speed permits accurate neuronal functioning. Any demyelinating disorder such as multiple sclerosis, or interference with normal myelination, results in slowed conduction velocity and incompetent functioning of the affected axons.

Microglia are very small phagocytes found in the CNS in response to an injury. They are the first glial cells to arrive at the injury and are found in abundance at the site for at least a week. As debris is removed, astrocytes move in and lay down fibrous scar tissue. The main task of microglia is removal of debris in the CNS.

Schwann cells are the supporting cells in the PNS. Their major functions are to separate, insulate, and myelinate axons. All peripheral axons have at least one layer of Schwann cell cytoplasm, called a *Schwann sheath*, surrounding them. Larger axons (greater than 2 μm) will have a complete myelin sheath formed from many concentric layers of Schwann cell membrane. Schwann cells can also respond to injury or to a degenerative process such as demyelination by phagocytosing debris. They can then divide and form new cells, which will remyelinate the axon. A Schwann cell can myelinate only one segment (one millimeter or so) of one peripheral axon, in contrast to oligodendroglia, which can myelinate one segment of many different central axons.

PERIPHERAL NERVOUS SYSTEM

Components

The extent of the peripheral nervous system (PNS) is easiest to define by exclusion: it comprises all the neural elements not in the brain and spinal cord. Because primary sensory, motor, and autonomic elements are all connected with the central nervous system (CNS), each has a peripheral as well as a central part. The peripheral parts can be subdivided into somatic and autonomic portions in the following manner:

Somatic Component

1. Sensory component, including receptors, primary sensory axons, and primary sensory cell bodies (found in the dorsal root ganglia).
2. Motor component, including the axons of lower motor neurons (LMNs) and the neuromuscular junction.

Autonomic Component

1. Sympathetic component, including preganglionic axons, ganglion cells, and their postganglionic axons.
2. Parasympathetic component, including preganglionic axons, ganglion cells, and their postganglionic axons.

Gross Anatomy of the PNS

There are two kinds of peripheral nerves, *spinal nerves* and *cranial nerves*. There are 31 pairs of spinal nerves. These are all mixed nerves containing more than one of the aforementioned sensory, motor, or autonomic components to the body. The cranial nerves supply these same functional components to the head and neck. The only difference, other than their area of supply, is that the individual cranial nerves are more specialized. Some of them are almost purely sensory, some are purely motor, and some are partially autonomic. Spinal nerves distribute to the body in a fairly regular pattern, based on their origin from the spinal cord. The 31 spinal nerves are distributed as follows: 8 cervical, 12 thoracic, 5 lumbar, 5 sacral, and 1 coccygeal.

The cervical nerves leave the spinal canal through the vertebral foramina rostral to their respective vertebrae except for cervical nerve 8, which leaves caudal to vertebra 7 (remember, there are only 7 cervical vertebrae). The rest of the spinal nerves leave the vertebral column caudal to their vertebrae. These nerves are numbered for their vertebral levels in the following manner: the first cervical nerve is designated C1; the second, C2, and so forth. The first thoracic is T1; the third lumbar is L3. The cervical nerves supply the shoulder and the upper limb. The thoracic nerves supply the body trunk in the thoracic and abdominal region. The lumbar and sacral nerves supply the lower limb and perineal region. Figure 1–13 shows the spinal nerves as they exit from the vertebral column.

Cranial nerves are designated by Roman numerals I through XII as well as by their individual names. Because their areas of distribution and their functions are not as regular as the spinal nerves, a brief summary has been provided in the section of this chapter on Regional Neuroanatomy (Table 1–4). These cranial nerves have been subdivided into their sensory, motor, and autonomic components. For a more complete and detailed review of these nerves as well as the precise distribution of the individual spinal nerves, one of the neuroanatomy textbooks listed in the bibliography should be consulted. Such detailed consideration is beyond the scope of this overview. Even though cranial nerves I (olfactory) and II (optic) have been included in the summary, they are really peripherally located tracts of the CNS, and should be considered part of the brain.

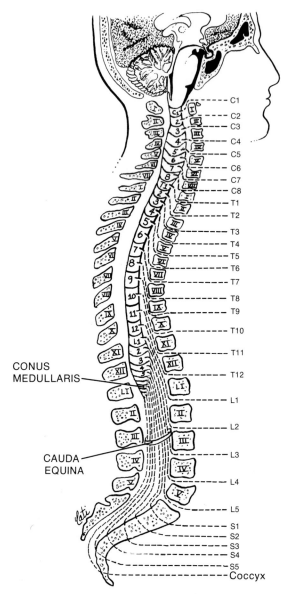

CONUS
MEDULLARIS

CAUDA
EQUINA

C1
C2
C3
C4
C5
C6
C7
C8
T1
T2
T3
T4
T5
T6
T7
T8
T9
T10
T11
T12
L1
L2
L3
L4
L5
S1
S2
S3
S4
S5
Coccyx

Figure 1–13. Spinal cord segments and their relationship to spinal nerves as they exit from the vertebral column.

Sensory Aspects of the PNS

There are many kinds of sensory receptors, but they all have one thing in common: They all act as transducers to convert various types of external stimuli into electrical impulses. We will not describe the anatomy of these receptors because we are more concerned with the kinds of information they can transform. For a detailed recounting of receptor anatomy, consult one of the major neuroanatomy textbooks cited at the end of the overview. Bear in mind that there is still no absolute correlation of morphological receptor types and the functional transductions they perform for specific modalities. For the body, these types of information (modalities) can be arranged as follows:

Epicritic Modalities (Somatic Sensation)

1. Fine, discriminative touch, vibration, two-point discrimination, stereognosis (the ability to determine the size, shape, and texture of an object by touch alone)
2. Proprioception, information concerning the action and position of muscles and joints
    (a) Conscious proprioception–joint position
    (b) Unconscious proprioception–muscle position and movement

Protopathic Modalities (Somatic Sensation)

1. Pain (both fast localized pain and slow, excruciating, poorly localized pain)
2. Temperature
3. Light moving touch

Special Senses

1. Vision
2. Olfaction
3. Audition
4. Vestibular proprioception, the position of the head in space (linear and angular acceleration)
5. Taste

Visceral Sensation

1. Painful sensation from the viscera
2. Nonpainful sensation from the viscera

Information transduced by the receptor is conveyed into the CNS by a primary sensory neuron. Its most distal part is the receptor and the initial segment immediately adjacent to the receptor. The initial segment is the portion of the axon in which the action potential is initiated, analogous to the axon hillock, except that it is not next to the cell body. The receptor can be

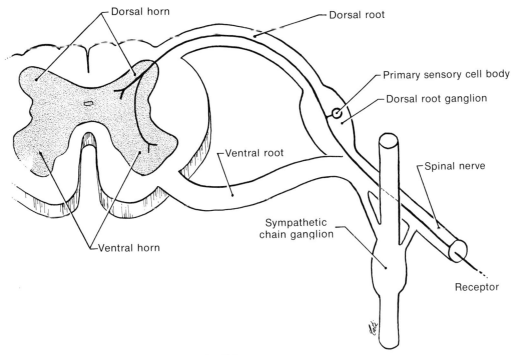

Figure 1–14. Primary somatosensory neuron.

functionally considered a dendrite. The rest of the process can be considered the axon, which continues into the spinal cord as part of a spinal nerve. The cell body of the primary sensory neuron is in the dorsal root ganglion, near the spinal cord. It does not have a part in carrying or initiating the action potential. The primary sensory cell body therefore mainly serves a trophic role to help nourish and maintain the process. After the axon passes through the dorsal root ganglion, it enters the spinal cord through the dorsal root (See Figure 1–14 for a summary of the anatomy and connections of a primary sensory neuron.) The central processing of the information conveyed by the primary sensory neurons will be discussed in more detail under the sections of spinal cord and sensory systems.

Motor Aspects of the PNS

The only component of the motor system found in the periphery is the axon of the LMN. Cell bodies of LMNs are found in the spinal cord anterior horn (*anterior horn cells*) and in *motor cranial nerve*

nuclei in the brain stem. The axon leaves the CNS with a cranial nerve, or with a spinal nerve after exiting through a ventral root. LMNs innervate skeletal muscle. Each motor axon innervates more than one muscle fiber and establishes a functional *motor unit*. When the axon carries an action potential to the terminals, all fibers of the motor unit contract together. In conditions in which LMNs are damaged or degenerating, aberrant discharges in LMNs lead to *motor unit twitches (fasciculations)*, which can be seen. The junctional complex, or synapse, between a LMN and the muscle is called a *neuromuscular junction* (NMJ), and the terminal of the LMN is called a *motor end plate*.

An action potential arriving at the terminal of a LMN depolarizes the terminal, causing the release of the neurotransmitter acetylcholine (ACh). ACh combines with a specific receptor on the muscle, causing it to depolarize, resulting in muscle contraction. In the total absence of ACh or other compounds that would bind with the receptor, the muscle will be unresponsive and flaccid. This is also true if the LMN itself is destroyed so that no neurotransmission can take place. The cholinergic (using ACh) receptors on the muscle also respond to the cutting of the nerve. Normally, receptors are clustered at the NMJ. When the nerve is lost, the receptors are then found all over the surface of the muscle, where they are sensitive to ACh circulating in the blood. Muscle twitches in this circumstance are not the result of normal neurotransmission from an intact nerve, but reflect the denervation hypersensitivity of the receptors. These twitches, called *fibrillations,* usually cannot be visually observed but can be detected by electrical recording, called *electromyography.*

ACh is removed from the receptor and is broken down by the enzyme acetylcholinesterase (AChE), also found on the muscle membrane. It is extremely important for normal nerve function that this enzyme be present and that it break down (hydrolyze) ACh. If it is not present and functioning properly, the ACh persisting in the synapse will cause continued stimulation of the receptor and continued contraction of the muscle that is no longer under complete neural control. With prolonged persistence of ACh in the cleft, the muscle membrane is chronically depolarized, resulting in total muscle paralysis.

Certain drugs have been developed that can be used to augment the action of ACh. For example, in the disease myasthenia gravis, either not enough ACh is produced or there are not enough receptors available to combine with the amount of ACh that is produced because of antibodies against the ACh receptors. A drug that blocks the action of AChE, called an *anticholinesterase,* is given so that the transmitter can persist in the synaptic cleft longer, increasing the chance that it will combine with receptors and cause muscle contraction. It should be clear that manipulation of the neurotransmitter — its synthesis, release, combination with a receptor, or its removal from the synapse and eventual metabolism — can be extremely important in controlling muscle activity. It should also be clear that without the presence of a LMN, the skeletal muscle cannot be made to function, no matter how much of a drug or manipulative therapy is used. Fortunately, peripheral nerves have the capacity to regenerate and repair themselves to some extent if the cell body has not been destroyed. In addition, other LMNs may be able to sprout and reinnervate muscles previously denervated. However, when the cell bodies have been destroyed, as in polio or a spinal cord crush injury at the level of total destruction, the neurons die and are not replaced. In these cases, no amount of treatment will help muscle tone or will restore even a small degree of movement.

Autonomic Aspects of the PNS

In general, the autonomic nervous system exists as a two-neuron chain. The first neuron has its cell body in the CNS and is called the *preganglionic cell.* Its axon, the preganglionic axon, is myelinated, leaves the CNS, and synapses in an autonomic ganglion. The ganglion contains cell bodies for the second neuron, called the *postganglionic neuron.* The postganglionic neuron synapses with the target tissue, which may be smooth muscle, cardiac muscle, or glands. The postganglionic axons are unmyelinated. The autonomic nervous system has two divisions, the sympathetic and the parasympathetic, which will be discussed separately.

Sympathetic Nervous System

The general action of the sympathetic nervous system is to cause arousal of the organism to prepare for "fight or flight" kinds of activity. The response of this system is widespread, preparing the whole body for activity. It is usually activated by the perception of stress and is not so much a reaction to a specific stimulus as a reaction to the nervous system's interpretation of that stimulus. It is particularly important for a therapist to realize, when working with a patient, that he may be responding to the manipulation as if it were stressful. The resultant activation of the sympathetics, with the concomitant tensing of muscles, increase in heart and respiration rate, and decrease in homeostatic mechanisms such as digestion may be undesirable and may interfere with therapy.

The anatomy of the sympathetic nervous system reflects its widespread effects. The preganglionic cell bodies are located in the spinal cord intermediate gray (Fig.

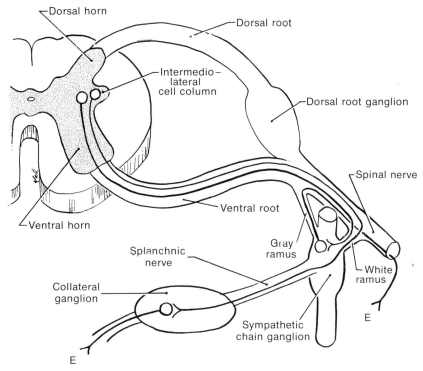

Figure 1–15. Sympathetic preganglionic neurons and ganglion cells.

1–15) of segments T1 through L2, also called the thoracolumbar region. These cell bodies are often described in the lateral horn, or intermediolateral cell column. However, recent evidence has demonstrated the presence of additional preganglionic sympathetic neurons in the medial regions of intermediate gray and in the dorsal commissural gray just above the central canal. The axons leave the spinal cord, traveling with the LMN axons through the ventral root, to a sympathetic chain ganglion that is attached to the spinal nerve near the vertebral column. The chain ganglion attaches to the spinal nerve by rami communicantes. The white ramus communicans (distal) contains myelinated preganglionic axons entering the ganglion, while the gray ramus communicans (proximal) contains unmyelinated postganglionic axons leaving the ganglion. There is a sympathetic chain ganglion for almost every spinal nerve, even though only the T1 to L2 segments of spinal cord have preganglionic sympathetic cells. This occurs because, while some of the preganglionic axons synapse on postganglionic cells located in the chain ganglion of the

same level, many preganglionic fibers go right through that ganglion and ascend or descend through connecting processes (rami) to another ganglion. Therefore, the chain ganglia are found from the neck all the way down to the pelvis. The chain ganglia supply specific structures in the head and neck and in the thoracic viscera, and also supply blood vessels (vasomotor fibers), arrector pili muscles (pilomotor fibers), and sweat glands (sudomotor fibers) in the periphery. These postganglionic fibers leave the chain ganglia through the gray rami communicantes and travel with the spinal nerves to their target structures, often hitchhiking along a blood vessel to reach their final destination.

Some preganglionic axons do not synapse in chain ganglia at all. They pass through the ganglia, forming bundles called *splanchnic nerves,* and eventually synapse in collateral, or paravertebral, sympathetic ganglia that are near the target organs. The postganglionic axons leave the ganglia to synapse on the target tissue directly. (See Figure 1–15 for a diagram of sympathetic neurons.) These synaptic structures are not like the usual nerve ter-

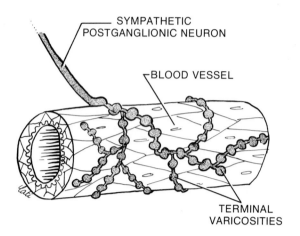

SYMPATHETIC
POSTGANGLIONIC NEURON

BLOOD VESSEL

TERMINAL
VARICOSITIES

Figure 1–16. Sympathetic terminal varicosities.

minal. They occur along the length of the terminal portion of the axon, as illustrated by Figure 1–16. The individual terminals are called *varicosities*, and this kind of synapse is called a *terminal en passage* because the axon does not end there. These synapses are different from the NMJ in that they have very wide synaptic clefts so that the neurotransmitter must diffuse over a much wider area. The presynaptic ending does not sit in close proximity to the postsynaptic site as does the cholinergic nerve ending to the NMJ.

Because the collateral ganglia are located near the organ innervated, the cell bodies are often intermingled with nerve terminals in this area. This combination of preganglionic axons and terminals, collateral ganglion cells, and postganglion axons and terminals, forms *plexuses*. A plexus also may contain both sympathetic and parasympathetic components. Therefore, the conglomeration of neural elements found on the ventral surface of the aorta and large blood vessels, and in or near many organs innervated, are located in plexuses. For details of the anatomy of the many peripheral plexuses, consult one of the major neuroanatomical textbooks cited at the end of this chapter.

The spreading out of the sympathetics from the relatively restricted preganglionic cells to the widely distributed ganglia, and the less specific nature of the synapses, provide anatomical evidence that the action of the sympathetic nervous system is widespread. In addition, the adrenal medulla, which produces mainly epinephrine (80 per cent) and some norepinephrine (20 per cent) for release

into the blood, can be considered a component of the SNS. The greater splanchnic nerves, arising from the thoracic chain ganglia (but not synapsing in them), contain preganglionic sympathetic axons that synapse on chromaffin cells of the adrenal medulla. Stimulation of these axons results in the release of epinephrine and norepinephrine into the blood, which carries these compounds to effector tissues, augmenting the action of the sympathetic nervous system. It should also be noted that adrenal corticosteroids, released by ACTH (adrenal corticotrophic hormone), a stress hormone from the anterior pituitary, can enhance production of catecholamines in the medullary chromaffin cells, further enhancing general sympathetic arousal.

The peripheral distribution of sympathetic nerves, once they leave the ganglia, usually follows blood vessels. For example, sympathetic supply to the head comes almost entirely from the superior cervical ganglion, the rostral-most ganglion of the sympathetic chain. Many of the postganglionic fibers travel along the surface of the carotid artery and its branches to reach their eventual terminations on smooth muscles (pupillary dilator muscle) and glands (mucosal glands) of the head. Some sympathetic fibers travel with nerves, but only rarely is a nerve entirely composed of postganglionic sympathetic fibers. (Remember that the splanchnic nerves are preganglionic sympathetic fibers.)

In general, the sympathetic nervous system functions as a single entity to prepare the body to cope with stress, particularly a dangerous or frightening situation. The pupils dilate, skin and gut blood vessels constrict, muscle blood vessels dilate, bronchioles dilate to allow passage of more air, heart rate increases, and more blood is pumped with each beat. Table 1–1 summarizes the actions of the sympathetic nervous system on various tissues. (Also consult the inventory in Chapter 2.)

The postganglionic sympathetic fibers achieve their effects on peripheral tissue by releasing the neurotransmitter norepinephrine (except for sweat glands, innervated by ACh). For this reason, they are called *noradrenergic* or *adrenergic neurons.* Many available drugs affect these neurons. The preganglionic cells use ACh as their neurotransmitter, as do the LMNs,

TABLE 1–1 SYMPATHETIC ACTIONS

Tissue	Action
Eye	
Pupil	Dilation by pupillary dilator muscle
Lens	Flattens lens for far vision by ciliary muscle relaxation
Eyelid	Elevation due to sympathetic nerve supply to levator palpebrae superioris muscle
Mucosal and salivary glands	Reduces blood flow through glands, produces small amounts of thick secretions
Blood vessels	
Skin	Constriction (causing pale skin)
Digestive system and other abdominal viscera	Constriction
Muscles	Dilation to provide increased nutrients and removal of metabolic wastes
Brain	Brain blood vessels normally respond more to presence or absence of oxygen in the blood, dilating when oxygen levels are low (and carbon dioxide levels are high). Brain regulates its own blood flow and does not have greatly increased nutritional demands during stress or sympathetic arousal
Heart	Increased rate, increased volume pumped per stroke, dilation of coronary blood vessels
Lungs	Dilation of bronchi and bronchioles
Digestive system	Decreased blood supply, decreased contractility and motility, decreased secretion of digestive enzymes
Liver	Increased release of glucose into blood
Thymus and spleen	Regulates immune responsiveness through transmitter influences on lymphocytes
Reproductive system	Ejaculation of semen, erection (actual engorgement of erectile tissue with blood is under parasympathetic control, but some sympathetic activity seems necessary for erection)
Urinary system	Inhibits urination by relaxing detrusor muscle of bladder
Skin	
Sweat glands	Secretion of sweat
Piloarrector muscles	Contraction, causing hair to stand on end
Adrenal medulla	Release of epinephrine and norepinephrine into blood

and are called *cholinergic neurons*. The difference is that the receptors on the postganglionic cells are different from those on muscles. They respond to the same transmitter, ACh, but they respond differently to other drugs that are applied to them. This is important pharmacologically because it allows the manipulation of one kind of receptor without necessarily causing the same effect on the other receptors. For example, a drug might be given that will partially block cholinergic receptors on muscle, causing relaxation of that muscle, but that drug will not block cholinergic preganglionic fibers from synapsing with ganglion cells of the autonomic nervous system. More details will be supplied concerning the pharmacological manipulation of the autonomic nervous system following the next section on the parasympathetic nervous system.

Parasympathetic Nervous System

The action of the parasympathetic nervous system is mostly homeostatic, allowing the maintenance and repair of the body. This is particularly true of the process of digestion, which depends extensively on the parasympathetic system. Sympathetic arousal virtually shuts digestion down. Parasympathetic stimulation is necessary for gut contractility, motility, and peristalsis, and secretion of digestive enzymes and other gut secretory products.

Anatomically, the parasympathetics are similar to the sympathetics in having a two-neuron chain, with preganglionic and postganglionic neuronal elements — but there the resemblance stops. The parasympathetic preganglionics have their cell bodies in two areas of the CNS. The first area, the cranial portion, is in the brain stem. Four cranial nerve nuclei contain parasympathetic preganglionic cells. These are: (1) the Edinger-Westphal nucleus, the parasympathetic portion of the oculomotor nucleus that sends fibers with cranial nerve III; (2) the superior salivatory nucleus that sends fibers with cranial nerve VII; (3) the inferior salivatory nucleus that sends fibers with cranial nerve IX; and (4) the dorsal motor (or efferent) nucleus of the vagus, whose fibers contribute to cranial nerve X. Figure 1–17 depicts a schematic view of the brain stem with the approximate locations of preganglionic cell bodies of the parasympathetic nervous system. The second area of preganglionic cell bodies is in the sacral spinal cord. These cells are located in the intermediomedial cell column of levels S2 to S4, the same zone of gray matter that contains some preganglionic sympathetics in the thoracolumbar regions. Because of the two locations of preganglionic cells, this portion of the autonomic system is often referred to as the craniosacral system.

The postganglionic neurons have their cell bodies in ganglia that are usually very close to, or actually part of, the organ innervated. In other words, preganglionic fibers of the parasympathetic nervous system are long, traveling to the organ innervated, while sympathetic preganglionic fibers are short, traveling to chain or collateral ganglia. As a result, the postganglionic parasympathetic fibers are rather short in comparison to the postganglionic sympathetic fibers that must travel to the organ innervated from their position closer to the spinal cord. In the head, there are specific ganglia associated with specific innervated structures. Most of the remaining postganglionic cell bodies are located in plexuses near the aorta or in the organs themselves. For example, the parasympathetic supply to the gut is located (1) in a plexus of cells between the longitudinal and circular smooth muscle layers of the gut wall (myenteric plexus, or Auerbach's plexus); and (2) in a submucosal plexus (Meissner's plexus). These particular arrangements allow coordinated constriction of the gut in order to pass its contents along. Table 1–2 gives the location of preganglionics, postganglionics, tissues innervated, and function of parasympathetic stimulation in that tissue.

Blood vessels are not supplied with parasympathetic fibers, but stimulation of the parasympathetic nervous system does affect the circulatory system by inhibiting the sympathetics. The result is dilation of gut and skin blood vessels, and dilation of the blood vessels involved in engorgement of erectile tissues.

Preganglionic parasympathetic cells are cholinergic (use ACh as a neurotransmitter) just like the preganglionic sympathetics; the postganglionic cells are also cholinergic, unlike the noradrenergic postganglionic sympathetics. But the postganglionic and effector tissue cholinergic receptors differ in their chemical and pharmacological characteristics.

Sympathetics and parasympathetics can exert their actions in one of two ways: They can cause primary effects by stimulating the target tissue or one can act to inhibit the other. This accounts for the effects of parasympathetics on blood vessels even though they have no parasympathetic innervation. In this case, parasympathetics inhibit sympathetic tone or constriction

and thereby cause dilation. In fact, both of these activities may occur at once. In the gut, sympathetics stop digestive processes partly by direct action and partly by inhibiting parasympathetic action. Often the sympathetics and parasympathetics oppose each other in action, but there are systems in which they complement each other, such as erection and ejaculation. In addition, during some behavioral states such as chronic stress, both systems may be active. The sympathetics may cause the release of catecholamines and a generalized arousal, while the parasympathetics cause increased gastric secretions, contributing to the production of stress ulcers.

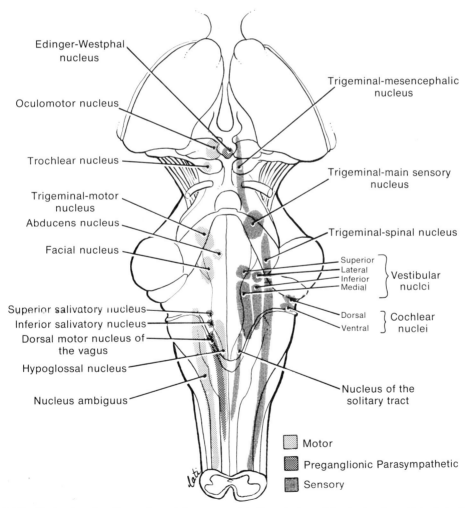

Figure 1–17. Brain stem locations of cranial nerve nuclei. Dorsal view of the brain stem. Note that all sensory nuclei are represented on the right side, and all motor and parasympathetic preganglionic nuclei are represented on the left side.

TABLE 1–2 PARASYMPATHETIC ACTIONS

Preganglionic Cell Bodies	Associated Cranial Nerve	Postganglionic Cell Bodies	Tissue Innervated	Function
Edinger-Westphal nucleus	III	Ciliary ganglion	Pupil Lens	Constriction of pupillary constrictor muscle; accommodation to near vision by contraction of ciliary muscle, causing thickening of lens
Superior salivatory nucleus	VII	Pterygopalatine ganglion	Lacrimal gland;	Increase secretions
			nasal mucosal glands	Increase secretions
		Submandibular ganglion	Salivary glands (submandibular sublingual)	Increase secretions
Inferior salivatory nucleus	IX	Otic ganglion	Parotid gland	Increase secretions
Dorsal motor nucleus of the vagus	X	Many plexuses around aorta and large blood vessels, in walls of innervated organs	Heart Lungs	Slow heart rate, decreases cardiac output Constricts bronchii
			Digestive system up to descending colon	Increase gut concontractility, mobility, peristalis; relax the sphincters; increase secretions of digestive enzymes
Sacral spinal cord intermediate gray (S2–S4)		Plexuses in many areas near the innervated organs	Digestive system below descending colon	Same as above
			Urogenital system	Increase motility of ureters, contraction of detrusor muscle for urination; erection of erectile tissue

Autonomic Neurotransmission

It is essential to have a general understanding of the actions of drugs on the autonomic nervous system, because many drugs given to patients affect autonomics either directly or indirectly. Terminology is a problem in discussing autonomic neurotransmission, so the following distinctions should be made before the details are given.

1. Adrenergic neurons are cells that use norepinephrine as a neurotransmitter.
2. Adrenergic receptors are receptors that recognize and respond to norepinephrine, epinephrine, or dopamine, such as the sympathetically innervated effector tissues.
3. Cholinergic neurons are cells that use ACh as a neurotransmitter.

4. Cholinergic receptors are receptors that recognize and respond to ACh, such as those on ganglion cells, on parasympathetically innervated effector tissue, or on skeletal muscles.

Even though all preganglionic autonomic axons, postganglionic parasympathetic axons, and LMN axons use ACh as a neurotransmitter to stimulate postsynaptic receptors, those receptors react differently to other drugs. It is known that nicotine will stimulate the cholinergic receptors normally stimulated by ACh from preganglionic autonomics and from LMNs, but not those normally stimulated by ACh from postganglionic parasympathetics. These postganglionic parasympathetic receptors are instead stimulated by muscarine and are called *muscarinic receptors*. Receptors sensitive to nicotine are called *nicotinic receptors*. This choice of designation is perhaps unfortunate because all nicotinic receptors are not equal. While they all respond to nicotine, they respond differently to still other drugs. For example, ganglionic blockers block the nicotinic receptors on ganglion cells normally stimulated by ACh but not the receptors at the NMJ, which are also nicotinic.

Adrenergic receptors are also of at least two different kinds. These are designated *alpha* and *beta receptors*. These types of receptors not only respond to different drugs, but they cause different effects on the postsynaptic site. In general, alpha receptors are excitatory except in the gut, where they are inhibitory; beta receptors are inhibitory except in the heart, where they are excitatory. Beta receptors can be further subdivided into beta$_1$ receptors (cardiac muscle, fat cells) and beta$_2$ receptors (bronchi, blood vessels). Recently alpha receptors have also been subdivided into at least two classes, alpha$_1$ (postsynaptic) and alpha$_2$ (presynaptic). These subdivisions are not rigid but may vary from one system to another.

The actions of many drugs are on the receptors. Drugs that block receptors are usually named for the kind of receptor they block (cholinergic blockers, ganglionic blockers, and adrenergic blockers). They are also called *antagonists*. Two very common antagonists for the cholinergic system are (1) the muscarinic blockers, atropine and scopalamine; and (2) the nicotinic blocker, curare. Common antagonists for the adrenergic receptors are: (1) alpha blockers, phentolamine and phenoxybenzamine, and (2) the beta blocker, propranolol. Drugs that mimic the affects of neurotransmitters are called *mimetics* (sympathomimetics, parasympathomimetics, and cholinomimetics). They are also called *agonists*.

Response of Peripheral Nerves to Injury

Peripheral neurons can be damaged in a number of ways: trauma, disease, toxic chemicals, and nutritional deficiencies. If the cell body is killed, no regeneration of the neuron can occur. After birth, peripheral neurons do not divide, and new neurons are not usually formed. However, if the injury occurs to the axon, if the damage is not too severe, and if the distal and proximal ends of the neuron are still close together, reinnervation can occur. The distal portion of the axon dies and is phagocytosed by Schwann cells (*Wallerian degeneration*), and sprouts extend from the proximal end of the damaged axons, grow into the intact "tube" left by the distal basement membrane, and travel to the target effector tissue, where reinnervation occurs. When the whole neuron is killed, it is possible that nearby neurons can sprout axonal processes and reinnervate the tissue. Sympathetic postganglionic axons (noradrenergic) are particularly able to sprout and reinnervate a denervated tissue.

Another kind of injury can occur to peripheral nerves. The neuron is dependent on the integrity of its myelin sheath for proper function. Demyelinating diseases can damage axons secondarily. If the Schwann cells cannot recover and cannot remyelinate the neuron, the neuron will first lose conduction velocity and eventually the unmyelinated segment will die. This problem can alter the function of sensory, motor, and autonomic nerves. However, since only the preganglionic autonomic axons are myelinated, this problem is mainly restricted to these neurons in the ANS.

SPINAL CORD

Gross Anatomy

The spinal cord lies in the vertebral canal, is surrounded by meninges, and is bathed in cerebrospinal fluid (CSF), as is the rest of the central nervous system (CNS). The spinal cord is divided into segments based on the spinal nerves associated with each segment. There are 31 segments grouped into four regions. From rostral to caudal these divisions are: (1) cervical spinal cord, with 8 segments; (2) thoracic spinal cord, with 12 segments; (3) lumbar spinal cord, with 5 segments; and (4) sacral spinal cord, with 5 segments, and a single coccygeal segment usually grouped with the sacral spinal cord.

During development, the vertebral column grows more rapidly than the spinal cord it encloses. Therefore, in the adult, vertebral levels do not correspond with spinal segments, even though they are often designated in the same way. For example, the designation C7 may refer to a vertebral level, to a spinal nerve, or to a segment of spinal cord. In this chapter we will use such a designation for the spinal segment only and will refer to the others more specifically as C7 vertebral level, or C7 spinal nerve. For example, it should be clear that an injury to a patient at the T8 vertebral level will injure the spinal cord at the T10 segment. It should also be clear that the spinal nerves are derived from cord segments of the same number. These nerves exit the vertebral column at the vertebral level of the same number. For instance, the T8 spinal nerve is derived from spinal cord segment T8 and must travel caudally within the vertebral canal to the T8 vertebral level (opposite T10 spinal cord segment) before it leaves the canal. In general, the cervical segments are about one segment different from the cervical vertebral levels. (The C5 vertebral level is approximately at the C6 spinal cord level.) The thoracic segments are about two segments different. (The T6 vertebral level is approximately at the T8 spinal cord level.) The T11 and T12 vertebral bodies correspond to the five lumbar spinal cord segments. The adult spinal cord ends at approximately the lower L1 vertebral level (see Fig. 1–13). The tapering end of the spinal cord in this area, composed of sacral spinal segments, is called the *conus medullaris.*

Caudal to the conus medullaris, the vertebral canal is filled with spinal nerves traveling to their appropriate vertebral levels of exit. This bundle of spinal nerves in the vertebral canal is called the *cauda equina* (or horse's tail). A spinal tap done to remove a sample of CSF is done in this region because entry of the needle will be unlikely to damage the spinal cord. The spinal nerves consist of components carrying both input and output. The input (sensory component) enters the spinal cord mainly through the dorsal roots. Output (motor and autonomic components) exit the spinal cord through the ventral roots. The dorsal and ventral root for each segment unite to form the spinal root for that segment. In actuality, the dorsal and ventral root for each segment is made up of six or more rootlets.

The spinal cord consists of two types of tissue, *gray matter* and *white matter,* as does the rest of the CNS. The gray matter consists of cell bodies arranged into clusters called *nuclei* (not to be confused with the nucleus of an individual cell). The white matter consists of axonal processes, appearing white because of the presence of myelin surrounding the larger fibers. Clusters of fibers are arranged into *tracts.* These tracts are variously called pathways, columns, channels, funiculi, fasciculi, lemnisci, and so on, but they are all axonal processes communicating with other cells at a distance.

In the spinal cord the gray matter is arranged in a butterfly, or "H," pattern in the center of the cord and can be further subdivided into a dorsal horn, a region of intermediate gray, and a ventral horn. In thoracic and upper lumbar segments, a lateral horn is present at the lateral edge of the intermediate gray. The white matter is arranged into dorsal, lateral, and ventral funiculi, anatomical zones of tracts subdivided by the dorsal and ventral horns. The gray matter can be further subdivided into 10 lamina, or layers, called *lamina of Rexed* (Fig. 1–18). In the dorsal horn, lamina I (marginal layer) is associated with spinothalamic projections, laminae II and

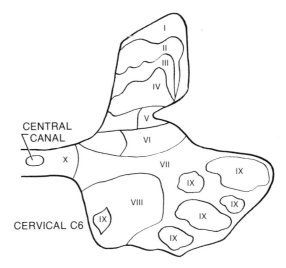

Figure 1-18. Spinal cord gray matter: Lamina of Rexed.

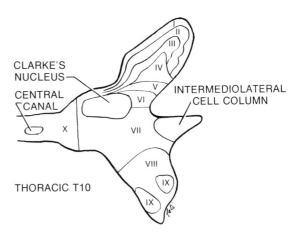

III (substantia gelatinosa) are associated with slow pain processing, and laminae IV and V (nucleus proprius) are associated with the processing of both slow and fast pain (see discussion p. 63). The dorsal horn is separated from the dorsolateral sulcus by the entrance zone of the dorsal root fibers, called *Lissauer's zone.* In the intermediate gray, laminae VI, VII, and VIII contain interneurons. In the ventral horn interneurons of laminae VII and VIII are present along with clusters of LMNs, which are collectively called *lamina IX.* Lamina X is found around the central canal, and in its dorsal portion contains some preganglionic autonomic cell bodies. See the atlas at the end of this chapter for the location of the aforementioned nuclei.

The spinal cord contains major process-

ing zones for sensory, motor, and autonomic portions of the CNS. Somatic input enters the spinal cord through the dorsal roots, and motor and autonomic output leave the spinal cord through the ventral roots. In addition, local neuronal processing in the dorsal, intermediate, and ventral gray matter regulates reflex activity in the spinal cord. Converging supraspinal influences from the brain regulate the final outflow from motor and autonomic neurons. The spinal cord also serves as a diverging channel for ascending sensory information, destined for both unconscious proprioceptive responses and conscious interpretation. These channels and components are most easily understood by subdividing them into their individual components, which include reflex channels, cerebellar channels, and lemniscal channels. Refer to

Table 1–3 for a summary of these components.

The tracts listed in Table 1–3, forming the spinal cord white matter, will be discussed under the heading *Systemic Neuroanatomy*. See the atlas at the end of the chapter for the location of these structures in cross section. Specific areas of cells in the gray matter will also be discussed as necessary with their functional descriptions.

Spinal Reflexes

Introduction

A spinal reflex is an appropriate motor response to a sensory stimulus, not requiring supraspinal input or higher processing. Such a reflex will occur even if supraspinal connections are removed or destroyed because of injury or disease. As long as sensory input and lower motor neuron

TABLE 1–3 SPINAL CORD CHANNELS AND COMPONENTS

1. Sensory input entering spinal cord through dorsal roots.
2. Lower motor neurons, located in ventral horn, whose axons leave spinal cord through ventral roots to innervate skeletal muscles.
3. Sympathetic and parasympathetic outflow from cell bodies in the intermediate gray of thoracic and the two upper lumbar segments (sympathetics) and the mid sacral segments, S2–S4 (parasympathetics). The axons leave the spinal cord through ventral roots to synapse in ganglia. These autonomic ganglia innervate smooth muscles and glands.
4. Interneurons for modulating both sensory input and reflex and supraspinal influences over lower motor neurons and preganglionic autonomic neurons.
5. Sensory channels from the body, carrying information from both outside and inside worlds into CNS.
   a. Reflex channels, conveying sensory input to local motor and autonomic outflow, and to distant outflow.
      (1) Monosynaptic muscle stretch reflexes
      (2) Polysynaptic reflexes, with spino-spinal connections
   b. Cerebellar channels, conveying unconscious proprioception to cerebellum to aid in smooth coordination of motor movements.
      (1) Dorsal spinocerebellar tract–carries information mainly from individual muscle fibers innervated by cord level T6 and below
      (2) Cuneocerebellar tract–carries information mainly from individual muscle fibers innervated by cord levels above T6
      (3) Ventral spinocerebellar tract–carries information mainly from tendons or whole muscles innervated by cord level T6 and below
      (4) Rostral spinocerebellar tract–carries information mainly from tendons or whole muscles innervated by cord levels above T6
   c. Lemniscal channels, conveying ascending sensory information to higher brain centers for conscious interpretation.
      (1) Dorsal column system–carries epicritic modalities
      (2) Spinothalamic and spinoreticular systems–carry protopathic modalities
      (3) Dorsolateral funiculus system–carries joint position, vibratory sensation, cutaneous sensation
6. Descending supraspinal motor pathways, which regulate the lower motor neurons and their control of skeletal muscles.
   a. Corticospinal tract–from both frontal and parietal cortex.
   b. Rubrospinal tract–from red nucleus in midbrain.
   c. Reticulospinal tracts–from brain stem reticular formation.
      (1) Medullary–from gigantocellular reticular nucleus
      (2) Pontine–from caudal and rostral pontine reticular nuclei
   d. Vestibulospinal tracts–from brain stem vestibular nuclei
      (1) Lateral–from lateral vestibular nucleus
      (2) Medial–from medial vestibular nucleus
   e. Bulbospinal tracts–from manoaminergic cell groups in medulla and pons.
      (1) Noradrenergic pathways–from locus coeruleus and medullary reticular formation nuclei in tegmentum
      (2) Serotonergic pathways–from raphe nuclei of medulla and pons.

(LMN) output are intact, a spinal reflex can occur. In fact, a spinal reflex may be hyper-responsive in a cord-injured patient (for example, mass reflexes). If LMNs are destroyed, as in polio, these reflexes cannot occur because no motor response is possible. Abolishing the sensory input is more difficult because it is often much more diffuse, but if all sensory input is destroyed, the reflex cannot occur. This can occasionally be seen in severe peripheral neuropathies.

The simplest example of a spinal reflex is the monosynaptic reflex. In this reflex, a sensory neuron synapses directly on a LMN. This reflex can be considered a holdover for the primitive two-neuron nervous system. It is fast and effective but not very flexible. In higher animals, upper motor neuronal control, especially through cortical regulation, can over-ride these reflexes or use this circuitry for performing complex movements. However, the supraspinal control present in intact animals makes the study of such reflexes difficult. In order to study spinal reflexes in isolation from upper motor neuronal or supraspinal control, experiments are often done on animals with lesions that cut off supraspinal input (such as spinal or decerebrate preparations). These experiments show what happens locally, both in an individual segment or in the whole spinal cord, but do not show how these reflexes are integrated into more complex motor behavior. The following discussion will include only spinal responses, but it should be remembered that upper motor neurons (UMNs) are extremely important for keeping LMNs and reflex pathways in a state of readiness for voluntary movements, as well as for initiating those movements.

There are basically two kinds of spinal reflexes, *cutaneous* (or *exteroceptive*) reflexes and *muscle reflexes.* The cutaneous reflexes are polysynaptic, while muscle reflexes may be polysynaptic (Golgi tendon organ [GTO] reflexes, reciprocal inhibition reflexes, distant responses to muscle stretch reflexes) or monosynaptic (the muscle stretch reflex). The cutaneous reflexes are a motor response to cutaneous stimulation. They are also called *withdrawal reflexes* or *flexor reflexes.* The term flexor reflex is actually a misnomer be-cause the motor response does not have to be flexion. The only requirement is that the motor response must be appropriate to the cutaneous stimulus. Most withdrawals are flexion movements, but the appropriate movement may also be carried out by an extensor muscle. The second kind of spinal reflexes, the muscle reflexes, adjust the tone and reactivity of muscles.

Cutaneous Reflexes

Cutaneous reflexes permit withdrawal from noxious or nocioceptive stimuli. The sensory input originates from receptors in the skin and deeper tissue. Because these receptors are on the exterior of the body rather than in the viscera, they are sometimes referred to as *exteroceptors* and the resultant cutaneous reflexes as *exteroceptive reflexes.* Exteroceptors are responsive to heat, cold, moving touch, and pain. There are several different morphological types of receptors, and it has been suggested that each type may report a different kind of stimulus. Unfortunately, the question of which receptor reports which stimulus has not been fully answered and will not be discussed further. Consult a major textbook for the many receptor types described by anatomists, and bear in mind that few absolute statements regarding modalities conveyed by these receptors can be made at present. It is likely that complex sensation, involved in stereognosis, requires processing of sensory information from many receptor types through complex sensory channels.

Painful or noxious stimulation of a receptor causes the withdrawal (usually by flexion) of the entire limb, and often of the entire body. Figure 1–19 shows a schematic of the simplest kind of polysynaptic reflex, with a receptor R, a primary sensory neuron S, synapsing on an interneuron I_1, which in turn synapses on LMN A. LMN A innervates a flexor muscle, F_1. Stimulation of the receptor causes an action potential to fire in the primary sensory neuron. The primary sensory neuron synapses on the interneuron I_1, exciting this neuron. The interneuron synapses on the LMN, causing it to fire an action potential in turn. The LMN action potential depolarizes its terminal at the motor end plate and releases acetylcholine as its neurotransmitter,

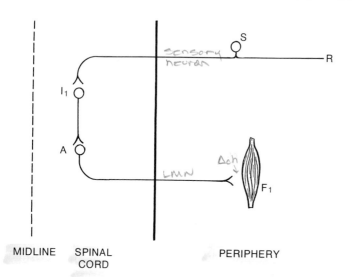

Figure 1–19. Simple polysynaptic reflex.

which crosses the neuromuscular junction and causes the muscle to contract, completing a cutaneous reflex.

The actual mechanism of the reflex is usually more complex than the simple reflex just described. When a finger is burned (a noxious cutaneous stimulus), the whole arm withdraws, not just the finger, or local flexor. Many muscles contract in a coordinated fashion to cause the withdrawal. This is done through interneurons that control the degree to which other LMNs will fire, and therefore the degree to which other muscles will contract. Generally speaking, the stronger the stimulus, the more interneurons will be recruited, and the more muscles will be involved in the reflex. Figure 1–20 illustrates this principle schematically. This schematic is similar to Figure 1–19, but to it has been added an additional excitatory interneuron, I_2 (remember that excitatory

neurons are represented by white or undarkened cell bodies and inhibitory neurons have black or darkened cell bodies); a second LMN, B; and a second flexor muscle, F_2, that represents a synergistic muscle, one that works with the first muscle. In this case, excitation of the receptor and the primary sensory neuron causes interneuron I_1 and subsequently LMN A to fire and muscle F_1 to contract; but it also causes the interneuron I_2 to fire, exciting LMN B, resulting in the contraction of muscle F_2. Adding more interneurons increases the possibility of greater responses and provides an appropriate response for a given stimulus. The whole body does not have to withdraw, like the sponge with the one-neuron nervous system does; only the part actually in danger must withdraw, but that withdrawal has to be both effective and quick.

Withdrawal reflexes affect more than

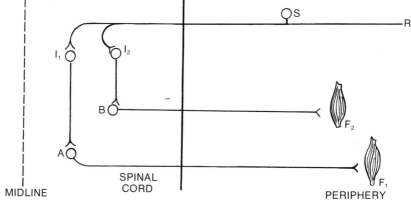

Figure 1–20. More complex polysynaptic reflex.

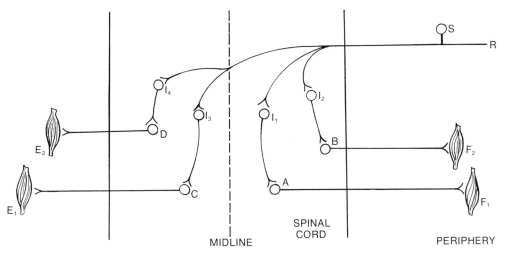

Figure 1–21. Flexion-crossed extension reflex.

just the muscles on the side of the body that receives the stimulus. Muscles on the opposite side of the body may respond as well, because of activation through interneurons. This is particularly true of withdrawal of the foot and leg, perhaps from stepping on a tack. The foot that steps on the tack withdraws by flexion of the leg, but in order to maintain balance, the other leg must extend to provide a strong pillar to keep the body from falling over. This kind of reflex is called a *flexion-crossed extension reflex.*

The processing that goes on in the spinal cord is diagrammed schematically in Figure 1–21. On the right side, Figure 1–21 is the same as Figure 1–20. The left side represents the left side of the spinal cord. Stimulation to receptor R will ultimately cause flexion of muscles F_1 and F_2 just as in Figure 1–20, but the primary sensory neuron also stimulates excitatory interneurons I_3 and I_4 on the left side of the

spinal cord. These interneurons excite LMNs C and D, which in turn cause the contraction of extensor muscle E_1 and its synergistic muscle represented by E_2. Any further processing diagrammed schematically in this manner will become too complex to follow, so the following simplification will be made. Figure 1–22 represents the same system as Figure 1–21. It is understood that the primary sensory neuron excites interneurons that in turn excite LMNs. The LMNs will be designated FLX for those exciting flexor muscles and EXT for those exciting extensor muscles. For simplicity, the muscles have been left out of the diagram.

Not only are flexors on the side of the stimulus and extensors on the side opposite the stimulus excited. In order for them to have optimal effect, the extensors on the side of the stimulus and the flexors on the opposite side from the stimulus are inhibited so that they will not be working

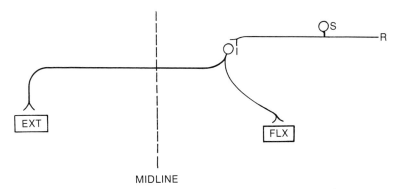

Figure 1–22. Flexion-crossed extension reflex simplified.

against the withdrawal reflex. This process is diagrammed in Figure 1–23. The inhibition of antagonist muscle groups is mediated through inhibitory interneurons (dark circle). If a stimulus is presented on the right, as it is in the diagram, the LMNs for flexor muscles on the right will be excited, while those for extensors on the right will be inhibited. LMNs for extensors on the left will be excited, while those for flexors on the left will be inhibited.

Maintaining balance while withdrawing a whole leg may require more than simply extending the other leg. Movement of the arms may be needed as well, to offset the loss of balance. Therefore, these reflexes can involve all four limbs and the trunk at once. These reflexes are often referred to as *long spinal reflexes,* but the movement of each limb is appropriate to withdrawal from the noxious stimulus and maintenance of balance during the movement, and will involve both flexion and extension.

The preceding discussion has considered what happens when one noxious stimulus is presented alone. It is important to note that when more than one such stimulus is presented, one stimulus may have priority over the others, preventing appropriate responses to the latter. Pain usually has precedence over other reflexes. For example, if a scratch reflex is being elicited from a dog, it will be stopped by pinching the dog's foot. The foot will be withdrawn. When the painful stimulus is stopped, the scratch reflex will resume.

Muscle Reflexes

Muscles have two specialized kinds of receptors: *muscle spindles* and *Golgi tendon organs* (GTOs). These receptors are responsible for reporting information about muscles to the spinal cord for spinal reflexes and to special nuclei in the spinal cord and medulla that relay the information to the cerebellum (see the discussion of cerebellar channels on pp. 60-62). Muscle spindles report static information concerning the length or amount of stretch of individual muscle fibers, and dynamic (phasic) information concerning the speed with which an active muscle fiber is being stretched. The GTO reports the amount of tension on a tendon from the passive stretch or contraction of the muscle. This information is called *proprioceptive information* and is necessary for two kinds of processing: (1) in the spinal cord, it provides input to LMNs and interneurons for local reflexes such as the muscle stretch reflex; and (2) in the cerebellum, via synapses in the spinal cord or medulla, it reports the state of the muscles so that the cerebellum can coordinate the superimpo-

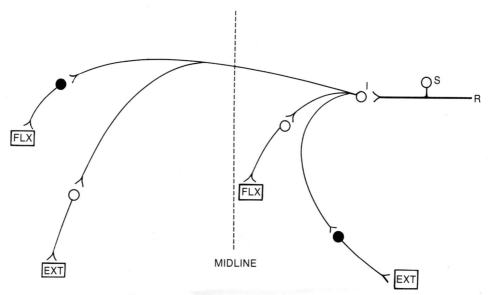

Figure 1–23. More complex reflex processing.

sition of voluntary movements directed by the cortex, or adjustments in tone and posture directed by brain stem UMNs.

Muscle Spindles

The muscle spindle is a sophisticated sensory receptor that reports sensory information from muscles to the CNS and has its own motor innervation through which it can be adjusted by the CNS. This mechanism assists the CNS by providing continuous sensory feedback from the muscles.

Anatomy of the Muscle Spindle. The muscle spindle is made up of special types of muscle fibers called *intrafusal fibers*, found in parallel with the skeletal muscle (extrafusal) fibers. It is attached at both ends to inelastic collagen tissue associated with a skeletal muscle fiber. The extrafusal fibers are responsible for generating the contractile power of the muscle (Fig. 1–24A). The muscle spindle is surrounded by a capsule that is attached at each end to the connective tissue of the skeletal muscle fiber about which it is re-

porting information. The spindle contains two types of intrafusal fibers attached to the capsule on the inside: chain fibers and bag fibers (Fig. 1–24B). These fibers have an equatorial or middle region that contains cell nuclei and a polar or end region that can contract in response to motor input to increase tension on the equatorial regions. The bag fiber has its nuclei arranged bag-like, in a central cluster, and the chain fiber has its nuclei arranged chain-like, in a row. Each muscle spindle usually has four to six chain fibers and one to two bag fibers. Fibers intermediate between the bag and chain fibers have been described, but their function is not well understood at present.

Innervation. The muscle spindle has both sensory and motor innervation (Fig. 1–25). The sensory innervation consists of group Ia fibers and group II fibers, which are sensitive to the tension of the equatorial regions of the bag and chain fibers. *Group Ia endings* wrap around the equatorial zone of the bag fibers. These Ia fibers are also called *primary endings*, or

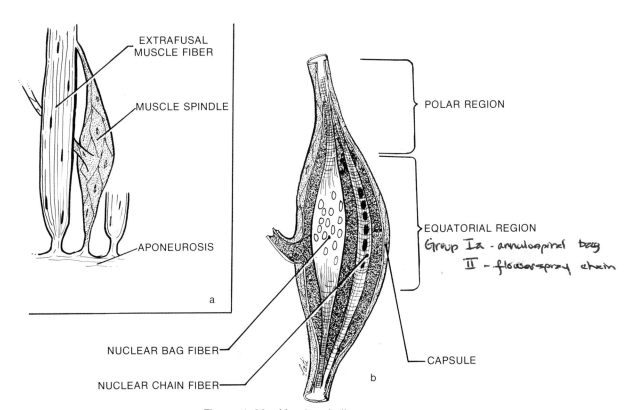

EXTRAFUSAL MUSCLE FIBER

MUSCLE SPINDLE

APONEUROSIS

a

NUCLEAR BAG FIBER

NUCLEAR CHAIN FIBER

POLAR REGION

EQUATORIAL REGION

Group Ia - annulospiral bag
II - flowerspray chain

CAPSULE

b

Figure 1–24. Muscle spindle.

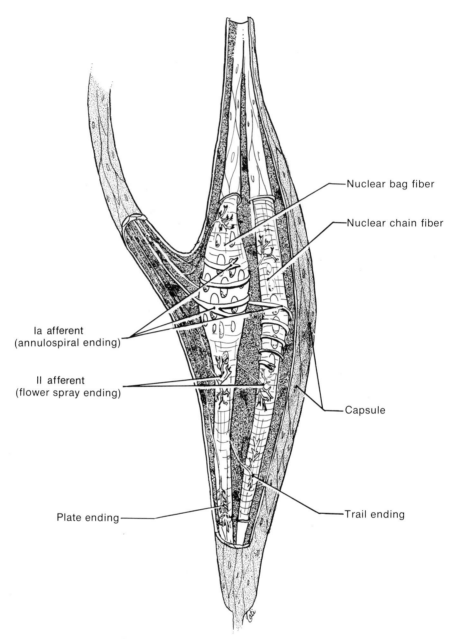

Nuclear bag fiber

Nuclear chain fiber

Ia afferent
(annulospiral ending)

II afferent
(flower spray ending)

Capsule

Plate ending

Trail ending

Figure 1–25. Muscle spindle innervation.

annulospiral endings. Group II endings innervate mainly the chain fibers. They are also called *secondary endings,* or *flower spray endings.* A stretch or tension on the equatorial region of the group Ia and II fibers will cause them to fire action potentials. The sensory input goes into the spinal cord, as discussed earlier, and synapses on LMNs or their interneurons, and on relay nuclei sending information to the cerebellum.

The motor innervation is also of two types called *gamma*$_1$ and *gamma*$_2$ *motor neurons,* or *fusimotor neurons* (to be distinguished from skeletomotor neurons). *Gamma*$_1$ *endings,* also called *plate endings,* innervate mainly the polar ends of the bag fibers, and *gamma*$_2$ *endings,* also called *trail endings,* end mainly on the chain fiber, near the polar region. Firing of these fusimotor neurons causes contraction of the polar region of the muscle spindle, stretching or putting tension on the equatorial region. Stretching of the equatorial region causes the sensory Ia and II fibers to fire. The resultant stimulation of skeletomotor neurons causes the skeletal muscle fibers to contract. Experimental stimulation of the fusimotor neurons causes fusimotor fibers to contract but adds no strength or power to the contraction of the skeletal muscle without the stimulation of skeletomotor neurons. Contraction of the muscle spindle is for the sole purpose of causing the Ia and II fibers to report specific kinds of sensory information to the CNS.

Function. Changes in skeletal muscle activity cause changes in the muscle spindle. Passively stretching the muscle by tapping on a tendon or experimentally stretching a muscle by hanging a weight on it will cause the muscle spindle to stretch. As the spindle stretches, tension is put on the equatorial regions, causing firing of Ia and II fibers. Increased activity in the Ia fibers results in contraction of the extrafusal muscle fibers, increasing the tension produced by the skeletal muscle fibers. This shortening of the extrafusal muscle fibers causes the spindle to slacken. Spindle slackening decreases tension on the equatorial region and decreases the firing of Ia and II fibers. In summary, the spindle reflex responds to a stretch on the muscle by contracting the extrafusal fibers, restoring the muscle to its original state before the stretch. The spindle reflex therefore is a mechanism for maintaining a muscle at a fixed state of contraction. Relaxation of a muscle that has been contracted is like stretching it; the sensory fibers increase their firing.

Gamma motor neurons act to modulate the length and consequently the tension in the muscle spindle so that the information reported to the CNS can be controlled. Contraction of a muscle causes slackening of the spindle so that little or no information goes into the CNS. Under these conditions, the spindle would fail to report sensory information whenever the muscle contracts. However, a resetting of spindle sensitivity is achieved by the gamma motor neurons. These neurons, when stimulated, contract the spindle by the $gamma_1$ and $gamma_2$ motor fibers and cause the resumption of sensory information report-

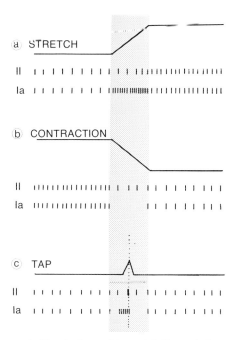

Figure 1–26. Actions of Ia and II fibers during various activities.

ing to the CNS. Figure 1–26 shows what happens to the firing of group Ia and group II fibers during various activities. Type II fibers report only static information; that is, they report the tension of the spindle, corresponding to the length of the extrafusal muscle fiber. Group Ia fibers also report static information to the CNS but are even more important in reporting dynamic information. In this capacity, they report the speed with which the extrafusal muscle fibers are changing their length.

In Figure 1–26A, the skeletal muscle is stretched, which also stretches the muscle spindle. The group II fibers respond to the new tension by increasing their base rate of firing to a new rate. The group Ia fibers also respond with a new rate of firing, but during the time the muscle fiber is changing its length there is a very rapid burst of activity that can be equated with velocity (or change in length with respect to time) of muscle stretch. When stretching stops and a new tension is reached, the group Ia fiber reports that new static tension with a new firing rate. In Figure 1–26B, the skeletal muscle is contracted, causing the muscle spindle to slacken. Group II fibers decrease their firing to report the new length. Group Ia fibers are silent during the period of collapse, then resume firing at a reduced rate corresponding to the new extrafusal fiber length. In Figure 1–26C, the muscle tendon is tapped in order to elicit a muscle stretch reflex. Group II fibers do not change their firing rate because the tap is too fast for them to respond. Group Ia fibers report a burst of firing during the stretch part of the tap. It is this quick burst of Ia fiber activity during the tap that causes the corresponding LMN to which it projects to fire. This causes contraction of the extrafusal fiber that was stretched originally.

The preceding discussion has not considered what happens when the fusimotor neurons fire. Stimulation of these neurons increases the responsiveness of the spindles. Stimulation of the gamma₁, or plate fibers, increases responsiveness to both static and phasic events, while stimulation of gamma₂, or trail fibers, increases responsiveness to static events. The fusimotor neurons are fired mainly by descending supraspinal channels, particularly those channels that are influenced by cerebellar outflow. On the other hand, stimulation of alpha motor neurons does not directly influence the contractile elements of the muscle spindle. These neurons cause the skeletal muscle extrafusal fibers to contract and indirectly influence the spindle through altered sensory activity caused by shortening of the extrafusal muscle fibers. Figure 1–27 shows a Ia afferent fiber synapsing directly on a LMN in the spinal cord. Ia stimulation is the single greatest driving force for firing LMNs and causing a muscle contraction or an increase in mus-

cle tension. This phenomenon is exploited clinically by vibration, which can tonically drive Ia afferents, enhancing the contraction of the associated muscle group. It should be clear that the fusimotor neurons, which can control the sensitivity or responsiveness of the Ia afferent fibers, are critical to the responsiveness of the alpha motor neurons and the control of muscle tone.

Most of the control of fusimotor neurons is from UMN systems that keep the fusimotor neurons in check (inhibited). Damage of these UMNs can cause a disinhibition of fusimotor neurons, increasing their firing. Increased stimulation causes the muscle spindle to become more sensitive, which produces more firing of Ia afferents and finally results in an increased stimulation of LMNs. This increased fusimotor activity and the resultant increased skeletomotor activity is called *spasticity.* Spasticity, an increased resistance of the muscle to passive stretch, is characterized by an increase in muscle tone caused by increased LMN firing and an exaggerated response to stretch reflexes owing to the increased sensitivity of the muscle spindle.

When UMN control is present during normal tone and posture, and during normal voluntary movements, both skeletomotor and fusimotor neurons are activated at the same time by the UMNs. This *alpha-gamma coactivation* prevents the muscle spindle from collapsing during the contraction of the skeletal muscle, so that information is continuously reported to the CNS. Therefore, both fusimotor and skeletomotor neurons act in concert to achieve

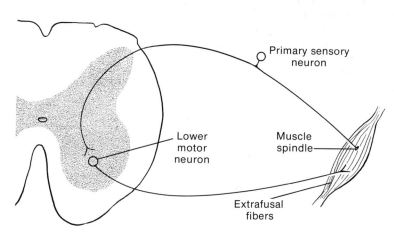

Figure 1–27. Monosynaptic reflex of Ia fibers on motor neurons.

Primary sensory neuron

Lower motor neuron

Muscle spindle

Extrafusal fibers

voluntary motor actions and provide optimum sensory information back to the CNS for maximum evaluation of current motor activity and for subsequent motor activity.

Golgi Tendon Organs

The Golgi tendon organ (GTO) is a receptor that is connected in series with the muscle so that contraction of the whole muscle increases tension on the tendon and excites the GTO. Primary sensory afferents from the GTO, called *Ib fibers*, enter the spinal cord and synapse on interneurons associated with LMNs, and in secondary sensory nuclei that relay unconscious proprioceptive information concerning the state of whole muscles to the cerebellum. The GTO is sensitive to tension on the tendon and is therefore active during both passive stretch and contraction. However, it is difficult to elicit a normal GTO response during a clinical examination. The Ib reflex associated with the GTO and the Ib afferent fiber is an inhibitory reflex that prevents the muscle tendon from being stretched too much from muscle contraction. Although the GTO is extremely sensitive to tension on the tendon, and may be involved with inibition necessary for alternating movements, no single specific reflex for the Ib fiber can be elicited as simply as can the Ia monosynaptic muscle stretch reflex. Ib reflex activity can be demonstrated best in a patient with spasticity who has greatly increased tone. Passive movement of the spastic limb will meet with considerable resistance at first, followed by a collapse of resistance as the passive movement is continued. The collapse is called a *clasp-knife reflex* (named after the collapsing of the blade in a pocket knife) and is thought to be the result of Ib inhibition, preventing firing of overactive LMNs so that the muscle will not be damaged because of excessive resistance of the spastic muscle.

Muscle Reflex Activity

Each of the three types of afferent fibers just discussed (Ia, II, Ib) has an effect on several groups of muscles through the LMNs supplying those muscles. LMNs supplying the muscle from which the af-

ferent fiber comes are called *homonymous LMNs*. LMNs to the muscles that work with the homonymous muscle are called *synergist LMNs*. LMNs to the muscle groups that work against or opposite to the homonymous muscle are called *antagonist LMNs*. Figure 1–28 shows schematically how these reflexes affect the appropriate LMNs. Ia afferents excite homonymous LMNs monosynaptically and synergist LMNs polysynaptically through interneurons. Ia afferents also inhibit antagonist muscle LMNs polysynaptically through an inhibitory interneuron. Ib afferents work in the opposite direction. They inhibit homonymous and synergist LMNs disynaptically through inhibitory interneurons and excite antagonist LMNs disynaptically. Group II reflexes do not work like Ia and Ib reflexes. The group II fibers respond as a unit with a flexor bias. That is, they consistently facilitate flexor LMNs and inhibit extensor muscle LMNs polysynaptically. However, most research on group II responses is conducted using nonprimate animal models. The actual role

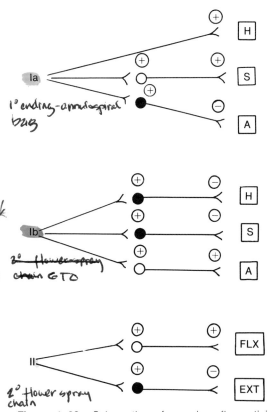

Figure 1–28. Schematics of muscle reflex activity from Ia, Ib, and group II afferent fibers.

of group II fibers in humans is not adequately understood at present, and definitive or dogmatic pronouncements about their role in normal or neurologically damaged patients are not possible.

REGIONAL NEUROANATOMY

Major Subdivisions of the Nervous System

The mammalian nervous system is divided into a peripheral nervous system (PNS) that is in contact with the outside world and a central nervous system (CNS) that provides integrated control of the periphery. The contacts between the outside world and the nervous system constitute the sensory and motor components of the nervous system. The sensory systems respond to stimuli from the external environment or the internal milieu of the body while the motor system causes skeletal muscles to contract, thus permitting movement and behavior in response to the environment. In addition, there is an autonomic nervous system that has components in both the CNS and PNS. This third functional component of the nervous system permits the regulation of smooth muscle, cardiac muscle, and glands, and operates as an internal visceral regulatory control system.

The PNS has the following components: (1) primary sensory cell bodies and axons, and associated receptors; (2) axons of lower motor neurons (LMNs) and their neuromuscular junctions (NMJs); (3) preganglionic axons, and ganglion cells and their postganglionic axons of the autonomic nervous system.

The CNS can be subdivided into the following major regions, based on the development of the brain:

Spinal cord
Rhombencephalon
  Myelencephalon–medulla
  Metencephalon–pons and cerebellum
Mesencephalon–midbrain
Prosencephalon (forebrain)
  Diencephalon (tweenbrain)–thalamus, hypothalamus, and minor components
  Telencephalon (endbrain)–olfactory system, limbic system, basal ganlia, neocortex

The human brain possesses surface landmarks that can be used to delineate these subdivisions (see Figs. 1–29 through 1–32). The spinal cord is distinguished from the medulla by the decussation (crossing) of the pyramids (corticospinal tract), seen on the ventral surface of the caudal-most portion of the medulla (Fig. 1–31). There are no clearly distinguishing features on the dorsal surface of the caudal medulla at its boundary with the spinal cord. The internal demarcation of the spinal cord–medulla transition is gradual. Therefore, by convention, an arbitrary division is made by a plane perpendicular to the *neuraxis* (long axis of the brain stem) passing through the spinal cord just above (rostral to) the first pair of cervical rootlets.

The demarcation of the rostral medulla from the caudal pons is both clear and consistent. It consists of a plane through the caudal boundary of the basis pontis of the ventral surface of the brain stem, perpendicular to the neuraxis (Fig. 1–31). This line of separation also marks the point where cranial nerves VII (facial) and VIII (vestibulocochlear) emerge from the brain stem at the *medullopontocerebellar (cerebellopontine) angle*.

The midbrain contains the *cerebral peduncles* on its ventral surface. The caudal boundary of the midbrain is the end of the basis pontis at its junction with the caudal-most beginning of the cerebral peduncles. The caudal boundary of the *mammillary bodies* in the hypothalamus delineates the rostral boundary of the mesencephalon. The dorsal surface of the midbrain contains two sets of small protrusions, or hillocks, the *inferior and superior colliculi* (Fig. 1–32). These colliculi are called the *quadrigeminal bodies*, which make up the midbrain tectum.

The diencephalon is a direct rostral continuation of the brain stem. The boundaries of the diencephalon include the mammillary bodies at the caudal end, located at the base of the brain, and the anterior commissure and lamina terminalis located at the rostral end of the third ventricle just above the optic chiasm (see Fig. 1–30). A plane passing perpendicular to the ventral surface of the brain at the rostral boundary of the hypothalamus separates the diencephalon caudally from the

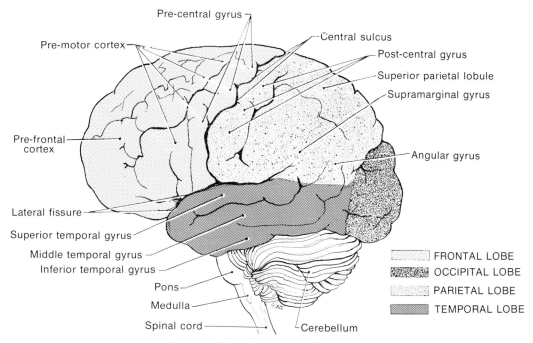

Figure 1–29. Lateral view of the brain.

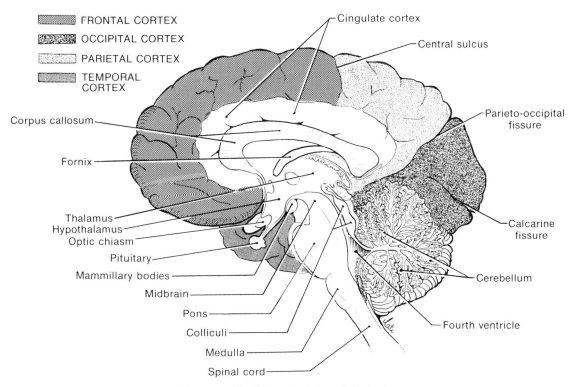

Figure 1–30. Midsagittal view of the brain.

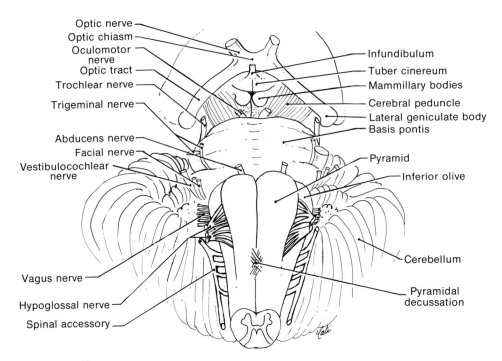

Figure 1–31. Ventral basal view of the brain stem and diencephalon.

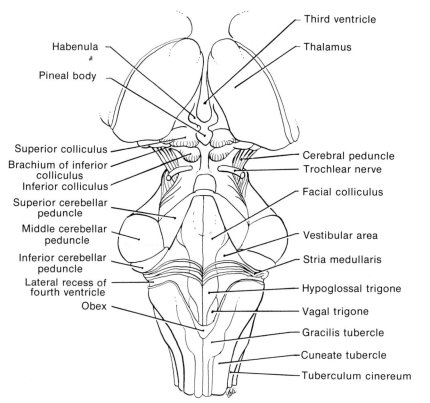

Figure 1–32. Dorsal view of the brain stem and diencephalon.

basal telencephalon rostrally. In addition, surrounding the diencephalon is an outer mantle of telencephalon containing both limbic forebrain and neocortical structures. In order to dissect specific regions of the thalamus and hypothalamus, it is necessary to remove or cut through an outer telencephalic shell of structures. Further subdivision of the telencephalon is based upon a functional parcellation of structures into the olfactory system, limbic system, basal ganglia, and neocortex.

Each of the regions just noted contains specific areas, tracts, and nuclei that will be considered in further detail. The spinal cord has been discussed in a previous section as a model for CNS organization. In the following section the brain stem (medulla, pons, midbrain, and cerebellum) and forebrain (diencephalon and telencephalon) will be discussed in a regional fashion. Even though regional neuroanatomy is the main focus of this portion of the chapter, it still contains a strong systemic orientation. With this approach, regional neuroanatomy makes more sense functionally, rather than merely being a recounting of innumerable anatomical structures.

Each structure discussed in this section is pictured in the atlas at the end of the chapter. The atlas and Figures 1–29 through 1–32 should be referred to contiually as this section is read so that the structures discussed can be visualized.

Brain Stem

General Organization of the Brain Stem

The brain stem is made up of the medulla, pons, midbrain, and cerebellum. These regions are so closely related that they are best considered as a functional unit. While some anatomists consider the diencephalon to be part of the brain stem, we definitely will not; the diencephalon is a highly specialized structure that will be considered separately. The nuclei and tracts of the brain stem are intermingled and appear scattered. However, they do follow functional patterns in the medulla, pons, and midbrain. These three major subdivisions contain six major components that form the basis for regional anatomy of each subdivision. There is obviously overlap, in some cases, of certain components (such as the sensory, motor, and autonomic cranial nerve nuclei).

Motor Systems

Lower Motor Neurons. The cell bodies are located in the brain stem and the axons exit through cranial nerves to innervate muscles of the head and neck.

Upper Motor Neurons. The cell bodies are located in the brain stem; the axons descend to the LMNs and associated interneurons, which they control.

Descending Motor Pathways. The pathways consist of axons of UMN systems that are passing through the region on the way to LMNs and associated interneurons at lower levels.

Autonomic Systems

Parasympathetic Preganglionic Cell Bodies. The cell bodies are located in the brain stem, and the axons exit through cranial nerves III, VII, IX, and X to terminate in parasympathetic ganglia near the smooth muscles and glands those ganglia supply (see Fig. 1–17).

Autonomic Centers. These centers regulate major visceral functions such as respiration, cardiac function, blood pressure, and gastrointestinal functions. These centers are sometimes viewed as reticular formation regions and can involve both motor and autonomic activities. The reticular formation will be discussed later in this section.

Descending Autonomic Pathways. The cell bodies from the hypothalamus send axons that descend through brain stem structures to terminate in preganglionic autonomic nuclei or associated limbic midbrain regions. These descending pathways can involve polysynaptic pathways, or can be direct connections from the hypothalamus to preganglionic autonomic cells.

Sensory Systems

Secondary Sensory Nuclei. The cell bodies receive input from primary sensory axons and send projections toward higher structures, particularly the thalamic sensory projection nuclei. Recall that all primary sensory cell bodies are found in ganglia associated with peripheral or cranial nerves, except for the mesencephalic nucleus of V, which is the only primary sensory cell group within the CNS. Primary sensory ganglion cells project to the secondary sensory nuclei through the peripheral and cranial nerves, and associated primary sensory tracts, such as the solitary tract, the descending tract of V, or fasciculi gracilis and cuneatus.

Ascending Pathways and Relay Centers. The pathways are mainly ascending secondary sensory (lemniscal) channels. The relay centers include tertiary nuclei or nuclei associated with sensory processing, and give rise to tertiary sensory channels.

Cerebellar Systems

Cerebellar Cortex. The cerebellar cortex includes three cell layers: molecular, Purkinje, and granular.

The Medullary Zone. This region consists of white matter deep to the cerebellar cortex.

Deep Cerebellar Nuclei. These outflow nuclei are located near the roof of the fourth ventricle.

Peduncles. These structures are the input and output axonal channels of the cerebellum, including the inferior, middle, and superior cerebellar peduncles.

Associated Cerebellar Insput Nuclei. The cell bodies are found in the brain stem, and the axons project through the peduncles to the cerebellum.

Reticular Formation

This general region, forming the core of the brain stem, includes nuclei, pathways, and centers. The reticular formation includes a medial two thirds (mainly motor), a lateral one third (mainly sensory), the midline raphe, and scattered catecholamine systems. It is responsible for maintaining consciousness, maintaining general muscle tone and posture, processing noxious stimuli, regulating major visceral functions, and providing a host of interconnecting links that are reflex in nature and allow quick and appropriate adjustments to disturbances in the external or internal environment.

Cranial Nerve Nuclei

These nuclei include components of the sensory, motor, and autonomic systems.

This category directly overlaps with categories 1, 2, and 3, and is best considered in these categories.

Medulla

Motor Systems

Lower Motor Neurons. Several motor cranial nerve nuclei are found in the medulla. The hypoglossal nucleus (Nucleus XII) is found near the midline and sends axons through the hypoglossal (XII) nerve to innervate the muscles of the tongue.

The nucleus ambiguus is located in the ventrolateral medulla and sends axons through the glossopharyngeal (IX), vagus (X), and spinal accessory (XI) nerves to innervate palatopharyngeal and laryngeal muscles.

The spinal accessory (XI) nucleus is located in the ventral gray matter of the upper cervical spinal cord; it sends axons through the XI nerve to the sternocleidomastoid and trapezius muscles. Although the LMNs are found in the spinal cord, the axons travel with a cranial nerve.

Upper Motor Neurons. The *gigantocellular reticular nucleus* in the medial reticular formation sends axons that run in the medullary (lateral) reticulospinal tract. This tract is mainly excitatory to flexor LMNs through interneurons and aids in the general maintenance of tone.

The *lateral vestibular nucleus* sends axons that run in the lateral vestibulospinal tract. This tract is mainly excitatory to extensor motor neurons, with a few direct connections and a predominance of indirect connections through interneurons. It aids in the maintenance of antigravity tone, particularly in response to vestibular stimulation.

The *medial vestibular nucleus* sends axons that run in the medial vestibulospinal tract. This tract terminates both directly and indirectly on cervical LMNs and regulates neck movements in response to vestibular input.

Raphe nuclei of the medulla (obscurus, pallidus, and magnus) send descending axons through scattered zones of the medulla and through the lateral and ventral funiculus of the spinal cord. These axons terminate in the ventral horn and aid in the maintenance of tone, perhaps enhancing or reinforcing the action of other neuro-transmitters on LMNs (neuromodulatory action). This descending pathway also influences sensory functions and is necessary for narcotic analgesia to occur.

Descending Motor Pathways. Several pathways descend through the medulla on their way to spinal cord interneurons and occasionally LMNs. The corticospinal tract arises in frontal and parietal lobes and descends through the internal capsule, cerebral peduncles, and basis pontis. Continuing its descent in the ventral medulla, 80 per cent of the fibers decussate at the caudal-most midline region of the medulla. The crossed portion continues into the spinal cord as the lateral corticospinal tract, while the uncrossed portion continues as the *anterior corticospinal tract* and then mainly crosses into the contralateral ventral horn through the anterior white commissure of the spinal cord. The corticospinal tract regulates fine skilled hand and finger movements, with a predominant influence on flexor LMNs.

The *rubrospinal tract* arises in the red nucleus of the midbrain, crosses the midline in the ventral tegmental decussation of the midbrain, descends through the ventrolateral medulla, and has a predominant influence on flexor LMNs.

The *pontine reticulospinal tract* arises in the pontine reticular formation, descends through the ventral medulla, and mainly influences extensor LMNs.

The *tectospinal tract* arises from the superior colliculus and to a lesser extent from the inferior colliculus, crosses the midline in the dorsal tegmental decussation, descends through the medial longitudinal fasciculus, and terminates mainly in the cervical spinal cord. This tract influences neck movements in response to visual and auditory stimuli.

The *noradrenergic bulbospinal tract* arises in the *locus coeruleus* (mainly) and to a lesser extent in the reticular formation of the medulla, descends in the lateral and ventral regions of the medulla, and influences general LMN tone in addition to autonomic functions.

Autonomic Systems

Parasympathetic Preganglionic Cell Bodies. The *dorsal motor nucleus of X* and related cells in the lateral reticular formation and commissural nucleus send preganglionic parasympathetic fibers through the X nerve to ganglia located near the visceral organs innervated. This system supplies the heart, lungs, and gastrointestinal viscera. Cell bodies supplying the heart are found in the lateral reticular formation around the nucleus ambiguus, while cell bodies supplying the lungs and gastrointestinal viscera are found in the main nucleus of the dorsal motor nucleus of X, the commissural nucleus of the caudal medulla, and dorsal lamina X of Rexed of the first six cervical spinal cord segments.

The *inferior salivatory nucleus* sends preganglionic parasympathetic fibers through the IX nerve to the otic ganglion. This ganglion supplies fibers to the parotid gland, producing a salivatory function.

Autonomic Centers. Numerous visceral centers have been described in regions of the reticular formation of the medulla. These centers act through the preganglionic autonomic cells and also influence some LMNs. These regions include centers for blood pressure regulation, heart rate and contractility, respiratory control, and emetic responses.

Descending Autonomic Pathways. Processes from cell bodies in the hypothalamus (paraventricular nucleus) descend directly to the dorsal motor nucleus of X; they also descend indirectly (anterior hypothalamus) through the dorsal longitudinal fasciculus to the dorsal tegmental nucleus and then to the dorsal motor nucleus of X. In the lateral aspect of the medulla, sympathetic fibers polysynaptically descend from the hypothalamus to the preganglionic sympathetic neurons in the thoracolumbar areas of the spinal cord.

Sensory Systems

Secondary Sensory Nuclei. *Nuclei gracilis* and *cuneatus* are found in the medial portion of the dorsal medulla at its caudal zone. These nuclei receive input from dorsal root ganglion cells carrying epicritic modalities (gracilis, T6 and below; cuneatus, above T6) via fasciculi gracilis and cuneatus, and send crossed fibers through a decussation in the caudal medulla to form the medial lemniscus. The medial lemniscus ascends to the ventral posterolateral (VPL) nucleus of the thalamus.

Nuclei gracilis and cuneatus also receive some information about vibratory sensation, joint position, and cutaneous sensation through projections of spinal cord neurons which travel in the dorsolateral funiculus.

The *nucleus of the solitary tract*, located in the dorsal medulla, receives cardiac and respiratory reflex afferents and taste fibers from the geniculate, petrosal, and nodose ganglia, via nerves VII (facial), IX, and X, respectively. This nucleus gives rise to a crossed projection, the solitariothalamic tract, which ascends to the ventral posteromedial (VPM) nucleus of the thalamus.

The *descending (spinal) nucleus of V* (trigeminal nerve), located at the lateral margin of the medulla, receives input from the trigeminal (Gasserion or semilunar) ganglion cells carrying protopathic modalities such as pain and temperature from the face and oral cavity. Some fibers carrying epicritic sensation (touch) from the face also terminate in this nucleus. This elongated longitudinal nucleus sends crossed fibers into the ventral trigeminothalamic tract (VTTT) which ascends toward the ventral posteromedial (VPM) nucleus of the thalamus. Some fibers from this tract also terminate in reticular formation and project toward nonspecific nuclei of the thalamus, as alternate routes for transmission of pain.

Vestibular nuclei (medial, lateral, inferior) are found in the medulla and continue into the pons *(superior)*. These nuclei receive vestibular input from Scarpa's ganglion via the VIII nerve (vestibular part of the vestibulocochlear nerve). This input carries information reporting angular acceleration from the semicircular canals and linear acceleration from the utricle and saccule. The secondary sensory afferents from the vestibular nuclei project to the spinal cord (medial and lateral vestibulospinal tract), to the cerebellum (along with some ganglion cell projections, through the medial portion of the inferior cerebellar peduncle, the juxtarestiform body), to the reticular formation through local reflex channels, and to the cranial nerve nuclei supplying extraocular muscles (III, oculomotor; IV, trochlear; VI, abducens) via the medial longitudinal fasciculus. These channels permit a coordi-

nate activation of extensor musculature of the body, neck musculature, and extraocular musculature in response to vestibular input.

Ascending Pathways and Relay Centers. Several ascending tracts arise in or pass through the medulla. The medial lemniscus carries epicritic modalities from the body. The spinothalamic tract carries protopathic modalities, particularly fast pain, from the body, while the spinoreticular tract carries slow pain from the body. The ventral trigeminothalamic tract and its additional projections to reticular formation carry protopathic modalities from the face, oral cavity, anterior two-thirds of the tongue, and sinuses. The solitariothalamic tract carries taste and visceral sensory information. The medial longitudinal fasciculus carries unconscious vestibular information to the extraocular cranial nerve nuclei.

Cerebellar Systems

The cerebellar cortex, deep nuclei, and peduncles will be considered separately in the section on the cerebellum. In the medulla, several tracts and nuclei project to the cerebellum.

Spinocerebellar tracts carry unconscious proprioceptive information to the cerebellum from the body. This information includes Ia afferents from individual muscle fibers (dorsal spinocerebellar tract from *Clark's nucleus* of the spinal cord for T6 and below; cuneocerebellar tract from the *medullary lateral [accessory] cuneate nucleus* for above T6) and Ib afferents from whole muscles (ventral spinocerebellar tract from spinal cord border cells for T6 and below; rostral spinocerebellar tract from spinal cord intermediate gray for above T6). These tracts enter the cerebellum through the inferior cerebellar peduncle, except for the ventral spinocerebellar tract, which enters through the superior cerebellar peduncle. For a schematic diagram of these cerebellar channels see Figure 1–34.

The *inferior olivary nucleus* is a large convoluted nucleus in the ventrolateral medulla that sends climbing fiber axons to the contralateral cerebellar cortex through the inferior cerebellar peduncle. This nucleus is an important motor feedback center and a spinal cord relay center for the cerebellum.

The *lateral reticular nucleus* of the ventrolateral medulla sends mossy fiber axons to the cerebellar cortex through the inferior cerebellar peduncle. This nucleus conveys spinal cord information from widely distributed sensory receptive fields to the cerebellum.

The medullary vestibular nuclei and the vestibular (Scarpa's) ganglion send vestibulocerebellar projections through the medial portion of the inferior cerebellar peduncle, the juxtarestiform body.

Thus, the inferior cerebellar peduncle is mainly a channel conveying information from the spinal cord and medulla to the cerebellum.

The inferior cerebellar peduncle carries some outflow from the cerebellar cortex and deep nuclei. Some Purkinje cell axons of the flocculonodular lobe and vermis project directly to the ipsilateral lateral vestibular nucleus. Purkinje cell axons from these areas also travel to the fastigial nucleus, which sends fibers through the ICP to vestibular and reticular nuclei of both sides of the brain stem.

Reticular Formation

The reticular formation is a collection of longitudinally oriented large neurons with numerous collaterals, giving rise to a tremendous amount of convergent and divergent sensory, motor, and autonomic information. In the medulla, the reticular formation contains several components. The lateral third is a sensory zone, part of the ascending reticular activating system, which receives widespread sensory input from numerous modalities and systems. This system aids in the maintenance of consciousness and attention through projections to the adjacent ascending portions into the medial reticular formation, which conveys this information to nonspecific nuclei of the thalamus. The medial two thirds is a motor zone that gives rise to the medullary reticulospinal tract. This zone aids in the maintenance of tone and posture and exerts a bias toward flexor LMNs.

The midline raphe nuclei and lateral noradrenergic cell bodies give rise to descending serotonergic and noradrenergic pathways. These tracts aid in the maintenance of tone and posture and also play a major role in sensory and autonomic functions. Autonomic centers regulating blood pressure, cardiac function, respiratory function, and emetic function are also found in the reticular formation.

Cranial Nerve Nuclei

Numerous cranial nerve nuclei are found in the medulla and are discussed in the sections on motor, autonomic, and sensory systems. These nuclei are associated with cranial nerves IX, X, XI, and XII, which leave or enter the medulla, and with cranial nerve VIII, found at the medullopontine junction at the cerebellopontine angle.

Pons

Motor Systems

Lower Motor Neurons. Three motor cranial nerve nuclei are found in the pons. The *facial nucleus* (VII) is found in a lateral position in the pontine tegmentum; it sends axons dorsomedially to loop around the abducens nucleus (genu of the facial nerve). These axons then exit through the caudal pons ventrolaterally and innervate the muscles of facial expression. The facial nucleus also innervates the stapedius muscle and aids in dampening the ossicles (stapes) in response to loud noises.

The *abducens nucleus* (VI) is found near the dorsal midline of the rostral pons. Its axons run ventrally through the pons and exit close to the ventral midline. This nucleus innervates the lateral rectus muscle of the eye and is responsible for turning the eye outward (lateral deviation).

The *trigeminal motor nucleus* (V) is found in the lateral region of the mid pons and sends axons laterally and a bit ventrally to exit through the mandibular division of the V nerve. This nucleus innervates the muscles of mastication and the tensor tympani muscle for additional dampening of the ossicles (malleus) in response to loud noises.

Upper Motor Neurons. The *caudal* and *rostral* (also called oral) *pontine reticular nuclei* are found in the medial two thirds of the pontine reticular formation. These nuclei send predominantly ipsilateral (uncrossed) axonal projections to the spinal cord, where they terminate on interneurons associated with extensor lower motor neurons (LMNs). This tract has a strong extensor bias; it augments and reinforces the extensor bias of the lateral vestibulospinal tract. The lateral vestibular nucleus and its lateral vestibulospinal tract are also present in the caudal pons. These were considered in the previous section on the medulla.

The *locus coeruleus* is a pigmented nucleus located just beneath the lateral portion of the fourth ventricle in the pons. This nucleus uses norepinephrine as its neurotransmitter and sends noradrenergic axons to the spinal cord through the ventral and lateral brain stem tegmentum. This pathway is augmented in part by axons of noradrenergic cells found in the lateral and dorsal medulla. These noradrenergic fibers aid in the maintenace of tone and posture through interneurons and LMNs and also contribute to the regulation of autonomic functions through preganglionic autonomic neurons.

Descending Motor Pathways. Major motor pathways descend through the pons on their way to interneurons and LMNs of the spinal cord. The corticospinal tract descends through scattered fascicles in the basis pontis. The rubrospinal tract and tectospinal tract descend through the tegmentum of the pons. These tracts also descend through the medulla. They were discussed in greater detail in that section.

Autonomic Systems

Parasympathetic Preganglionic Cell Bodies. The *superior salivatory nucleus* is located in the dorsomedial pons as a rostral continuation of the dorsal motor nucleus of X and the inferior salivatory nucleus. This nucleus sends fibers through the facial nerve to the pterygopalatine ganglion and the submandibular ganglion. The pterygopalatine ganglion cells supply postganglionic parasympathetic fibers to the lacrimal glands (tear production) and to glands of the nasal mucosa. The submandibular ganglion supplies postganglionic parasympathetic fibers to the submandibular and sublingual salivary glands.

Autonomic Centers. A few additional autonomic centers are found in the pontine reticular formation, rostral to the medullary centers. Some respiratory functions are directed through pontine respiratory centers.

Descending Autonomic Pathways. Hypothalamic autonomic pathways, discussed in the previous section on the medulla, descend through the pontine tegmentum on their way to sympathetic and parasympathetic preganglionic neurons in the spinal cord and rhombencephalon.

Sensory Systems

Secondary Sensory Nuclei. Sensory nuclei associated with the V and VIII nerves are found in the pons. The dorsal and ventral cochlear nuclei are located at the extreme lateral portion of the dorsal zone of the caudal pons. They receive auditory input from the cochlea through the spiral (auditory) ganglion and its projections through the VIII nerve. The *dorsal and ventral cochlear nuclei* send principally contralateral (crossed) fibers through acoustic stria to innervate accessory nuclei or to form ascending sensory channels. The upper part of the dorsal cochlear nucleus gives rise to the dorsal acoustic stria; the lower part of the dorsal nucleus and upper part of the ventral cochlear nucleus give rise to the intermediate acoustic stria, and the lower (anterior) part of the ventral cochlear nucleus gives rise to the *ventral acoustic stria*, also called the *trapezoid body*. These stria form the *lateral lemniscus*, the major ascending auditory pathway. Some fibers of the trapezoid body terminate in the *superior olivary nuclei*. One portion of this nucleus (dorsal accessory superior olivary nucleus) receives input from both sides and is responsible for localization of sound in space. The superior olivary nuclei contribute fibers to both the ipsilateral and contralateral lateral lemniscus. In addition, some lateral lemniscus fibers terminate in accessory auditory nuclei (nuclei of the lateral lemniscus, nuclei of the trapezoid body). These nuclei also contribute both ipsilateral and contralateral fibers to the lateral lemniscus. The lateral lemniscus ascends to the nucleus of the inferior colliculus. This entire auditory system is clearly a bilateral system, accounting for the failure of a lesion in this system to produce deafness with a discrete localization.

The main sensory nucleus of V is found just lateral to the motor nucleus of V in the lateral portion of the midpons, and receives input from trigeminal semilunar ganglion cells carrying epicritic modalities from the face, oral cavity, and anterior two thirds of the tongue via all three divisions (V_I, ophthalmic; V_{II}, maxillary; V_{III}, mandibular) of the trigeminal nerves. The dorsal portion of this nucleus gives rise to the *dorsal trigeminothalamic tract* (DTTT), which travels ipsilaterally to the ventral posteromedial (VPM) nucleus of the thalamus. This system carries fine discriminative modalities of the face for conscious interpretation. Some cells of the main sensory nucleus of V send crossed projections into the VTTT.

The descending nucleus of V is also partially found in the pons and has been discussed in the section on the medulla, where the main portion of this nucleus is found. This nucleus gives rise to the *ventral trigeminothalamic tract* (VTTT), which carries mainly protopathic modalities from the face toward nucleus VPM of the thalamus.

The superior vestibular nucleus is located in the pons. It contributes to the same extraocular, reticular formation, and cerebellar channels as the other medullary vestibular nuclei (inferior, lateral, medial). These channels are discussed in further detail in the section on the medulla.

Ascending Pathways and Relay Centers. Several sensory tracts ascend through the pons. The medial lemniscus carries epicritic modalities from the body. The spinothalamic tract carries protopathic modalities, particularly fast pain, from the body, while the spinoreticular tract carries slow pain from the body. The ventral trigeminothalamic tract carries mainly protopathic modalities from the face, oral cavity, anterior two thirds of the tongue, and sinuses. The dorsal trigeminothalamic tract carries epicritic modalities from the same regions. The solitariothalamic tract carries taste and visceral sensory information. The lateral lemniscus carries auditory information. The medial longitudinal fasciculus carries unconscious vestibular information to the extraocular cranial nerve nuclei.

Cerebellar Systems

The basis pontis contains clusters of neurons located in pontine nuclei. These nuclei act as a cerebral-cerebellar relay channel. The pontine nuclei receive input from all regions of the cerebral cortex and send axonal projections to the cortex of the contralateral cerebellar hemispheres in the form of mossy fibers. These pontocerebellar fibers enter the cerebellum through their own peduncle, the middle cerebellar peduncle. This relay pathway coordinates voluntary motor activity, apparently initiated by the cortex, with tone and position of the muscles at any given moment. This relay pathway is concerned mainly with fine coordinated movements.

The pons also contains passing fibers of the ventral spinocerebellar tract (VSCT), which enters the cerebellum through the superior cerebellar peduncle, and trigeminocerebellar fibers, which enter the cerebellum through both the superior and inferior cerebellar peduncles.

Reticular Formation

The pontine reticular formation contains the same motor (medial two thirds) and sensory (lateral third) divisions as the medullary reticular formation. The motor division aids in the maintenance of tone and posture, and the sensory division aids in the maintenance of attention and consciousness.

In addition, ascending monoamine pathways arise from reticular formation nuclei of the pons. The locus coeruleus sends ascending noradrenergic fibers to the hypothalamus, thalamus, limbic forebrain, and cerebral cortex through the brain stem tegmentum and the medial forebrain bundle. This system aids in the regulation of neuroendocrine functions and visceral functions (feeding, drinking, temperature regulation) of the hypothalamus, emotional or affective behavior, and cognitive and intellectual functions. Dysfunction of this noradrenergic system has been implicated in depressive illness. The dorsal raphe nucleus and central superior nucleus send ascending serotonergic axons to the hypothalamus, thalamus, limbic forebrain, basal ganglia, and cerebral cortex through the brain stem tegmentum and the medial forebrain bundle. This ascending serotonergic system closely overlaps the ascending noradrenergic system. The serotonergic system has been implicated in neuroendocrine and visceral hypothalamic function, emotional behavior, and cognitive functions. These noradrenergic and serotonergic pathways and their terminals are the major sites of action of the drugs used to treat depressive and other affective disorders.

Cranial Nerve Nuclei

Numerous cranial nerve nuclei are found in the pons, and they are discussed in the sections on motor, autonomic, and sensory systems. These nuclei are associated with cranial nerves VII and VIII at the cerebellopontine angle and with cranial nerves V and VI of the pons.

Midbrain

Motor Systems

Lower Motor Neurons. Two motor cranial nerve nuclei of the extraocular system are found in the midbrain. The trochlear nucleus (IV) is found near the midline of the caudal midbrain and innervates the superior oblique muscle of the contralateral side. The fibers of the trochlear nerve cross before exiting the brain stem. The IV nerve is the only cranial nerve to exit the brain stem from its dorsal surface. The superior oblique muscle depresses the eye (moves the eye downward) when it is turned inward. The oculomotor nucleus (III) is found near the midline in the central gray just rostal to the IV nucleus. It innervates the ipsilateral inferior oblique muscle and the medial, superior, and inferior rectus muscles. The inferior oblique muscle elevates the eye when it is turned outward, while the inferior rectus muscle depresses the eye when it is turned outward. The medial rectus moves the eye medially, while the superior rectus elevates the eye. The oculomotor and trochlear nuclei work with the abducens nucleus to coordinate the six extraocular muscles of each eye for coordinated conjugate movements of the eyes.

Upper Motor Neurons. The *red nucleus* is a large cell group found in the medial portion of the ventral midbrain tegmentum. This nucleus sends fibers that cross in the ventral tegmental decussation at the level of the red nucleus and descend as the *rubrospinal tract*. This tract descends in the lateral brain stem tegmentum and the lateral funiculus of the spinal cord and terminates at all levels of the spinal cord. The rubrospinal tract has a flexor bias and terminates mainly on interneurons. It aids the corticospinal tract in overcoming antigravity tone and in achieving skilled flexor movements.

The *superior colliculus,* and to a lesser extent the inferior colliculus, send descending fibers across the midline of the central gray of the midbrain in the dorsal tegmental decussation, to descend as the *tectospinal tract*. This tract terminates in the cervical cord on interneurons related to LMNs responsible for neck movements. The tectospinal tract conveys visual stimuli and to a minor extent auditory stimuli, to elicit reflex movement of the head and neck in response to these stimuli.

Descending Motor Pathways and Other Motor Structures. Cortical efferent fibers descend through the midbrain on their way to lower brain stem and spinal cord structures. These cortical fibers are respectively called *corticobulbar* and *corticospinal tracts*. The corticospinal and corticobulbar tracts descend through the middle three fifths of the cerebral peduncles on the ventral surface of the midbrain.

The *substantia nigra,* a dopamine-containing nucleus in the ventral midbrain tegmentum just above the cerebral peduncle, is a motor structure mainly associated with the basal ganglia. The substantia nigra has reciprocal connections with the caudate nucleus and putamen and helps to regulate the motor activities of these structures. The basal ganglia enhance wanted movements and suppress unwanted movements, working in concert with the cerebral cortex. The importance of the substantia nigra in motor functions has been underscored by the finding of degeneration and depletion of dopamine in this structure in Parkinson's disease, a motor disorder characterized by a resting tremor, muscular rigidity, and an inability to initiate voluntary movements (bradykinesia).

Autonomic Systems

Parasympathetic Preganglionic Cell Bodies. The *nucleus of Edinger-Westphal* is found in the midline of the central gray in the rostral midbrain, as a rostral component of the oculomotor complex. The nucleus of Edinger-Westphal sends axons ventrally, where they exit from the interpeduncular fossa at the ventral surface of the midbrain in the III nerve. These preganglionic parasympathetic fibers terminate in the ipsilateral ciliary ganglion. The ciliary ganglion supplies postganglionic fibers to the pupillary constrictor muscle and the ciliary muscle. These fibers produce pupillary constriction and accommodation to near vision, respectively.

Descending Pathways. Pathways descending from the hypothalamus to preganglionic neurons of the parasympathetic and sympathetic nervous systems traverse the midbrain as well as the pons and medulla. These systems were discussed in the section on the medulla.

Sensory Systems

Sensory Nuclei. The midbrain colliculi are major visual (superior colliculus) and auditory (inferior colliculus) relay centers. The *superior colliculus* receives visual input from the optic (II) nerve, and gives rise to both ascending and descending channels. The ascending channel projects to the pulvinar of the thalamus, which in turn conveys the visual information to associative visual cortex (areas 18, 19) of the occipital lobe. The descending channels travel to the spinal cord via the tectospinal tract and to the cerebellum via tectocerebellar projections. The superior colliculus is also involved in some pain processing via input from spinoreticular projections. The *inferior colliculus* sends auditory information to the medial geniculate body (MGB) of the thalamus via the brachium of the inferior colliculus. The MGB in turn projects to the auditory cortex of the temporal lobe.

The *mesencephalic nucleus of V* is found scattered throughout the mesencephalon at the lateral edge of the periaqueductal gray. Some neurons are also found in the rostral pons just lateral to the lateral portion of the rostral fourth ventricle. These neurons are the only primary sensory cell bodies found within the CNS. Their peripheral processes are Ia afferent fibers that innervate muscle spindles in facial, masticatory, and extraocular muscles. These primary sensory axons enter the CNS through the three divisions of the trigeminal nerve and then travel as primary sensory axons in the tract of the mesencephalic nucleus of V. This unconscious muscle spindle information is then conveyed to other central structures such as the motor nucleus of V, forming the basis for the jaw jerk monosynaptic reflex.

The periaqueductal gray of the midbrain is involved in sensory processing of protopathic modalities. The periaqueductal gray receives input from the reticular formation through polysynaptic spinoreticular channels. In addition, very high levels of endogenous narcotics, the *enkephalins*, are found in the periaqueductal gray, further suggesting a role for this structure in pain processing and analgesia. Stimulation of specific portions of the periaqueductal gray with electrical current can produce long-lasting analgesia, perhaps through the enhanced activity of the enkephalin neurons in that area.

Ascending Pathways. The ascending pathways in the midbrain include those tracts that ascend through the pons; they are summarized in the section on the pons. In addition, tectal sensory pathways are found. The brachium of the inferior colliculus carries auditory information from the inferior colliculus to the MGB. The tectopulvinar fibers carry visual information from the superior colliculus to the pulvinar of the thalamus.

Cerebellar Systems

The *superior cerebellar peduncle* (SCP) connects the cerebellum with the midbrain. This fiber bundle is mainly an outflow system for the cerebellum but also conveys some input to the cerebellum. The input comes from the ventral spinocerebellar tract and some trigeminocerebellar fibers. The output comes from the deep nuclei, which are in turn regulated by Purkinje cells in the cerebellar cortex. Purkinje cells in the paravermal region of the cerebellum project to the globose and emboliform nuclei, which in turn project through the SCP to the red nucleus and to a lesser extent to the ventrolateral (VL) nucleus of the thalamus. Purkinje cells in the lateral cerebellar hemispheres project to the dentate nucleus, which in turn projects through the SCP to the ventrolateral (VL) nucleus of the thalamus and to a lesser extent to the rostral third of the red nucleus.

These projections from globose, emboliform, and dentate nuclei cross the midline in the middle of the caudal midbrain tegmentum through the decussation of the SCP. In addition, these deep cerebellar nuclei also project fibers to the reticular formation. The outflow from the deep cerebellar nuclei permits the cerebellum to regulate motor activity through the control of UMN systems, such as the motor cerebral cortex (through the ventrolateral nucleus of the thalamus), the red nucleus, and the brain stem reticular formation.

Reticular Formation

The midbrain reticular formation conveys axons of the ascending noradrenergic and serotonergic pathways to the forebrain structures, previously described in the section on the pons. In addition, an ascending mesolimbic and mesocortical dopamine pathway arises from the ventral tegmental area found in the midline of the midbrain surrounding and above the interpeduncular nucleus. This dopamine pathway ascends to nucleus accumbens and the olfactory tubercle (mesolimbic pathway to limbic forebrain structures), and to cerebral cortex, particularly the frontal and cingulate cortex (mesocortical pathway). This latter pathway has been implicated in emotional and cognitive behavior; some investigators believe that dysfunction of this dopaminergic system characterizes schizophrenia, since the antischizophrenic drugs, the phenothiazines, mainly alter this system. This hypothesis awaits further substantiation.

Several midbrain nuclei that are intimately associated with the hypothalamus and limbic forebrain structures have been described. These midbrain nuclei collectively are called the limbic midbrain area of Nauta; they are the interpeduncular nucleus, the ventrolateral periaqueductal

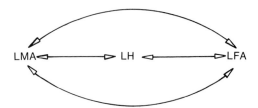

Figure 1–33. Relationship of limbic midbrain, lateral hypothalamus, and limbic forebrain.

gray, the dorsal raphe nucleus, the central superior nucleus, and the dorsal and ventral tegmental nuclei. These nuclei have reciprocal connections with the hypothalamus (mainly the lateral portion) and in turn with the limbic forebrain structures or area (LFA). A schematic of these relationships is found in Figure 1–33. These connections permit an integration of both midbrain and forebrain limbic structures through the hypothalamus.

Several midbrain structures are also concerned with processing of pain. These regions include the lateral third of the reticular formation, the central (periaqueductal) gray, and part of the tectum, or colliculi. These structures receive input from the polysynaptic spinoreticular system for protopathic modalities and help to integrate the extremely complex and diverse perception of pain. The periaqueductal gray contains high levels of the newly discovered opioid peptides, the *enkephalins* and *β-endorphin*. The enkephalins are found in small neurons in this structure, while the *β*-endorphin is found in nerve terminals whose cell bodies are found in the periarcuate region of the ventrobasal hypothalamus. These endogenous narcotic systems have a predilection for pain-processing areas and may mediate analgesic effects of chronic pain or pain associated with highly stressful, life-threatening circumstances. In addition, the lateral third of the midbrain reticular formation is important in the maintenance of attention and consciousness through projection into the medial reticular formation, conveying the ascending reticular activating system. Destruction of this system results in an irreversible comatose state.

Cranial Nerve Nuclei

Several cranial nerve nuclei are found in the midbrain and are discussed in the sections on motor, autonomic, and sensory systems. These nuclei are associated with cranial nerves III and IV of the midbrain, and to a lesser extent with cranial nerve V of the midpons.

Cerebellum

The cerebellum is responsible for modulating coordinated and smoothly integrated motor behavior. The major sensory input to the cerebellum consists of: (1) unconscious proprioceptive information channeled through the spinal cord via the four spinocerebellar tracts, (2) vestibular information from the vestibular nuclei and directly from Scarpa's ganglion through the vestibular nerve, and (3) reticular formation projections from prominent medullary reticular nuclei and some pontine reticular nuclei. These inputs inform the cerebellum of the position and state of contraction of the musculature and the tension on the tendons throughout the body, the position of the head in space, and the general activity of total-body sensation from the reticular formation, respectively. They enter the cerebellum through the inferior cerebellar peduncle, except for the ventral spinothalamic tract, which enters through the superior cerebellar peduncle. In addition, trigeminal information (trigeminocerebellar fibers) enters the cerebellum through the inferior and superior cerebellar peduncle and visual and auditory information (tectocerebellar fibers) enters the cerebellum mainly through the superior peduncle. Information from the cerebral cortex also enters the cerebellum, synapsing first in the pontine nuclei, which in turn send axons into the contralateral cerebellar cortex through the middle cerebellar peduncle. This corticopontocerebellar input informs the cerebellum of movements that have been initiated through the descending supraspinal systems such as the corticospinal and corticobulbar tracts. The cerebellum can then coordinate and interpret these planned movements and integrate them with movements already in progress, whose feedback channels relay back to the cerebellum through sensory-cerebellar input systems. It should be noted that each side of the cerebellum receives information from the ipsilateral side of the body. This is the opposite of the cerebral cortex, which receives sensory input from the contralateral side of the body.

The input to the cerebellum distributes to specific layers of the cerebellar cortex (molecular, Purkinje, and granular cell layers) in the form of climbing fibers (from the inferior olivary nucleus), direct noradrenergic fibers (from the locus coeruleus), and mossy fibers (from all other input nuclei). The climbing fibers synapse on the dendrites of the Purkinje cells, the main output neurons of the cerebellum, in a manner comparable to a vine adhering to the branches of a tree. The mossy fibers terminate on granular cells of the cerebellum, which in turn project parallel fibers into the molecular layer to synapse consecutively on the dendrites of many Purkinje cells arranged perpendicular to the parallel fibers. These parallel fibers pass the orderly parallel plate arrangement of the Purkinje cell dendrites in a manner similar to telephone wires running across hundreds of telephone poles, all arranged in a straight row. In addition, complex local neurons (basket, stellate, and Golgi II cells) modulate the cerebellar input and processing to achieve a single coordinated and integrated output through the Purkinje cells. The basket cells in the molecular layer mainly inhibit Purkinje cell bodies, the stellate cells in the molecular layer mainly inhibit Purkinje cell dendrites, and Golgi cells in the granular layer mainly inhibit mossy fiber input to granular cells. The output from the cerebellar cortex arises solely from the Purkinje cells and projects to the four deep cerebellar nuclei (fastigial, globose, emboliform, and dentate nuclei) and to the lateral vestibular nucleus. The projections of these nuclei leave the cerebellum mainly through the superior cerebellar peduncle and the medial portion of the inferior cerebellar peduncle (juxtarestiform body). The cerebellar outflow from the deep nuclei provides control over UMN systems such as the corticospinal, rubrospinal, vestibulospinal, and reticulospinal tracts. The cerebellar outflow does not directly regulate LMNs; it influences these neurons only through the UMN pathways.

The cerebellar cortex is thrown into a series of convolutions, with gyri and sulci.

The gyri are called *folia of the cerebellum*. Grossly, the cerebellar cortex consists of three longitudinal zones: (1) the vermis, in the midline; (2) the paravermis, on either side of the vermis; and (3) the lateral hemispheres, accounting for the bulk of the cerebellar cortex in primates.

The vermal Purkinje cells project mainly to the fastigial nucleus, which in turn regulates reticulospinal and vestibulospinal systems through projections that travel in the ICP. Some Purkinje cell axons project directly to the lateral vestibular nucleus. The paravermal Purkinje cells project mainly to the globose and emboliform nuclei, which in turn regulate the rubrospinal system. The lateral hemispheric Purkinje cells project mainly to the dentate nucleus, which in turn regulates the corticospinal system through the ventrolateral nucleus of the thalamus and its motor cortical connections. The outflow of the globose, emboliform, and dentate nuclei travels contralaterally to these target structures through the SCP.

An older system of anatomical description divides the cerebellum into anterior, posterior, and flocculonodular lobes. The flocculonodular lobes are phylogenetically the oldest part of the cerebellum and evolved mainly to aid vestibular processing. In general, coordination of movements of the extremities is mediated by the paravermis and hemispheres of the anterior and posterior lobes. The lateral hemispheres are particularly important for the coordination of complex hand and finger movements. It is therefore no surprise that the cerebellar hemispheres increase in size and importance as the motor portions of the cerebral cortex increase in size and importance throughout phylogeny. Control of trunk musculature and vestibular responses are mediated through the vermis and the flocculonodular lobe.

The cerebellum performs several vital tasks. During normal posture, the cerebellum must aid in the coordination of trunk and proximal limb muscles to permit smooth tone and posture, a stable upright position of the body, and error correction for minor shifts in posture. The cerebellum must also smooth and coordinate complex movements of the distal extremities, must carry out sophisticated feedback control of dexterous motor activity, and must adjust moment-to-moment motor movements through sensory feedback. The cerebellum must be recruited to achieve control of UMN systems through the initiation of specific neuronal cerebellar "subroutines" before skilled motor acts can be learned and perfected. These numerous tasks account for the need of the cerebellum to receive both multimodal sensory input and cortical input through the pontine nuclei.

A Summary of the Cranial Nerves, Cranial Nerve Nuclei, and Their Associated Ganglia

Cranial Nerves. The cranial nerves contain only three major functional components: sensory (S), motor (M), and autonomic parasympathetic (A). While other classification systems subdivide these components into numerous categories based upon developmental considerations, they do nothing to enhance the functional understanding of the cranial nerves. Rather, they obscure a rather simple system with an archaic and confusing exercise in terminology. A summary is given in Table 1–4 based on a straightforward functional classification.

To summarize further, the cranial nerves are mainly sensory, mainly motor, or mixed nerves:

Sensory nerves: I, II, VIII

Motor nerves: III, IV, VI, XI, XII

Mixed sensory and motor nerves, V, VII, IX, X

Nerves carrying preganglionic parasympathetic fibers: III, VII, IX, X

Motor Nuclei (Brain Stem Lower Motor Neurons). For a summary of cranial nerve motor nuclei see Table 1–5.

Sensory Nuclei. A summary of the cranial nerve sensory nuclei is given in Table 1–6. Nuclei associated with the olfactory and optic nerves are not included in this summary because nerves I and II are CNS tracts and not true peripheral nerves, as are cranial nerves III through XII.

Cranial Preganglionic Parasympathetic Nuclei. Table 1–7 contains summary of the cranial preganglionic parasympathetic nuclei.

TABLE 1-4   CRANIAL NERVE SUMMARY

Cranial Nerve	Component	Function
I–Olfactory	S	Olfaction
II–Optic	S	Vision
III–Oculomotor	M	Innervation of inferior oblique muscle, and medial, inferior, and superior rectus muscles of eye.
	A	Innervation of ciliary ganglion, which regulates pupillary constriction (pupillary constrictor muscle) and accommodation to near vision (ciliary muscle).
IV–Trochlear	M	Innervation of superior oblique muscle of eye.
V–Trigeminal	S	Sensation (epicritic and protopathic) from face, nose, mouth, nasal and oral mucosa, anterior two thirds of the tongue, and meningeal sensation, through all three divisions (ophthalmic, maxillary, mandibular).
	M	Innervation of muscles of mastication and the tensor tympani muscle (through the mandibular division, V_{III}, only).
VI–Abducens	M	Innervation of lateral rectus muscle of eye.
VII–Facial	S	Taste from anterior two thirds of the tongue.
	M	Innervation of muscles of facial expression and the stapedius muscle.
	A	Innervation of pterygopalatine ganglion, which innervates lacrimal gland and nasal mucosal glands, and submandibular ganglion, which innervates submandibular and sublingual salivary glands.
VIII–Vestibulocochlear	S	Hearing (cochlear division); linear and angular acceleration, or head position in space (vestibular division).
IX–Glossopharyngeal	S	Taste and general sensation from posterior third of the tongue; sensation (epicritic and protopathic) from pharynx, soft palate, and tonsils; chemoreception from carotid body and baroreception from carotid sinus (unconscious reflex sensory information).
	M	Innervation of pharyngeal muscles.
	A	Innervation of otic ganglion, which supplies parotid gland.

Table continued on following page

TABLE 1–4 CRANIAL NERVE SUMMARY (*Continued*)

Cranial Nerve	Component	Function
X–Vagus	S	Visceral sensation (excluding pain) from heart, bronchi, trachea, larynx, pharynx, and GI tract to level of descending colon; general sensation of external ear; taste from epiglottis.
	M	Innervation of pharyngeal and laryngeal muscles, and muscles at base of tongue.
	A	Innervation of local visceral ganglia, which supply smooth muscles in respiratory, cardiovascular, and GI tract to level of descending colon.
XI–Spinal Accessory	M	Innervation of trapezius and sternocleido-mastoid muscles.
XII–Hypoglossal	M	Innervation of muscles of tongue.

TABLE 1–5 CRANIAL NERVE MOTOR NUCLEI

Nucleus	Lower Motor Neuron Location
Oculomotor nucleus (III)	Midbrain
Trochlear nucleus (IV)	Midbrain
Trigeminal motor nucleus (V)	Pons
Abducens nucleus (VI)	Pons
Facial nucleus (VII)	Pons
Nucleus ambiguus	Medulla
Hypoglossal nucleus (XII)	Medulla
Spinal accessory motor nucleus (XI)	Upper Cervical Cord

TABLE 1–6 CRANIAL NERVE SENSORY NUCLEI

Sensory Nucleus	Cranial Nerves Projecting to Nucleus	Ganglion Cells of Origin
Main sensory nucleus of V	V	Semilunar ganglion
Descending nucleus of V	V	Semilunar ganglion
Mesencephalic nucleus of V	V (carries primary sensory fibers)	None
Nucleus of solitary tract	VII	Geniculate ganglion
	IX	Petrosal ganglion
	X	Nodosa ganglion
Vestibular nuclei (inferior, superior, lateral, medial)	VIII	Scarpa's (vestibular) ganglion
Cochlear nuclei (dorsal, ventral)	VIII	Spiral (auditory) ganglion

TABLE 1–7 CRANIAL NERVE PREGANGLIONIC PARASYMPATHETIC NUCLEI

Nucleus	Cranial Nerve of Exit	Innervated	Ganglion Target
Nucleus of Edinger-Westphal	III	Ciliary ganglion	Pupillary constrictor muscle and ciliary muscle
Superior salivatory nucleus	VII	Pterygopalatine ganglion	Lacrimal and nasal mucosal glands
		Submandibular ganglion	Submandibular and sublingual salivary glands
Inferior salivary nucleus	IX	Otic ganglion	Parotid gland
Dorsal motor nucleus of X	X	Ganglia near viscera	Trachea, bronchi, heart, great vessels, GI tract to the descending colon

Prosencephalon (Forebrain)

Diencephalon

The diencephalon consists of two major parts, the *thalamus* and the *hypothalamus.* In addition, the epithalamus and subthalamus are also classified as part of the diencephalon. The subthalamus is most properly an accessory nucleus associated with the basal ganglia, while the epithalamus, particularly the habenulae, is associated with limbic system connections. These two minor components of the diencephalon will not be considered further in this section.

Thalamus. The thalamus is the major sensory relay station to the cerebral cortex, acting as the gateway to neocortex for ascending lemniscal systems. All sensory information except olfactory input must pass through the thalamus and synapse before further processing by the cerebral cortex for conscious interpretation of the outside world. (Table 1–8 contains a summary of thalamic nuclei.) The sensory lemniscal input to the thalamus terminates in four major nuclei. The *ventral posterolateral* (VPL) *nucleus* receives epicritic somatosensory input from the body via the medial lemniscus and the fast component of pain via the direct spinothalamic tract. Nucleus VPL then projects this information to the postcentral gyrus of the parietal lobe of the cerebral cortex (except to the lateral portion). The *ventral posteromedial* (VPM) *nucleus* receives epicritic and fast pain sensory information from the head via the trigeminothalamic tracts and taste information via the solitariothalamic projections. Nucleus VPM projects this information to the lateral portion of the postcentral gyrus of the parietal cortex. The lateral geniculate body (LBG) receives visual input from the ganglion cell layer of the retina via the optic tract and conveys this information to the primary visual cortex on the banks of the calcarine fissure of the occipital cortex. The medial geniculate body (MGB) receives auditory input via the brachium of the inferior colliculus and conveys this information to the transverse gyrus of Heschl of the temporal lobe at the edge of the lateral fissure. An additional thalamic nucleus, the pulvinar, has part of its projection directed to a sensory cortical structure. The pulvinar receives visual input from the superior colliculus and projects to the visual association cortex of the occipital lobe.

The thalamus also projects motor and autonomic information to the cortex. The *ventrolateral* (VL) *nucleus* receives information from the dentate nucleus of the cerebellum and from the globus pallidus of the basal ganglia and projects fibers to the motor cortex on the precentral gyrus of the frontal lobe. The *ventral anterior* (VA) *nucleus* receives input mainly from the globus pallidus and projects fibers to the premotor cortex of the frontal lobe. The precentral gyrus and the premotor cortex are major regions of origin of the corticospinal and corticobulbar tracts, and cortical outflow to brain stem UMN sys-

TABLE 1–8   THALAMIC NUCLEI

Name	Category	Input	Region of Termination
Ventral Postero-lateral (VPL)	Sensory relay	Medial lemniscus, spinothalamic tract	Areas 3, 1, 2 (medial postcentral gyrus)
Ventral Postero-medial (VPM)	Sensory relay	Trigeminothalamic and solitariothalamic tracts	Areas 3, 1, 2 (lateral postcentral gyrus)
Lateral geniculate body (LGB)	Sensory relay	Optic tract	Area 17 (calcarine fissure)
Medial geniculate body (MGB)	Sensory relay	Brachium of the inferior colliculus	Areas 41, 42 Transverse gyrus of Heschl
Pulvinar	Sensory relay and association relay	Frontal eye fields; superior colliculus; other thalamic nuclei	Areas 18–19 (visual association cortex) Inferior parietal lobule
Ventrolateral (VL)	Motor relay	Dentate nucleus, globus pallidus; substantia nigra	Area 4 (precentral gyrus)
Ventral Anterior (VA)	Motor relay	Substantia nigra, globus pallidus	Area 6 (premotor cortex)
Anterior (ANT)	Limbic relay	Mammillothalamic tract; fornix	Cingulate gyrus anterior portion
Medial dorsal (MD)	Association relay	Amygdala, temporal neocortex; hypothalamus; other thalamic nuclei, basal ganglia	Prefrontal cortex
Lateral dorsal (LD)	Association relay		Cingulate gyrus posterior portion
Lateral posterior (LP)	Association relay		Superior parietal lobule
Intralaminar nuclei	Nonspecific nuclei	Brain stem reticular formation	Specific thalamic nuclei, diffuse cortical areas
Centromedian (CM) nucleus		Cerebral cortex, globus pallidus	Caudate nucleus, putamen Diffuse cortical areas
Reticular nucleus		Globus pallidus; colliculi; other thalamic nuclei, hypothalamus	Specific thalamic nuclei

tems such as the red nucleus. The anterior nuclei (ANT) receive input from the limbic system (particularly the mammillary bodies of the hypothalamus) and project axons carrying visceral information to the anterior cingulate cortex.

In addition to major sensory, motor, and visceral-autonomic projection nuclei, the thalamus also contains association nuclei that project to association areas of the cerebral cortex. The pulvinar projects to widespread areas of parietal, occipital, and temporal cortex near the supramarginal and angular gyri. The *lateral dorsal* (LD) *nucleus* projects fibers to the posterior cingulate cortex, while the lateral posterior (LP) nucleus projects fibers to the posterior portion of the parietal cortex. The medial dorsal (MD) nucleus sends fibers to the prefrontal cortex and plays an important role in maintaining the social, intellectual, and personality-related functions of prefrontal cortex. All of the projection nuclei of the thalamus, including the association nuclei, receive reciprocal projections from the region of cortex to which they themselves project. Therefore, the cerebral cortex can monitor and influence its own thalamic input.

Finally, the thalamus contains nonspecific nuclei that project only diffuse and sparse fibers to the cortex. They receive input from the reticular formation of the brain stem and from each other and are associated with maintenance of consciousness. They are also instrumental in the conscious interpretation of painful stimuli of deep, long-lasting nature. The main nuclei in this category are the centromedian nucleus, intralaminar nuclei, parafascicular nucleus, posterior nuclei, and reticular nucleus of the thalamus. These nuclei can arouse the cerebral cortex through local connections to the specific projection nuclei and perhaps also through very sparse cortical connections. These nuclei, along with nucleus MD, contain enkephalins and β-endorphin and may mediate the affective or interpretative aspects of pain.

Hypothalamus. The hypothalamus lies ventral to the thalamus and surrounds the third ventricle. The nuclei of the hypothalamus fall into two main groups: nuclei that are part of the neuroendocrine system and nuclei that regulate autonomic and visceral activities such as feeding, drinking, reproduction, and thermoregulation. The neurosecretory nuclei, the supraoptic and paraventricular nuclei, send axons into the posterior pituitary, where they release the hormones vasopressin (anti-diuretic hormone, ADH) and oxytocin into the general circulation. Additional nuclei from widespread areas of hypothalamus and other CNS regions release hormonal-releasing factors (or hormones) and inhibiting factors into the hypophyseal portal system at the contact zone of the median eminence. These factors either increase or decrease the release of anterior pituitary hormones into the blood. The arcuate and periventricular nuclei project dopaminergic fibers to the median eminence, where they may influence the release of releasing factors. In addition, dopamine itself may act as the prolactin inhibitory factor. Numerous other fiber systems (serotonin, substance P, other peptide systems) also converge on the median eminence to influence the release of the releasing factors. β-Endorphin cell bodies in a zone adjacent to the arcuate nucleus (periarcuate region) send opioid-containing terminals to widespread regions of the CNS, where β-endorphin may mediate a wide range of humoral, visceral, affective, or cognitive functions.

Visceral regulatory areas are not always organized into discrete nuclei, and are therefore called *areas*. The anterior hypothalamic area regulates the parasympathetic nervous system, while the posterior hypothalamic area regulates the sympathetic nervous system. Hunger and thirst and satiety in eating and drinking are controlled by the dorsomedial, ventromedial, and lateral hypothalamic nuclei or areas. The preoptic area regulates body temperature and sexual function, along with the anterior hypothalamic area. In addition, the suprachiasmatic nucleus and the medial preoptic area regulate cyclic activity of the hypothalamus, particularly associated with hormonal outflow. The mammillary nuclei in the caudal hypothalamus are major integrative centers for limbic system connections, receiving input from the hippocampus and projecting to the anterior thalamic nucleus. The hypothalamus also participates in reproductive and social behavior through limbic connections with the amygdala, the septum, limbic midbrain structures, and regions of cortex. This places the hypothalamus in a role as the final zone of limbic convergence.

Telencephalon

The telencephalon is made up of four major systems: (1) the olfactory system, (2) the limbic system, (3) the basal ganglia, and (4) the neocortex.

The olfactory system is represented by the olfactory nerve (called *cranial nerve I*, despite the fact that it is actually a CNS tract and not a nerve), the olfactory bulb, the olfactory tract, and an associated area of primitive cortex called the *olfactory cortex of the temporal lobe*. In addition, several limbic forebrain subcortical nuclei receive olfactory input, such as the amygdala, septum, anterior perforated substance, and anterior olfactory nucleus. The additional connections are extremely numerous and complicated and are beyond the scope of a neuroanatomical overview. Olfaction is the only sensory system that bypasses the thalamus to enter cerebral cortex directly. Olfaction evolved as a system with important direct connections to limbic forebrain structures. Olfaction plays an important role in feeding and reproductive behavior in many animals and has retained these connections in the course of evolution of the human brain.

The limbic system consists of the following groups of structures:
1. Midbrain tegmental structures, called the *limbic midbrain area.*
2. The lateral hypothalamus and selected thalamic nuclei in the diencephalon.
3. Limbic forebrain structures, including noncortical (amygdala, septum, and anterior perforated substance, also called the *olfactory tubercle*) and cortical (hippocampus, parahippocampal cortex and periamygdaloid cortex that make up the entorhinal cortex, cingulate cortex, and prefrontal cortex) areas.

The limbic system controls emotional responsiveness and expression, short-term memory, and responsiveness of the visceral and endocrine hypothalamus. The limbic system provides an individual interpretive response to the outside world and the inside world, releasing the animal from mandatory, built-in, stereotyped responses to stimuli. This system works in concert with other areas of the cerebral cortex to achieve complex behavioral activity and responses. The nuclei and tracts of the limbic system function as a single, holistic system. It is difficult, if not impossible, to specify an exact function for each component of the limbic system. The nuclei and tracts simply do not function autonomously but depend upon activity in the total limbic circuitry for any part of the system to function properly. However, a few limbic forebrain structures have been implicated as playing a major role in a few specific functions. The hippocampus is necessary for consolidation of short memory. The amygdala can regulate emotional responsiveness in the form of docility on one hand or rage on the other. The periamygdaloid cortex can regulate sexual responsiveness. However, these structures still interact with other limbic structures, and utilize limbic-hypothalamic connections to achieve the expression of such forms of behavior.

The basal ganglia (nuclei) form a phylogenetically old motor system often described as being involved in maintenance and programming of stereotyped, repetitive, and routine motor behavior. The basal ganglia consist of the *striatum*, made up of the caudate nucleus and the putamen, and the *pallidum*, consisting of the globus pallidus. The striatum and pallidum have close, reciprocal relationships with the substantia nigra and the subthalamus, respectively. The subthalamus and substantia nigra are often considered to be nuclei associated with the basal ganglia. The basal ganglia outflow, directed from the globus pallidus, influences motor activity through UMN systems, particularly through projections to the ventrolateral thalamic nucleus, which projects to cells of origin in the precentral gyrus of the corticospinal system. The basal ganglia also work in concert with the cerebral cortex to achieve control over voluntary motor activities. The basal ganglia suppress unwanted movements and enhance desired patterns of movement. The basal ganglia therefore work closely with the neocortex, and indeed have evolved to a highly complex and sophisticated level in the human brain. It is probably best not to think of the basal ganglia as an old system merely concerned with stereotyped and repetitive movements. Rather, the highly evolved structure and function of the basal ganglia and their role in aiding neocortical motor activity should be kept in mind.

The *neocortex* is a mantle of gray matter containing six sheets of cells in a laminated pattern. The entire cortical mantle consists of four major lobes: (1) frontal lobe, (2) parietal lobe, (3) temporal lobe, and (4) occipital lobe (see Figs. 1–29 and 1–30). An additional region of cortex, the insula, is sometimes considered to be a fifth lobe of cerebral cortex, but its reported visceral functions are presently poorly understood. The neocortex is the highest center for both voluntary motor activity and sensory integration and interpretation. It is a center for both understanding and initiating speech and written language. The neocortex enables humans to anticipate the future and to remember the distant past, including the ability to pass information from generation to generation. In addition, the neocortex is the neurological source of personality and is also thought to be the source of the highest mental capabilities and intellectual achievements of the human brain. The ability to describe perfectly the function of neocortex would require a perfect understanding of the complexity of human personality, human behavior and its pathology, and interaction of humans with each other, spanning the range of disciplines from psychology to sociology and history. This represents perhaps the most complex and frustrating task of neurobiology, to explain human behavior and its pecularities and alterations in terms of neuronal structure, function, and chemistry.

SYSTEMIC NEUROANATOMY

As with the regional neuroanatomy section, all structures discussed in the systemic consideration are labeled in the atlas at the end of this chapter. In addition, many of the systems described in this section are also summarized in schematic diagrams, the purpose of which is to provide the reader with an overall representation of the connections and flow of information in that system.

Sensory Systems

Somatosensory System

Sensory information enters the nervous system when a receptor in the periphery is stimulated sufficiently to send an electrical impulse into the central nervous system (CNS). The receptor is a sensory transducer that changes mechanical, heat, or light energy into electrical energy in the form of an electrical potential in the sensory neuron. Information passes along the primary afferent axon toward the CNS. The cell bodies of these primary sensory neurons are found in sensory ganglia located outside the CNS. For spinal nerves, these ganglia are the dorsal root ganglia, located on the dorsal root near the spinal cord. The sensory cranial nerves have sensory ganglia that are also peripheral, located on the cranial nerve either close to the brain stem or at a distance, near the sensory receptors. These ganglia will be discussed in the appropriate sensory sections. The axons of primary somatosensory neurons enter the spinal cord, synapse with secondary sensory neurons, and form three types of functional secondary sensory connections, called channels: (1) reflex channels (2) cerebellar channels, and (3) lemniscal channels.

Reflex Channels. Reflexes exist in several forms. The simplest is the monosynaptic reflex. In this reflex, the incoming primary sensory axon terminals, whose cell bodies are in the dorsal root ganglia, synapse directly on a lower motor neuron (LMN) in the anterior horn of the spinal cord. The deep tendon reflex (muscle stretch reflex) is an example of a monosynaptic reflex, in which the stretch of a tendon (quadriceps tendon in the knee jerk reflex) excites a primary sensory group Ia axon, which synapses on a lower motor neuron innervating the muscle whose tendon was stretched (quadriceps), resulting in the contraction of that muscle (the knee jerk). Other reflexes in the spinal cord are polysynaptic, requiring the participation of interneurons. These reflexes may function within the same segment of the spinal cord as the sensory input or may involve many segments. For example, withdrawal reflexes elicited by touching a hot object require participation of many interneurons at both local and distant spinal levels compared to the input. These reflexes can even extend upward into the neuraxis to influence LMNs of the motor cranial nerve nuclei. An example of this is stepping on a tack, resulting in the entire body withdrawing from the stimulus, requiring the movement of skeletal muscles in the body and in the head and neck.

Cerebellar Channels. Information going to the cerebellum from the somatosensory system (Fig. 1–34) comes mainly from proprioceptive receptors in the muscles and tendons but can arise from virtually all types of sensory receptors. Information concerning the state of contraction of individual muscle fibers travels mainly along Ia afferent fibers from muscle spindles into the spinal cord, where it synapses with cells of origin of the dorsal spinocerebellar tract (DSCT) in Clarke's nucleus and with the cells of origin of the cuneocerebellar tract in the lateral (accessory) cuneate nucleus of the medulla. Information reporting the state of contraction of whole muscles (tension on tendons) travels mainly along Ib afferent fibers from

Golgi tendon organs (GTOs) into the spinal cord, where it synapses with the cells of origin of the ventral spinocerebellar tract (VSCT) and the rostral spinocerebellar tract (RSCT) in the dorsal and intermediate spinal gray. Proprioceptive information from the body at level T6 and below travels in the dorsal spinocerebellar tract and the ventrospinal cerebellar tract. Proprioceptive information from the body above level T6 travels in the cuneocerebellar tract and the rostral spinocerebellar tract.

Cells of the dorsal spinocerebellar tract receive primary sensory afferents mainly from muscle spindle Ia afferents from levels T6 and below. These afferents enter the spinal cord and synapse in Clarke's nucleus in the gray matter at the medial base of the dorsal horn of the thoracic spinal cord. (This nucleus is actually present from levels T1 to L2.) Cells of Clarke's nucleus send ipsilateral projections (to the same side) that ascend in the peripheral zone of the dorsal half of the lateral funiculus of the spinal cord and enter the cerebellum through the inferior cerebellar peduncle.

KEY TO ABBREVIATIONS IN FIGURES 1–34 — 1–52

DRG	– dorsal root ganglion		V³	– third (mandibular) branch of the trigeminal nerve
ICP	– inferior cerebellar peduncle			
X	– crossed fiber connection		ARAS	– ascending reticular activating system
UX	– uncrossed fiber connection			
SCP	– superior cerebellar peduncle		Coll	– colliculus
AWC	– anterior white commissure		MLF	– medial longitudinal fasciculus
1°	– primary		Tr.	– tract
Aδ	– A-delta fiber class (small myelinateds)		Subs.	– substantia
			Int.	– intermediate
STT	– spinothalamic tract		RF	– reticular formation
VPL	– ventral posterolateral thalamic nucleus		Asc.	– ascending
			LSCT	– lateral corticospinal tract
C	– c fiber class (unmyelinateds)		ACST	– anterior corticospinal tract
CTX	– cortex		FUN	– funiculus
CNN	– cranial nerve nuclei		LVST	– lateral vestibulospinal tract
VPM	– ventral posteromedial thalamic nucleus		MVST	– medial vestibulospinal tract
			INH	– inhibitory
DTTT	– dorsal trigeminothalamic tract		VL	– ventrolaterolateral nucleus of the thalamus
VTTT	– ventral trigeminothalamic tract			
cortical area numbers – according to Brodmann			DA	– dopamine
			5HT	– 5 hydroxytryptamine
CBL	– cerebellum		SUB P	– substance P
SCG	– superior cervical ganglion		VA	– ventral anterior nucleus of the thalamus
OT	– optic tract			
SC	– superior colliculus		CM	– centromedian nucleus of the thalamus
INC	– interstitial nucleus of Cajal			
EW	– nucleus of Edinger-Westphal			

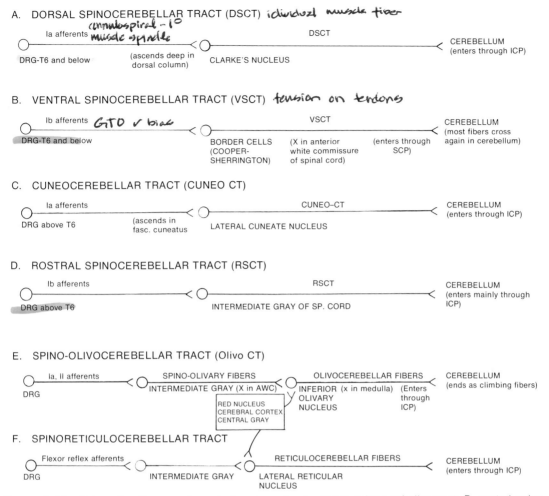

Figure 1–34. Schematic diagram of cerebellar channels. A, dorsal spinocerebellar tract; B, ventral spino-cerebellar tract; C, cuneocerebellar tract; D, rostral spinocerebellar tract; E, spino-olivocerebellar tract; F, spino-reticulocerebellar tract. These connections represent only the main pathways and contributors of these systems.

Cells of the ventral spinocerebellar tract receive primary sensory afferents mainly from GTO Ib afferents from levels T6 and below. These afferents enter the cord and synapse with cells in the lateral portion of the intermediate gray known as border cells (of Cooper-Sherrington). These cells send projections across the midline of the spinal cord in the anterior white commissure at the level of entry of the primary sensory fiber. The crossed secondary sensory fibers ascend in the peripheral zone of the ventral half of the lateral funiculus of the spinal cord and in the lateral white matter of the rhombencephalon to the level of the rostral pons, where most of them enter the cerebellum through the superior cerebellar peduncle. A majority of these fibers then recross the midline to terminate ipsilateral to the source of the primary sensory input.

Cells of the cuneocerebellar tract receive mainly primary sensory muscle spindle Ia afferent fibers from levels above T6. These afferents enter the cord and ascend ipsilaterally in the dorsal funiculus to the lateral cuneate nucleus of the medulla, where they synapse. The cells of the lateral cuneate nucleus project fibers ipsilaterally through the cuneocerebellar tract into the cerebellum through the inferior cerebellar peduncle.

Cells of the rostral spinocerebellar tract receive mainly primary sensory GTO Ib afferents from levels above T6, which enter the spinal cord and synapse with scattered cells in the intermediate gray matter. These cells give rise to fibers of the rostral spinocerebellar tract, which ascends ipsilaterally and enters the cerebellum through the inferior cerebellar peduncle.

In addition to the four direct spinocerebellar pathways, there are two indirect spinocerebellar pathways, a spino-olivo-cerebellar system and a spinoreticulo-cerebellar system. In the inferior olivary system, some primary sensory Ia, II, and Ib afferents enter the spinal cord and synapse in the intermediate gray. Fibers from the intermediate gray cross the midline and ascend to the inferior olivary nucleus, where they synapse. Inferior olivary cells send olivocerebellar fibers across the midline, where they enter the cerebellum through the inferior peduncle. It should be kept clearly in mind that the inferior olivary nucleus receives input from areas other than the spinal cord, such as the red nucleus and cerebral cortex. The inferior olivary nucleus therefore serves as a feedback mechanism for the cerebellum, integrating a wide range of sensory and motor information from widespread areas of the CNS (see Fig. 1–51).

In the lateral reticular system, flexor reflex afferents and a wide variety of cutaneous information from all four extremities enter the cord and synapse in the intermediate gray. The intermediate gray cells then project ascending fibers to the lateral reticular nucleus. The lateral reticular nucleus sends reticulocerebellar fibers into the ipsilateral cerebellum through the inferior peduncle. The lateral reticular nucleus also receives input from sources other than the spinal cord; therefore it is also an integrating system. The large receptor fields (from all four extremities) of these cells also emphasize the integrative nature of this nucleus.

It should be noted that the vast majority of cerebellar input from spinal sources is ipsilateral. Therefore, cerebellar lesions result in symptoms on the same side as the lesion. With truncal ataxia, the patient will fall toward the side of the cerebellar lesion (if the lesion is only unilateral). A lesion of one cerebellar hemisphere or one superior cerebellular peduncle will result in an ipsilateral intention tremor, ipsilateral dysmetria, loss of coordination, and past-pointing (the inability to accurately reach for, or point directly to, a target).

Lemniscal Channels. Conscious sensory information is processed through lemniscal pathways from the periphery to secondary sensory nuclei and then via lemniscal pathways to the thalamus. These thalamic nuclei then convey this information to the cortex, either by direct projections (from the ventral posterolateral nucleus [VPL]) or indirectly through nonspecific nuclei of the thalamus. Both light moving touch and pain sensations are considered lemniscal even though most of their projections do not travel in discrete pathways through the brain stem and do not actually reach the thalamus directly.

Epicritic modalities from the body such as fine discriminative touch, pressure, joint position, two-point discrimination, and vibratory sensation travel in a true lemniscal system called the *dorsal column system* (Fig. 1–35). Primary sensory afferents come mainly from skin, hair follicles, pacinian corpuscles, joints, joint capsules, and menisci of joints. These fibers enter the spinal cord through the dorsal roots and travel in the dorsal columns of

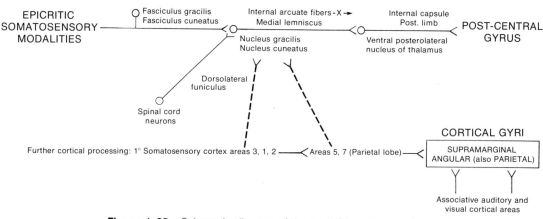

Figure 1–35. Schematic diagram of the medial lemniscus system.

the dorsal funiculus, where they ascend toward their secondary sensory nuclei in the medulla. Fibers entering the spinal cord below T6 ascend in the fasciculus gracilis, and fibers entering at T6 and above ascend in the fasciculus cuneatus. The primary sensory input is somatotopically arranged, with input from the feet ascending most medially and input from the cervical region ascending most laterally. In the medulla, primary sensory afferents from below T6 traveling in fasciculus gracilis synapse in nucleus gracilis, while those from T6 and above traveling in fasciculus cuneatus synapse in nucleus cuneatus. Additional sensory information processed through dorsal horn interneurons is conveyed to nuclei gracilis and cuneatus through the dorsolateral funiculus, providing an additional route through the spinal cord white matter for joint position, vibratory sensation, and cutaneous sensation to reach the dorsal column nuclei. Nuclei gracilis and cuneatus give rise to axons that decussate in the medulla, just rostral to the decussation of the pyramids, as the internal arcuate fibers; these crossed fibers then ascend toward the thalamus as the medial leminiscus. Medial lemniscus fibers synapse in the ventral posterolateral (VPL) nucleus of the thalamus. This nucleus projects to the central and medial portions of the postcentral gyrus of the parietal lobe. Thus the entering information terminates in the contralateral parietal lobe. This entire lemniscal system remains somatotopically arranged all the way from the spinal cord to the cortex. In the cortex, information from the feet terminates most medially, in the paracentral lobule, while information from cervical levels terminates more laterally, on the convexity of the postcentral gyrus.

The very specific and direct lemniscal pathway of the dorsal column system contrasts with most of the spinothalamic-spinoreticular pathway (Fig. 1–36) carrying protopathic information (pain, temperature, light moving touch). Protopathic receptors are generally free nerve endings or small myelinated fibers. Some small myelinated fibers (A-delta fibers) enter the spinal cord in the dorsal roots and terminate on cells of laminae I and V. These spinal cord cells send fibers across the midline in the anterior white commissure that ascend in the spinothalamic tract in the ventrolateral white matter of the spinal cord. These secondary sensory axons ascend to the nucleus VPL of the thalamus, which in turn sends fibers to the postcentral gyrus. This direct lemniscal portion of the protopathic system reports so-called fast pain. Fast pain is the first sensation of injury or pain, is accurately localized, and does not last longer than the duration of the stimulus. The slow, excruciating pain, outlasting the stimulus, travels by a more polysynaptic route. It is this pain that is so dismaying and difficult to relieve in medical practice.

Unmyelinated axons (C-fibers) of the primary sensory cells, conveying slow pain, enter the spinal cord through the medial portion of the dorsal roots, traverse Lissauer's zone above the dorsal horn, and either enter the gray matter and synapse at the level of entry, or ascend or descend for a segment or two before entering the gray matter and synapsing. The primary afferents synapse in the dorsal horn, mostly in substantia gelatinosae (laminae II and III). Cells of substantia gelatinosae project to deeper layers of the dorsal horn called the *nucleus proprius* (laminae IV and V). Fibers from nucleus proprius and fibers from cells of the intermediate gray (lamina VII), to which nucleus proprius cells project, cross the midline in the anterior white commissure and ascend in the spinal cord in the ventrolateral (anterolateral) funiculus as the spinothalamic-spinoreticular tracts. The cells of origin of those systems are the target of considerable convergence and divergence in the spinal cord. The spinothalamic tract projects to the ventral posterolateral nucleus of the thalamus, but most of the fibers never reach the thalamus directly. Instead, they end in the reticular formation.

After many synapses with interneurons of the spinal cord, which tend to diffuse the stimulus, the fibers eventually enter the spinoreticular portion of the spinothalamic-spinoreticular system and ascend toward the reticular formation. In the reticular formation, many collaterals are given off, further diffusing the signals. From the reticular formation, the information is carried to the inferior colliculus, periaqueductal gray, other mesencephalic "pain-processing" regions, and nonspecific nuclei of the thalamus. The pain information may be transmitted to the cortex directly via the diffuse projections from the nonspecific nuclei and also may reach the cortext indirectly through intrathalamic connections with direct projection nuclei of the thalamus. The cortex then interprets activation of the reticular formation as dull, aching, long-term pain. In addition to the crossed spinoreticular fibers that synapse in the reticular formation, ipsilateral fibers also enter the reticular formation. C-fibers enter the spinal cord and synapse in substantia gelatinosa. Polysynaptic channels carry the information diffusely into the ipsilateral reticular information. Thus, the reticular formation receives diffuse input from both ipsilateral and contralateral projections that derive from a variety of spinal cord neuronal pools. This accounts for the futility and ineffectiveness of tractotomies and lesions induced to alleviate chronic pain in humans in all but terminal patients. Despite severing of the ventrolateral white matter of the cord to alleviate contralateral intractible pain, the pain returns in several months. Pain has perhaps the most widespread and diffuse ascending channels to the forebrain of any sensory modality. A system that evolved for quick, adaptive responses to noxious stimuli has carried forward such a strong evolutionary legacy that it often defies even the best efforts of medical technology today.

A final comment about the spinothalamic-spinoreticular system is warranted. Some textbooks describe a separate lateral spinothalamic tract carrying pain and a ventral spinothalamic tract carrying light moving touch and temperature. This subdivision is somewhat artificial and results from a partial separation of both modalities and somatotopic levels. It is therefore best to think of the protopathic channel in the ventrolateral funiculus as the combined spinothalamic-spinoreticular system. This system conveys the direct fast pain fibers (spinothalamic), some

1. FAST PAIN: SST

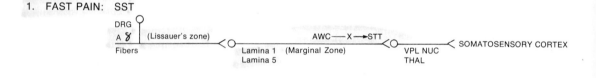

2. SLOW PAIN

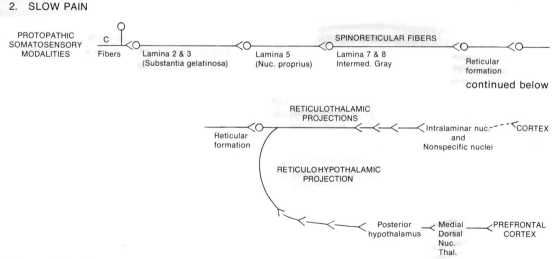

Figure 1–36. Schematic diagram of the spinothalamic-spinoreticular system; pain pathways, temperature sensation and light moving touch follow the same pathway as fast pain.

of the diffuse slow pain fibers (spinoreticular), fibers conveying temperature, and fibers conveying light moving touch. This last modality was noted in patients with lesions of the dorsal funiculus. When this epicritic system was destroyed, patients could still detect touch from a light wisp of cotton moved across the body.

Trigeminal Sensory System

The trigeminal sensory system (Fig. 1–37) is a rostral continuation of the somatosensory system. All trigeminal primary sensory cell bodies, except those innervating muscle spindles, are located in the trigeminal, or semilunar, ganglion, outside the brain stem. Reflexes mediated through this system are both monosynaptic and polysynaptic. The monosynaptic reflexes

travel via Ia muscle spindle afferents of cranial nerve V (for example, for the jaw jerk reflex). Polysynaptic reflexes include those mediated through other cranial nerve motor nuclei, such as the blink reflex mediated through afferents of cranial nerve V and through LMNs of the facial nerve (VII) nucleus. There is also a cerebellar channel for the trigeminal system. Primary afferents synapse in the main sensory nucleus and the descending nucleus of V and then enter the cerebellum, mainly through the inferior peduncle. A few trigeminocerebellar fibers also enter through the superior cerebellar peduncle.

The primary sensory afferent fibers conveying epicritic information for conscious interpretation have their cell bodies in the semilunar ganglion just outside the mid pons. The primary sensory axons project to a secondary sensory nucleus, the main

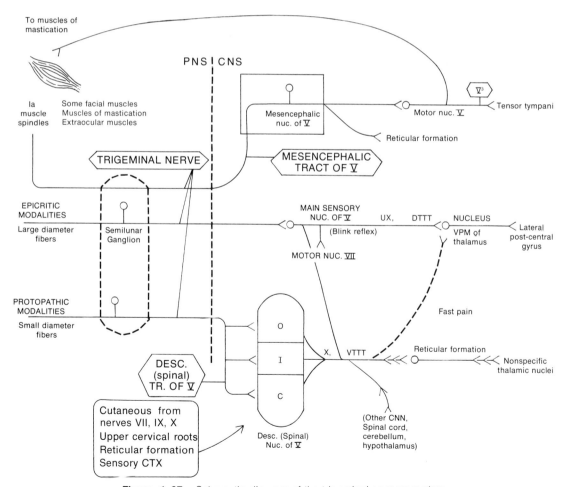

Figure 1–37. Schematic diagram of the trigeminal sensory system.

sensory nucleus of V. Fibers from the main sensory nucleus ascend ipsilaterally as the dorsal trigeminal thalamic tract (DTTT) to the ventral posteromedial nucleus of the thalamus (VPM). The fibers of nucleus VPM then project to the most lateral aspect of the postcentral gyrus of the parietal lobe just lateral to the region of postcentral gyrus receiving fibers from the upper extremity through nucleus VPL of the thalamus.

Primary sensory afferent fibers projecting protopathic information for conscious interpretation also have their cell bodies in the semilunar ganglion. They project mainly to the descending nucleus of V, especially the most caudal portion of it. This nucleus extends from the mid pons caudally to the upper few levels of spinal cord. Cells of this nucleus send fibers carrying sensations of fast pain, temperature, and some cutaneous information to nucleus VPM of the thalamus in the crossed ventral trigeminothalamic tract (VTTT). Some additional crossed projections from cells of the main sensory nucleus of V convey epicritic trigeminal information to nucleus VPM via the VTTT. Many axonal projections of neurons in the descending nucleus of V terminate in the reticular formation and never reach the thalamus directly, and, like the spino-thalamic-spinoreticular system, send diffuse information into the lateral reticular formation, where it is joined by sensory input from all other sensory systems. The somatosensory system and the trigeminal sensory system are therefore similar in the projection of fibers for conscious interpretation of cutaneous sensation to the thalamus via direct lemniscal channels and to the reticular formation via poly-synaptic connections for the processing of slow pain.

The modalities that travel in the trigeminal system arise from receptors found in the face, the oral cavity, the anterior two thirds of the tongue (general sensation, not taste), the teeth, the nasal cavity, the paranasal sinuses, and part of the meninges.

Visual System

The retina, in the inner posterior curve of the eye, contains the primary sensory cells — the *photoreceptor rods* and *cones* — that process visual information. The cones transduce color vision and the rods transduce black and white images. Light enters the eye by passing through the transparent cornea then continues through the anterior chamber of the eye, which contains aqueous humor, passes through the lens where it is further refracted and passes through the vitreous body, which contains a gelatinous but transpaent fluid. The light passes through all the layers of the retina and strikes the visual pigments in the photoreceptors, which are protected by a melanin-pigmented layer to avoid dispersion and back-scatter. The cones cluster in the central region of the retina, the *macula*, the region struck by light from an object fixed by the eye. These cones are responsible for color images for daylight vision (photopic vision). The rods are particularly abundant in the peripheral zones of the retina and are responsible for night vision (scotopic vision). When light strikes a photoreceptor, it alters the conformational structure of the visual pigment in the outer segment of the photoreceptor, resulting in a change in ionic conductance in the photoreceptor. In the case of rods, the 11-cis retinal portion of the pigment rhodopsin is transformed to all trans-retinal, which alters the Ca^{++} conductance in the rod. This in turn alters the Na^+ conductance, setting up a receptor potential. The photoreceptor actually hyperpolarizes when light transduction occurs, resulting in a decrease in neurotransmission compared to the constant transmitter release apparently occurring in the dark. The pigments are located in stacked discs in the outer segment of the photoreceptor.

From the retina, the visual message is sent through a vertical arrangement of cells. The photoreceptors communicate with bipolar cells, which in turn project to the ganglion cells in the innermost layer of the retina. An additional horizontal organization of horizontal cells and amacrine cells adds local processing of visual information in the retina. Many of the retinal elements communicate with graded potentials rather than action potentials and can produce either depolarization or hyperpolarization in the next neuron in line. Only in ganglion cell axons, the main outflow of the retina, are action potentials consistently seen. The ganglion cells give rise to the optic nerve, optic chiasm, and optic tract, successively (Figs. 1–38 and 1–39). Optic tract fibers project directly to the lateral geniculate body (LGB) of the thalamus The patterns of crossed and uncrossed fibers depend on the area of the retina in which the ganglion cell is located.

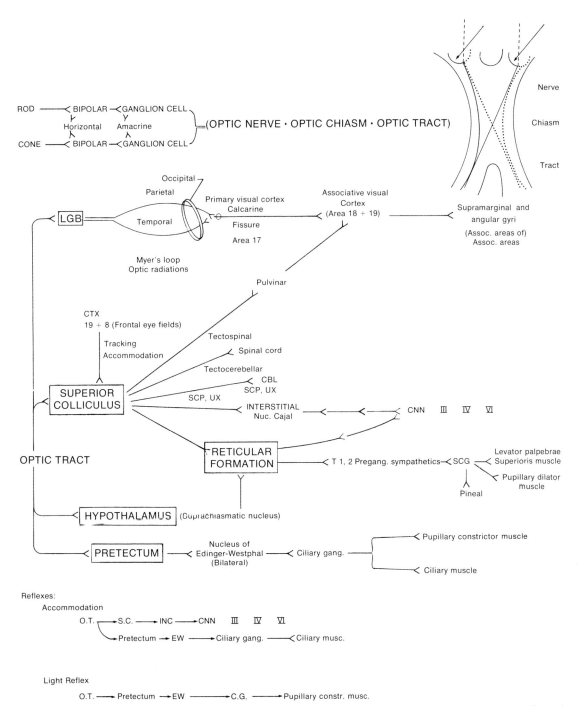

Figure 1–38. Schematic diagram of the visual system. The pathway from the retina into the optic tract is indicated at the top of the diagram. Connections of the optic tract to target structures are drawn from left to right in the main body of the diagram. Pathways for some visual reflexes are indicated at the bottom of the diagram.

Ganglion cells on the temporal (outside) half of the retina project uncrossed fibers to the ipsilateral lateral geniculate body (Fig. 1–38). Ganglion cells on the nasal (inside) half of the retina project crossed fibers to the contralateral lateral geniculate body. The area of crossing fibers is a prominent landmark on the ventral surface of the hypothalamus, called the *optic chiasm.* The tracts leaving the chiasm are called the *optic tracts.* The optic tract therefore contains projections carrying visual information from the contralateral half of the visual world (visual field) (Fig. 1–39). The LGB then projects to the primary visual cortex (area 17) in the occipital lobe on the banks of the calcarine fissure through the optic radiations in the posterior-most portion of the posterior limb of the internal capsule. The optic radiations spread out through the parietal and temporal lobes as they pass around the lateral ventricles. Fibers carrying information from the upper retina (lower visual fields) project through the parietal lobe, while fibers carrying information from the lower retina (upper visual fields) project through the temporal lobe in Myer's loop. Each of these zones of upper or lower visual information in the cortex can be selectively damaged, producing a contralateral visual quadrant deficit.

The optic tract also projects fibers to the superior colliculus, which is primarily responsible for visual reflex responses by sending information to the cervical spinal cord via the tectospinal system in the descending limb of the medial longitudinal fasciculus. The superior colliculus also sends tectocerebellar fibers through

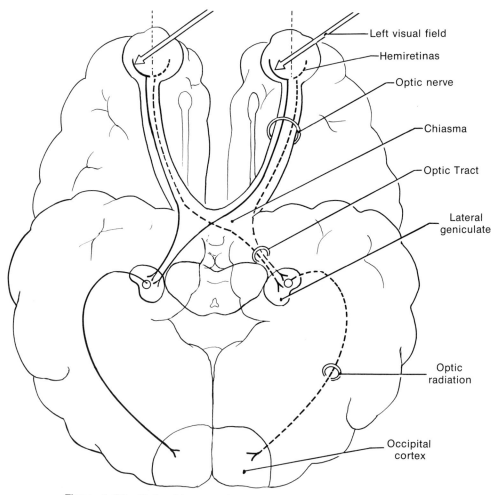

Left visual field

Hemiretinas

Optic nerve

Chiasma

Optic Tract

Lateral geniculate

Optic radiation

Occipital cortex

Figure 1–39. Optic chiasm as viewed from the basal surface of the brain.

the superior peduncle to the cerebellar cortex. In addition, the superior colliculus sends fibers to the pulvinar of the thalamus, which in turn projects to associative areas of visual cortex in the occipital lobe, areas of 18 and 19. These projections are thought to tell *where* an object is in the visual field, while the lateral geniculate body projections are thought to tell *what* that object is. The optic tract also projects to the pretectum, which conveys fibers bilaterally to the nucleus of Edinger-Westphal, resulting in the pupillary light reflex through the efferent III nerve projections to the ciliary ganglion and the ciliary ganglion projections to the pupillary constrictor muscle. Additional optic tract input synapses in the suprachiasmatic nucleus of the hypothalamus, where circadian light-dark rhythms may be influenced, and in the mesencephalic tegmentum, where light-dark cycles influence sympathetic catecholamine activity in the superior cervical ganglion through polysynaptic supraspinal projections to the T1–T2 intermediolateral cell column. The superior cervical ganglion in turn influences the output of the hormone melatonin from the pineal gland, influencing gonadal maturation.

Auditory System

The auditory system transduces mechanical energy of sound waves into electrical signals, which are then analyzed by the CNS for not only tone, loudness, and mechanical phenomena but for content related to speech and complex interpretation of the outside world. The peripheral apparatus for transduction of mechanical energy (Fig. 1–40) is a system of membranes, small bones called *ossicles*, fluid-filled ducts, and sensitive hair cells. The outer ear funnels the sound waves to the *tympanic membrane*, which vibrates at a specific frequency according to the energy of the sound wave striking it. This tympanic membrane separates the outer ear from the middle ear.

The middle ear contains a chain of three small bones, the ossicles, which connect the tympanic membrane with the oval window of the inner ear. The malleus is attached to the tympanic membrane and is moved by vibration of that membrane. The malleus in turn attaches to the incus, which moves the stapes. The stapes inserts on the oval window and transfers the energy conducted to it through the other ossicles to the oval window. This ossicular chain amplifies the original vibration of the tympanic membrane and provides for a distinct and interpretable movement of the oval window in response to a given frequency of sound waves. Two muscles, the tensor tympani and the stapedius, insert on the malleus and the stapes, respectively. These muscles, innervated by the V and VII nerves, respectively, are controlled through auditory reflex mechanisms that contract the muscles in response to loud noises. These muscles dampen the movement through the ossicular chain and prevent physical damage to the peripheral auditory apparatus.

Movement of the oval window sets up a fluid wave in the *scala vestibuli*, a cavity at the base of the cochlea filled with perilymph. The cochlea is a coiled structure in the inner ear, supported by the bony modiolus, with fluid-filled canals running through it; the hair cells, the true auditory transducing cells, are located in a special region of this cochlea called the *organ of Corti*. The fluid wave through the perilymph starts at the base of the scala vestibuli, travels to the apex (called the *helicotrema*) and at this point is directly continuous with the second perilymph-filled cavity, the *scala tympani*. At the base of the cochlea, the scala tympani ends at the round window. Thus the perilymph wave moves to the helicotema and back to the base. Between these two perilymph-filled channels, in cross section, runs the cochlear duct, called the *scala media*. This duct is filled with endolymph, a fluid high in potassium. The basilar membrane of the cochlear duct separates this duct from the scala vestibuli; on the basilar membrane sits the organ of Corti. Another membrane, Reissner's membrane, separates the scala tympani from the cochlear duct. On the basement membrane sits the organ of Corti, which contains rows of hair cells. There is an inner row of inner hair cells and three to five outer rows of outer hair cells. Attached to the bony part of the cochlea is an additional membrane, the tectorial membrane, whose distal portion moves with endolymph fluid waves. The perilymph fluid wave results in movement of the basilar membrane and sets up a fluid wave through the endolymph.

The basilar membrane widens toward the helicotrema. Each specific portion of the basilar membrane, from the base to the helicotrema, responds best, with maximal displacement, to a specific frequency of sound. The base responds best to high-frequency sounds, while regions toward the helicotrema respond best to low-frequency sounds. This specific differential movement is called *tonotopic organization*. As a specific region of the basilar membrane is displaced, the hair cells of the organ of Corti move with the basilar membrane according to mechanical forces that are different from those acting on the tectorial membrane. The hairs of the hair cells extend away from the direction of the basilar membrane into the tectorial membrane. The tectorial membrane movement in response to the endolymph fluid waves exerts a sheering force against the hairs bending them. The tectorial membrane contacts the hairs either directly or sets up fluid movement that displaces the hairs. The deflection of the hairs sets up a charge in electrical conductance in the hair cell. This change in conductance, producing a graded electrical potential,

releases a neurotransmitter from the base, which excites the primary sensory endings (corresponding to dendrites) of the primary sensory ganglion cells.

The ganglion cells are found in the spiral of the cochlea and are called the *spiral* or *auditory ganglion*. These cells are bipolar neurons, with the peripheral process innervating the hair cells and the central process entering the CNS through the auditory or cochlear division of the VIII nerve. (See Figure 1–41 for a schematic diagram of the auditory system.) These primary afferent fibers of the VIII nerve project ipsilaterally to the dorsal and ventral cochlear nuclei in the pons through the cochlear portion of the VIII cranial nerve. The dorsal cochlear nucleus gives rise to fibers that cross the midline in the dorsal and intermediate acoustic stria and ascend in the lateral lemniscus. The ventral cochlear nucleus projects fibers that cross in the ventral acoustic stria through the trapezoid body and ascend in the lateral lemniscus. The cochlear nuclei also send uncrossed fibers, which either synapse with the suprior olivary nucleus or ascend into the lateral lemniscus. The lateral lemniscus fibers synapse in the inferior colliculus. The inferior colliculus projects through the brachium of the inferior colliculus to the medial geniculate

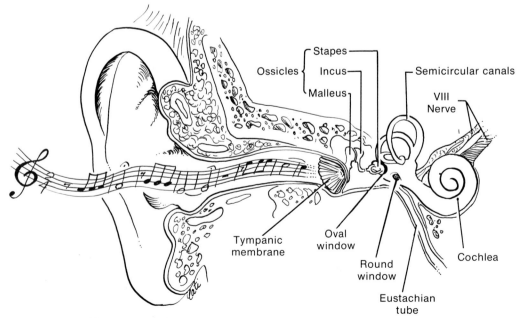

Figure 1–40. Schematic of the auditory system peripheral apparatus.

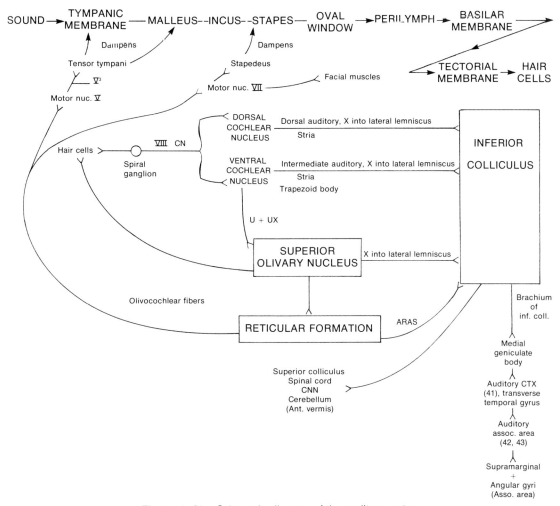

Figure 1–41. Schematic diagram of the auditory system.

body of the thalamus, which in turn projects to the primary auditory cortex in the temporal lobe on the transverse gyrus of Heschl. Other brain stem nuclei are interposed in the projection system of the lateral lemniscus.

One nucleus of particular importance is the superior olivary nucleus in the pons. The medial portion of this nucleus has rabbit-ear cells that receive information from both sides of the cochlear apparatus and act to integrate the temporal sequence of sound striking each ear at a slightly different time. Nuclei of the lateral lemniscus and nuclei of the trapezoid body also receive indirect auditory projections and send fibers into both the ipsilateral and contralateral lateral lemniscus. Therefore the auditory lemniscal channel is both

crossed and uncrossed and shows repeated recrossing at each level of auditory connections. This explains why a unilateral lesion in the ascending auditory pathway does not produce contralateral deafness but only decreased hearing in general. However, auditory nerve damage or cochlear damage will produce unequivocal one-sided deafness ipsilateral to the lesion.

At each step of the auditory pathway, reciprocal descending projections are found. One particularly prominent connection runs from the superior olivary nucleus to contact the hair cells or primary afferent endings on the hair cells. This system, the olivocochlear bundle, can modulate the transmission of auditory information that enters the CNS.

Vestibular System

The vestibular system consists of two sets of receptors in the inner ear that communicate information about angular acceleration and linear acceleration into the CNS. This information aids the brain in the interpretation of the direction of gravitation and the direction of movements through space. One set of receptors is found in the cristae ampullares of the semicircular canals (or ducts), while the other set is found in the maculae of the utricle and saccule (Fig. 1–42). There are three semicircular canals on either side of the body in the inner ear: a lateral canal, a posterior canal, and an anterior canal. These canals are all at right angles to each other, like the X, Y, and Z planes in solid geometry. If a patient's head is tilted forward 30 degrees, the lateral canals are parallel to the ground. This pair of lateral canals work together. The anterior canal of one side works in conjunction with, and is parallel to, the posterior canal of the other side. The canals are filled with endolymph and are in continuity with the endolymph of the cochlear duct through a thin ductus reuniens. Each canal has an enlarged region called the *ampulla.* Hair cells sit in the base of the ampulla and are collectively called the *crista.* The hairs of the hair cells protrude upward into a gelatinous wedge, called the *cupula.* The cupula extends approximately one third of the way into the ampulla. As the head moves, the endolymph drags behind as the canal moves (much like a driver is pushed back into the car seat during acceleration and is thrown forward with braking). As the endolymph moves differentially with regard to the canal, the cupula is bent and the hairs are moved. This movement produces a change in hair cell conductance, which is communicated to the primary sensory nerve endings through use of a neurotransmitter. This information reported by the canals is angular acceleration and is transient. During a slow banking of a plane, a pilot has differential endolymph movement only for 20 seconds or so. After this period, the endolymph and canals are rotating at the same velocity, interpreted by the CNS as a stationary position. Therefore the canals report changes in the position of the head and are transient sensory receptors. All six canals must operate properly for correct interpretation of head movements; one side balances, and works together with, the other side. Damage to the canals or the vestibular nerve reporting this information on one side will produce a vestibular imbalance. The patient will often feel as if he or his environment is moving abnormally or inappropriately, using in a spinning motion (called *vertigo*).

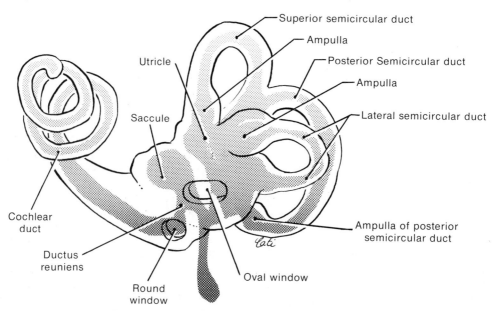

Figure 1–42. Vestibular system peripheral apparatus.

The second type of vestibular receptor is found in two enlarged sac-like structures, the *utricle* and the *saccule*. These sacs are filled with endolymph, also connected with the endolymph in the semicircular canals. In the base of these sacs are maculae, containing hair cells. Sitting on these hairs are calcium carbonate structures, similar to small pebbles, called *statoliths*, or *otoconia*. These statoliths produce pressure on the hairs, with resultant alterations in ionic conductance in the hair cells, which is in turn transmitted to the primary sensory nerve endings. The utricle is oriented so that maximal stimulation occurs with upright posture. The saccule is oriented so that maximal stimulation occurs in a supine position. In addition, some investigators believe that the saccule responds to low-frequency vibrations. These stimuli report the direction of the gravitational field (linear acceleration) through statolith stimulation of the hair cells. These hair cells do not adapt to statolith stimulation and are therefore different from the transient and adaptable hair cells in the cristae ampullares of the semicircular canals. The utricle and saccule report linear acceleration continuously, as long as the statoliths stimulate the hairs of the hair cells.

The primary sensory information concerning angular acceleration from the semicircular ducts, and linear acceleration from the utricle and saccule, travels through cranial nerve VIII, the vestibular portion. (See Figure 1–43 for a schematic diagram of the vestibular system.) The cell bodies of these bipolar primary sensory afferents are located in Scarpa's ganglion. These ganglion cells send peripheral processes to innervate the hair cells in the cristae ampullares of the semicircular canals and the maculae of the utricle and saccule; they also send central axonal processes to the four vestibular nuclei and directly to the flocculonodular lobe of the cerebellum. The vestibular nuclei send projections to the cerebellum through the medial portion of the inferior cerebellar peduncle, the *juxtarestiform body*. These projections coordinate the position of the body in space with the state of contraction and tension on the muscles. Other secondary sensory vestibular projections ascend in the medial longitudinal fasciculus to the motor nuclei of cranial nerves III, IV, and VI, for coordinated control of eye movements during changes in head position. Distortion of one side of the vestibular input results in an imbalance in the MLF system, producing a rhythmic oscillatory

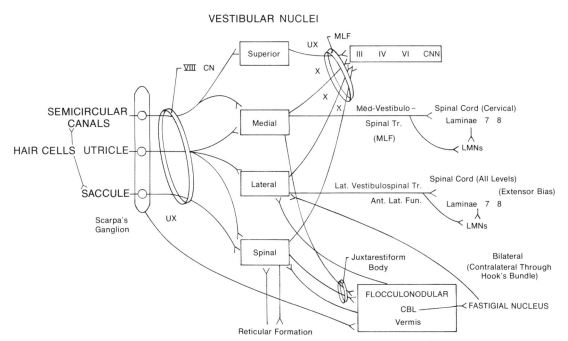

Figure 1–43. Schematic diagram of the central connections of the vestibular system.

movement in the eyes, called *nystagmus*. It is also possible that conscious sense of vestibular stimulation can be detected through projections from the vestibular nuclei to the medial geniculate body and subsequent MGB projections to regions of temporal cortex. The vestibular nuclei also send fibers into the reticular formation, where reflex responses related to nausea, vomiting, and other characteristics of vestibular malfunction are initiated.

Two of the vestibular nuclei also send UMN projections to the spinal cord. The lateral vestibular nucleus conveys ipsilateral control over extensor muscles of the body via the lateral vestibulospinal tract. The medial vestibular nucleus conveys control over muscles of the neck that maintain the head in space through the medial vestibulospinal tract projections to LMNs in the upper cervical spinal cord.

Visceral Sensory System

The primary sensory afferents carrying taste information (Fig. 1–44A) from taste buds (which contain chemoreceptors responsive to molecular stimulation) travel through the following cranial nerves: (1) nerve VII through projections of the geniculate ganglion from the anterior two thirds of the tongue, (2) nerve IX through projec-

tions of the petrosal ganglion from the posterior one third of the tongue, and (3) nerve X through projections of the nodosa ganglion from the epiglottis. This information is conveyed through the solitary tract in the medulla into the nucleus of the solitary tract, a secondary sensory nucleus. This nucleus in turn projects crossed fibers to nucleus VPM of the thalamus through the solitariothalamic tract. Nucleus VPM of the thalamus projects to the lateral aspect of the postcentral gyrus of the parietal lobe, overlapping the trigeminal system projections through this same thalamic nucleus. As a result, taste information from the tongue and epiglottis overlaps the cortical zone of projection of facial and oral cavity sensation. Some reflex visceral information (Fig. 1–44B) is also sent to the nucleus of the solitary tract, particularly through the IX and X nerves. For example, chemoreceptive information from the carotid body and baroreceptive information from the carotid sinus travel via the IX nerve and the solitary tract in the medulla to the synapse in the nucleus of the solitary tract. The nucleus of the solitary tract in turn conveys this reflex information to preganglionic autonomic neurons for reflex regulation of cardiovascular and respiratory responses.

Visceral pain information (Fig. 1–44C) is

A. VISCERAL PAIN

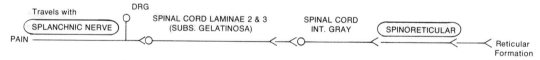

B. PROPRIOCEPTION–TONGUE

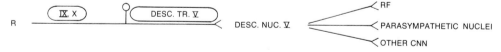

C. TASTE

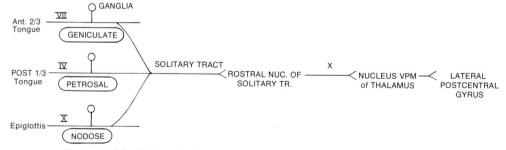

Figure 1–44. Schematic diagram of the visceral sensory systems.

not associated with the nucleus of the solitary tract. It enters the spinal cord and is processed in the same way as other pain sensation, through both crossed and uncrossed spinoreticular projections. It should also be noted that general sensation of the pharynx and posterior palate is conveyed to the descending nucleus of V and not the solitary nucleus.

The olfactory system is also considered to be a visceral sensory system. However, this system has intimate association with the limbic system, is not processed through the brain stem and thalamus, and is most appropriately discussed in the section on the limbic system.

Motor Systems

Lower Motor Neurons

LMNs send axons through the ventral roots and peripheral nerves directly to striated muscles, where the release of acetylcholine regulates the contraction of the muscle. These neurons depend upon two kinds of input to maintain their activity and subsequent muscle tone: (1) sensory input via reflex connections; (2) UMN supraspinal regulation of tone, posture, and voluntary movements. LMNs innervating muscles of the body are located in the ventral horn of the spinal cord and are subdivided into two categories. The large alpha-motor neurons directly innervate extrafusal striated muscle fibers and are under control of both sensory input and supraspinal systems. The smaller gamma-motor neurons innervate intrafusal fibers

of the muscle spindles and are mainly under control of supraspinal systems. LMNs innervating skeletal muscles of the head and neck are located in the motor cranial nerve nuclei. These nuclei are the motor nuclei of III, IV, and VI for extraocular muscles, V for muscles of mastication, VII for muscles of facial expression, nucleus ambiguus for palatopharyngeal and laryngeal muscles, XI for trapezius and sternocleidomastoid muscles, and XII for muscles of the tongue.

Upper Motor Neurons

UMNs communicate with LMNs either directly through monosynaptic connections or indirectly through interneurons located near the LMNs (Fig. 1–45). These upper motor neurons direct and control the lower motor neurons, individually or in groups, and achieve behavioral responses through an integrated activity.

The cortex is the source of the two UMN systems. The first is the corticospinal tract (Fig. 1–46). It originates in the cerebral cortex from premotor cortex of the frontal lobe (30 per cent), from the motor strip of the precentral gyrus (30 per cent), and from the sensory cortex of the postcentral gyrus of the parietal lobe (40 per cent). Cells of these cortical areas send fibers through the corona radiata, a fan-like array of fibers, into the posterior limb of the internal capsule in the forebrain, and through the middle three fifths of the cerebral peduncles of the mesencephalon. In the basis pontis, the fibers are broken up into numerous small bundles. They recondense in the pyramids of the medulla. At

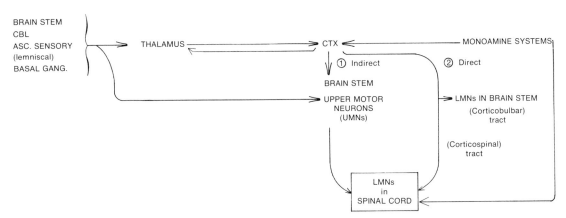

Figure 1–45. Schematic diagram of upper motor neuron systems and their relationship to lower motor neurons. Other central systems influencing UMNs are included in the diagram.

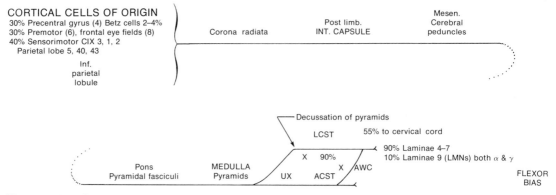

Figure 1–46. Schematic diagram of the corticospinal tract. The dotted lines (from upper to lower) indicate a continuation of the tract.

the caudal-most end of the medulla, 80 to 90 per cent of the fibers cross the midline as the decussation of the pyramids. The crossed fibers continue as the lateral corticospinal tract in the lateral funiculus of the spinal cord. The uncrossed portion of the fibers descend in the anterior corticospinal tract in the anterior (or ventral) funiculus down to all levels of the spinal cord. A majority of these fibers then cross through the anterior white commissure and synapse contralateral to the cortical cells of origin. Perhaps it is the small percentage of corticospinal tract fibers that remain ipsilateral all the way to their terminations that therapeutic intervention utilizes in rehabilitation of stroke patients and recovery from forebrain injuries. The corticospinal tract terminates heavily in cervical spinal cord segments (about 55 per cent), corresponding to control of LMNs that innervate hand and finger musculature. The corticospinal control heavily influences fine flexor movements associated with skilled hand and finger movements. The thoracic, lumbar, and sacral spinal cord levels receive the other 45 per cent of the

corticospinal connections. In the human, 90 per cent of the corticospinal fibers synapse indirectly on interneurons, while the other 10 per cent synapse directly on LMNs. In nonprimates, the corticospinal tract synapses entirely with interneurons. Direct corticospinal connections with LMNs are a recent evolutionary development seen in primates only and appear to confer a greater control over finger and thumb musculature. These movements are essential for tool use and fine dexterous motor acts.

The corticobulbar system (Fig. 1–47) arises from the lateral regions of the same cortical areas as the corticospinal system and travels along with the corticospinal system to the brain stem. However, corticobulbar fibers pass through the genu of the internal capsule rather than the posterior limb. This tract distributes crossed fibers to the lower part of the facial nucleus, supplying muscles of the lower face, distributes both crossed and uncrossed fibers to nuclei of cranial nerves V and XII, and distributes both crossed and uncrossed fibers to the upper

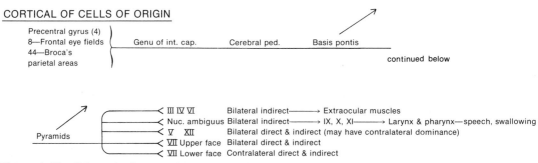

Figure 1–47. Schematic diagram of the corticobulbar tract. The tract continues directly from upper right to lower left.

AFFERENTS TO RED NUCLEUS

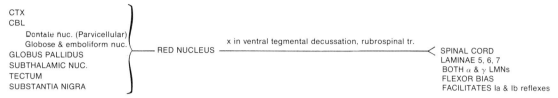

Figure 1–48. Schematic diagram of the rubrospinal tract.

half of the facial nucleus, supplying muscles of the upper face, and to the other motor cranial nerve nuclei. The result of this system of corticobulbar fibers supplying many of the motor cranial nerve nuclei is bilateral cortical control of most of these motor nuclei. Therefore, damage to descending corticobulbar fibers on one side of the brain (genu of internal capsule) usually results in a palsy of only the lower facial muscles, because the other LMNs of the cranial nerve nuclei can still be controlled by connections from the undamaged side. In some individuals, the V and XII nerve nuclei also receive mainly crossed corticobulbar fibers; damage to corticobulbar fibers on one side will result in deviation of the tongue or the jaw, when protruded, to the side opposite the lesion. Only bilateral corticobulbar damage will leave all of the motor cranial nerve nuclei with loss of UMN control (called *Pseudobulbar palsy*).

A major flexor UMN system originates in the brain stem. The rubrospinal tract (Fig. 1–48) arises from the red nucleus in the ventral tegmentum of the midbrain. The rubrospinal fibers cross the midline in the ventral tegmental decussation, at the level of emergence from the red nucleus, and synapse indirectly through interneurons with LMNs throughout the spinal cord.

The rubrospinal tract exerts a bias toward LMNs to flexor skeletal muscles. In this way, it reinforces and augments the flexor bias of the corticospinal tract, particularly in movements of the extremities.

The vestibulospinal system (Fig. 1–49) consists of two tracts. The first tract is the lateral vestibulospinal tract (Fig. 1–49A) that originates in the lateral vestibular nucleus. It synapses both directly and indirectly with ipsilateral LMNs throughout the cord and exerts a powerful extensor bias. This tract is important in the maintenance of antigravity tone and upright posture. The second tract is the medial vestibulospinal tract (Fig. 1–49B). It originates in the medial vestibular nucleus and synapses directly with ipsilateral LMNs of the cervical region of the spinal cord, which innervates muscles of the neck.

Two reticulospinal tracts (Fig. 1–50) originate in the rhombencephalon. Cells of origin of the pontine reticulospinal tract (Fig. 1–50A) reside in the reticular formation in the caudal and rostral pontine reticular nuclei. This tract projects to interneurons in the spinal cord mainly on the ipsilateral side and aids the lateral vestibulospinal system in maintaining extensor tone. The medullary reticulospinal tract (Fig. 1–50B) originates in the reticular formation of the medulla in nucleus

A. LATERAL VESTIBULAR SYSTEM

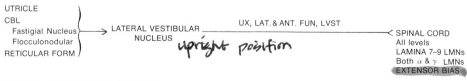

B. MEDIAL VESTIBULAR SYSTEM

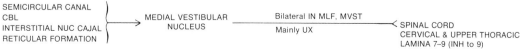

Figure 1–49. Schematic diagram of the vestibulospinal system.

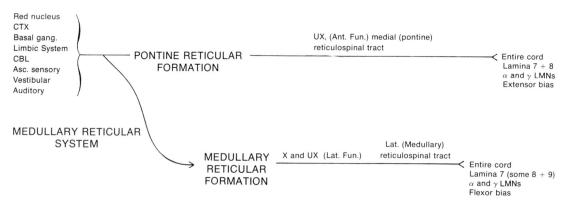

Figure 1–50. Schematic diagram of the reticulospinal system.

reticularis gigantocellularis, synapses with interneurons of the spinal cord mainly on the ipsilateral side, and aids in the maintenance of flexor tone, thus augmenting the effects of the rubrospinal and corticospinal tracts. Both of the reticulospinal tracts are mainly ipsilateral; they are the only UMN tracts that are not specifically somatotopically organized.

The bulbospinal systems are important in maintaining basic muscle tone and posture through the LMNs. In the pons, the fibers come principally from locus coeruleus and in the medulla a lesser number of fibers arise from the lateral and dorsal tegmentum. These fibers use norepinephrine as a transmitter. Additional pontine and medullary fibers come from the raphe nuclei (nuclei raphe magnus, obscurus, and pallidus) and use serotonin as a transmitter. The exact role of these noradrenergic and serotonergic fibers in maintaining the activity of LMNs has not yet been worked out. However, they do seem to be important for the proper functioning of the LMNs in maintenance of tone, perhaps acting as neuromodulators.

All of the brain stem UMN systems receive either direct (rubrospinal, reticulospinal) or indirect (vestibulospinal, bulbospinal) input from the cerebral cortex. The red nucleus may mediate influences from high structures on the lateral vestibular nucleus. Thus the cerebral cortex influences LMNs not only through the corticospinal and corticobulbar tracts, but also through corticorubrospinal, corticoreticulospinal, and corticobulbospinal connections.

Cerebellum

The cerebellum functions by comparing existing motor behavior with newly initiated behavior and smooths and coordinates the resulting movement through connections with the cells of origin of the UMN systems (Fig. 1–51). The cerebellum receives its sensory input mostly through the inferior peduncle; these enter from the dorsal, rostral, and cuneocerebellar tracts, from the inferior olive and the lateral reticular nuclei, and from the vestibular and reticular nuclei. Cortical input synapses first in the pontine nuclei, which send projections to the contralateral cerebellar cortex through the midline cerebellar peduncle. A few inputs from the ventral spinocerebellar tract and from trigeminocerebellar and tectocerebellar projections enter the cerebellum through the superior cerebellar peduncle. The cerebellum integrates this sensory and motor input to smooth and coordinate muscle activity through communication with upper motor neurons.

Purkinje cells in the vermis of the cerebellum project to the fastigial nucleus and also directly project to the lateral vestibular nucleus at the medullopontine junction. The fastigial nucleus sends projections through the juxtarestiform body to the vestibular and reticular nuclei that send upper motor neuronal projections to the spinal cord lower motor neurons.

Purkinje cells in the paravermis project to the globose and emboliform nuclei, which in lower animals are merged into a single interpositus nucleus. These nuclei

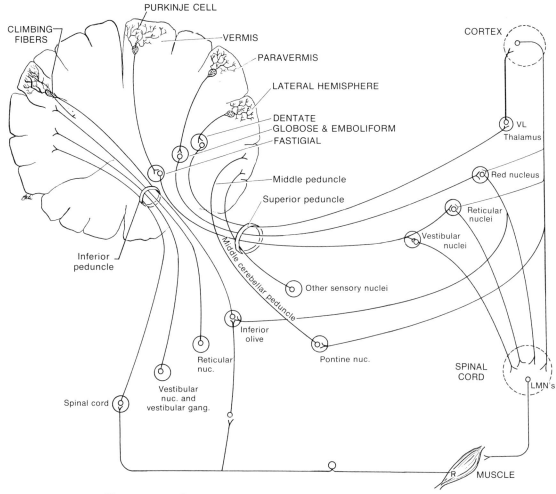

Figure 1–51. Schematic diagram of the cerebellum and its connections.

send projections through the superior peduncle principally to the red nucleus, and also to the ventrolateral nucleus of the thalamus and reticular nuclei of the brain stem.

Purkinje cells in the cerebellar hemispheres project to the dentate nucleus, which sends its outflow through the superior peduncle to the ventrolateral nucleus of the thalamus. Additional dentate fibers terminate in the red nucleus. Nucleus VL of the thalamus then directly regulates the cortical cells, which give rise to some of the cells of origin of the corticospinal and corticobulbar systems, as well as the corticorubrospinal, corticoreticulospinal, and corticobulbospinal systems. Thus the outflow of the entire cerebellum is heavily directed toward the UMNs through the outflow of the deep nuclei. The cerebellum achieves control of movement through

regulation of these brain stem and cortical systems, which have direct control over the LMNs.

Basal Ganglia

The basal ganglia are composed of the caudate nucleus, the putamen, and the globus pallidus (the pallidum). The caudate nucleus and putamen together make up the *striatum*. These nuclei are developmentally, anatomically, and neurochemically quite similar. The striatum (see Fig. 1–52 for a schematic diagram) receives input from all lobes of the cerebral cortex, from the centromedian nucleus of the thalamus, from the pars compacta of the substantia nigra via the nigrostriatal pathway, a dopamine pathway, and from the raphe nuclei of the midbrain via an ascending serotonergic pathway. The striatum has reciprocal connections with the substantia nigra via a striatonigral pathway that uses GABA and perhaps Substance P as its transmitters, terminating in pars reticulata of substantia nigra. The main output of the striatum terminates in the globus pallidus. Some of these striatal projections use enkephalins as their transmitters. The globus pallidus also receives input from the subthalamus via the subthalamic fasciculus and communicates back to the subthalamus via the pallidosubthalamic pathway. Thus two caudally placed nuclei have reciprocal interactions with the basal ganglia—the substantia nigra with the striatum and the subthalamic nucleus with the pallidum. These connections are apparently important in suppressing unwanted activities of the basal ganglia. When substantia nigra is damaged in humans, Parkinson's disease results, with muscular rigidity, a resting tremor, and *bradykinesia* (a slowness of initiating voluntary movements). When the subthalamic nucleus is damaged in humans, *ballismus* (wild uncontrolled flailing movements of the limbs) results.

The major output of the basal ganglia is directed through the pallidum. The globus pallidus projects to the ventrolateral and ventral anterior nuclei of the thalamus, as well as to the nonspecific centromedian nucleus of the thalamus. These pallidothalamic projections travel via the ansa lenticularis and the lenticular fasciculus, which then join the thalamic fasciculus. The globus pallidus also sends polysynaptic descending projections into the brain stem through the pallidotegmental tract.

The activity of the basal ganglia is integrated with the thalamus, cerebellum, and cortex to regulate motor movements. The thalamus, particularly the ventrolateral nucleus, receives communication from the globus pallidus, the dentate nucleus of the cerebellum, and the red nucleus. The thalamus then sends information to UMNs of the cortex, which modulate the outflow of the vital cortical motor neurons. Therefore both the cerebellum and the basal ganglia influence motor outflow only through connections with UMNs. The basal ganglia are reported to participate in the initiation and control of stereotyped, repetitive movements. However, the function of the

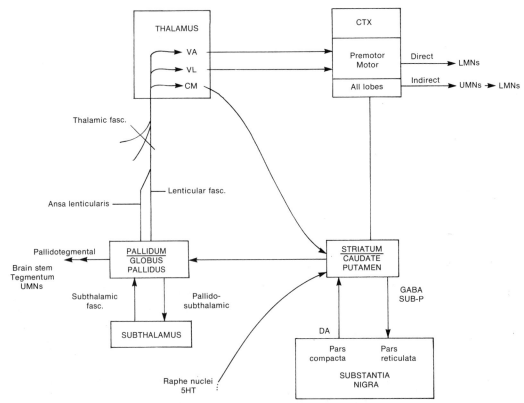

Figure 1–52. Schematic diagram of the basal ganglia and their connections.

basal ganglia is best considered as an adjunct to the cortex, through which they can maintain a focus on desired voluntary movements and can suppress superfluous unwanted movements. The basal ganglia are so thoroughly integrated with other motor components of the CNS that it is easier to explain dysfunction than function. Damage to the cerebellum or the basal ganglia and its associated nuclei results in involuntary motor disorders such as tremor, rigidity, incoordination, and involuntary movements. These motor phenomena result from altered activity in the affected structure, which in turn alters the activity of the UMNs to which it projects, and the subsequent LMNs under the regulation of those altered UMN systems. Pathology of the cerebellum and basal ganglia clearly illustrate the point that neuronal damage can often be reflected in a patient's actions or activities only through subsequent altered activity or dysfunction of long chains of neurons. For example, substantia nigra damage results in motor problems of the limbs through the dysfunction of a chain of at least six neurons.

Visceral and Neuroendocrine Systems

Pituitary and Median Eminence

The pituitary gland is composed of two major lobes, the anterior lobe and the posterior lobe. The posterior pituitary contains the terminals of neurosecretory cells from the supraoptic and paraventricular nuclei, which release vasopressin and oxytocin directly into the blood. The anterior pituitary has few direct neuronal connections from the hypothalamus; instead, the median eminence of the hypothalamus acts as a zone (hypophyseotrophic zone) in which releasing and inhibitory factors are secreted into primary capillaries of the hypophyseal-portal system, which transports these factors to the anterior pituitary where they activate or inhibit the release of hormones into the blood.

The median eminence is controlled by hypothalamic inputs that influence the release of these factors and by other brain stem and forebrain systems whose projections influence the outflow of the releasing or inhibitory factors. The other regulatory systems influencing the median eminence include peptide systems, catecholamine systems, serotonin systems, and many other transmitter systems.

Hypothalamus

The nuclei and areas of the hypothalamus can be divided into two functional but overlapping groups, the neuroendocrine centers and the visceral regulatory centers. The neuroendocrine centers include the supraoptic and paraventricular nuclei, which release vasopressin and oxytocin from terminals in the posterior pituitary, and the arcuate and periventricular nuclei, which send dopaminergic fibers to the contact zone of the median eminence to influence the release of releasing or inhibitory factors. Some neurons that manufacture releasing or inhibitory factors and send projections to the contact zone of the median eminence may have their cell bodies in the hypothalamus.

The visceral regulatory nuclei of the hypothalamus include the posterior hypothalamic area, the anterior hypothalamic area, the mammillary nuclei, the dorsomedial and ventromedial nuclei, the lateral hypothalamic area, the preoptic nuclei, and the suprachiasmatic nucleus. The posterior hypothalamic area regulates the sympathetic nervous system through the descending projections of the medial forebrain bundle. The anterior hypothalamic area regulates the parasympathetic nervous system via projections to the midbrain through the dorsal longitudinal fasciculus. Both of these autonomic regulatory areas of the hypothalamus are regulated by input from the limbic forebrain.

The mammillary nuclei of the hypothalamus form a major connection in the limbic system. They receive input from the hippocampus via the fornix. These nuclei also receive input from the mesencephalic tegmentum through the mammillary peduncle. The mammillary nuclei send information to the anterior nucleus of the thalamus via the mammillothalamic tract, forming part of Papez's circuit of limbic activity. The mammillary nuclei also send outflow to the mesencephalic tegmentum through the mammillotegmental tract, which it is integrated with other descending hypothalamic influences that terminate in the mesencephalic tegmentum and exert control over the autonomic nervous system and motor nuclei.

The dorsomedial and ventromedial nuclei have been implicated in feeding behavior. The input to this area comes from the limbic forebrain. Output goes through both the medial forebrain bundle and the dorsal longitudinal fasciculus to autonomic and motor nuclei in the brain stem. There are also numerous intrahypothalamic projections interconnecting the dorsomedial and ventromedial nuclei with areas such as the lateral hypothalamic area.

The lateral hypothalamic area is associated with feeding and drinking behavior. It is also the main interconnecting zone between the limbic forebrain and the limbic midbrain areas. Major input from the mesencephalic tegmentum and from brain stem monoamine nuclei arrives via the medial forebrain bundle. The lateral hypothalamic area also receives input from olfactory structures, orbitofrontal cortex, and septal nuclei via descending projectioning of the medial forebrain bundle.

The preoptic area receives input from the amygdala via the stria terminalis, from the orbitofrontal cortex via the medial forebrain bundle, and from other hypothalamic nuclei. The preoptic output goes mainly to other hypothalamic nuclei, where it is thought to regulate circadian and cyclic rhythms, particularly in association with sex hormones. Both the suprachiasmatic and the preoptic nuclei have been implicated in control of circadian rhythms.

In summary, it is clear that the hypothalamus, as both the neuroendocrine and visceral regulatory system, is an important region of influence of the limbic system and its connections. This relationship is further discussed below.

Limbic System

The limbic system controls emotional responsiveness and affective behavior through the utilization of the visceral and neuroendocrine systems of the hypothalamus. The limbic system consists of a midbrain portion situated in the midbrain tegmentum. The limbic midbrain includes the dorsal and ventral tegmental nuclei, the interpeduncular nucleus, the serotonergic central superior and dorsal raphe nuclei, the ventrolateral periaqueductal gray, and the ventral tegmental area. These areas receive integrated sensory and visceral information from the reticular formation. The limbic midbrain conveys the actual state of the body, both internally and externally, to the hypothalamus and to the limbic forebrain. The limbic forebrain projects back to the limbic midbrain, placing the hypothalamus in a strategic position for integrating information going in both directions. The lateral hypothalamus subserves this major integrative position within the hypothalamus. In addition, the limbic midbrain structures project to many limbic forebrain areas, including the septum, amygdala, olfactory tubercle, nucleus accumbens, cingulate cortex, and hippocampus.

The limbic forebrain consists of both cortical and subcortical structures. The subcortical structures include the septum, amygdala, and basal olfactory nuclei such as the olfactory tubercle (anterior perforated substance), nucleus accumbens, and anterior olfactory nucleus. The cortical structures include the hippocampus, the cingulate cortex, entorhinal cortex (including parahippocampal and periamygdaloid cortex), and prefrontal cortex. Most of the limbic forebrain connections channel into the hypothalamus, where they influence both visceral hypothalamic and neuroendocrine outflow. The individual structures making up the limbic forebrain are difficult to describe functionally because they act as an integrated whole. The entire limbic forebrain must act together to achieve the regulation of affective behavior that is normally seen. However, a few pathways are of particular importance. The hippocampus sends information to the mammillary bodies, the septum, and the preoptic hypothalamus via the fornix. The amygdala interconnects with many visceral and neuroendocrine centers of the hypothalamus via the stria terminalis and the direct amygdalofugal pathway (diagonal band of Broca). The septum has a major output to the hippocampus through the fornix and also interconnects with the hypothalamus. The cingulate cortex also has a major influence over the hippocampus through polysynaptic connections. Prefrontal cortex sends projections to the anterior and preoptic hypothalamus via the descending portion of the medial forebrain bundle. Both cerebral neocortex and the olfactory system play a major controlling role over limbic forebrain structures.

Thalamus and Neocortex

The thalamus is the major relay center to the cortex for all sensory systems except the olfactory system, for motor systems, particularly the cerebellum and basal ganglia, and for autonomic-visceral systems through the anterior nuclei. A discussion of the thalamic nuclei and the portions of cortex to which they project was presented in the section on regional neuroanatomy. Since the thalamus and cortex have reciprocal connections and act in concert to maintain the overall activity of the cerebral cortex, only a few functional aspects of the cortex will be further discussed in this section.

The cerebral cortex receives information from specific projection nuclei of the thalamus, from a few fibers of nonspecific thalamic nuclei, from the olfactory system, and from brain stem noradrenergic, dopaminergic, and serotonergic nuclei. The output of the cortex includes projection fibers, commissural fibers, and association fibers. The projection fibers have been partially discussed with motor systems. The major projection fibers of the cerebral cortex include the following systems:

1. Corticospinal tract
2. Corticobulbar tract
3. Corticorubrospinal system
4. Corticoreticulospinal system
5. Corticobulbospinal system (polysynaptic)
6. Corticotectal fibers regulating visual reflex responses
7. Corticopontine fibers
8. Corticostriate fibers
9. Corticonuclear fibers to secondary nuclei for regulation of sensory input
10. Corticothalamic connections with all projection nuclei and with nonspecific thalamic nuclei
11. Cortical connections to other brain stem nuclei such as the inferior olivary nucleus

It can therefore be seen that the cortical outflow projects to virtually every subdivision of the CNS and regulates major functions of the brain and spinal cord.

In addition to projection fibers, the cortex has many cortical intercommunications. These connections are of two types: commissural bundles that cross the midline, and association, or arcuate, fibers that interconnect cortical areas of a single hemisphere. The commissural bundles (see Fig. 1–30) are the corpus callosum and the anterior commissure. The corpus callosum interconnects the frontal lobes (through the rostrum and genu), the parietal lobes (through the body) and the temporal and occipital lobes (through the body and splenium). The anterior commissure mainly interconnects limbic forebrain structures of the temporal lobes. Arcuate fibers are either short arcuate fibers, interconnecting adjacent gyri, or long arcuate fibers, interconnecting more distant areas of cortex.

One particularly interesting feature of the cortex is lateralization of function. The two hemispheres are not identical. One of the hemispheres, the dominant hemisphere, controls both the understanding and the interpretation of speech and the motor initiation of speech. In 98 per cent of humans, the dominant hemisphere is the left hemisphere. Broca's area in the frontal lobe is the area of motor control, or expressive control of speech. Also, on the parietotemporal border of the dominant hemisphere is Wernicke's area, the receptive area for speech. Loss of these areas renders a person unable to initiate speech or to understand speech, respectively. Although Broca's area and Wernicke's area are described as separate regions, they really represent a continuum of cortex involved in language function. Control of writing and reading of language is also under principal control of the dominant hemisphere, in more posterior areas of parietotemporal cortex. Damage here may result in dyslexia or dysgraphia. The nondominant hemisphere processes geometric and spatial relationships. Recent data also suggest that the dominant auditory cortex emphasizes processing of spoken language while the nondominant auditory cortex plays a major role in musical interpretation and appreciation. Thus, both the dominant and nondominant (or the conversant or nonconversant) hemispheres must work together to achieve a final interpretation of the outside world and to achieve a full complement of human skills and behavior.

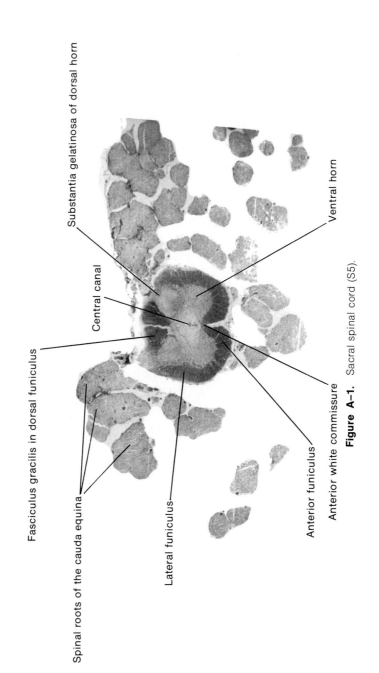

Figure A–1. Sacral spinal cord (S5).

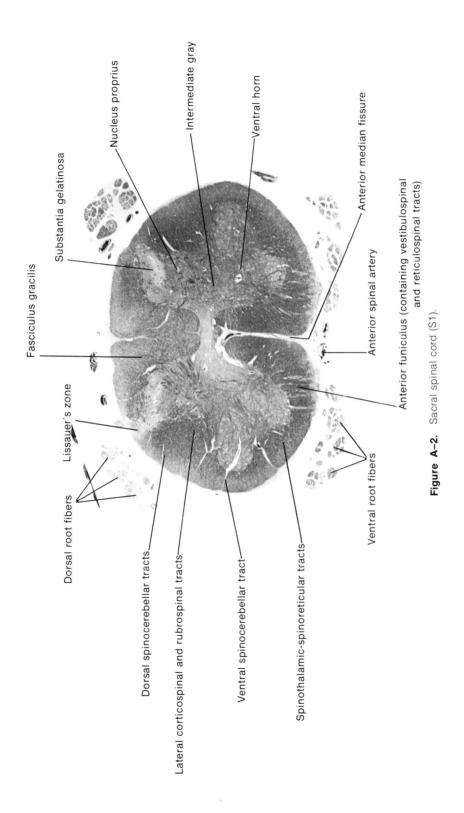

Figure A–2. Sacral spinal cord (S1).

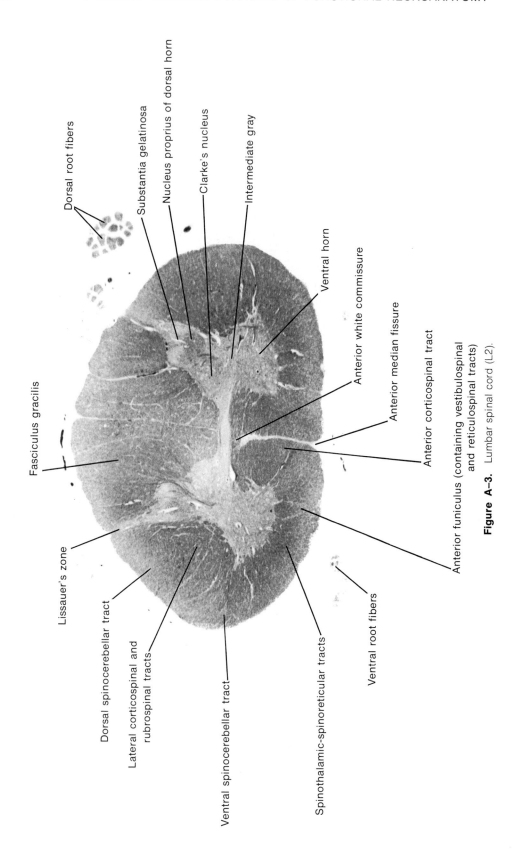

Figure A–3. Lumbar spinal cord (L2).

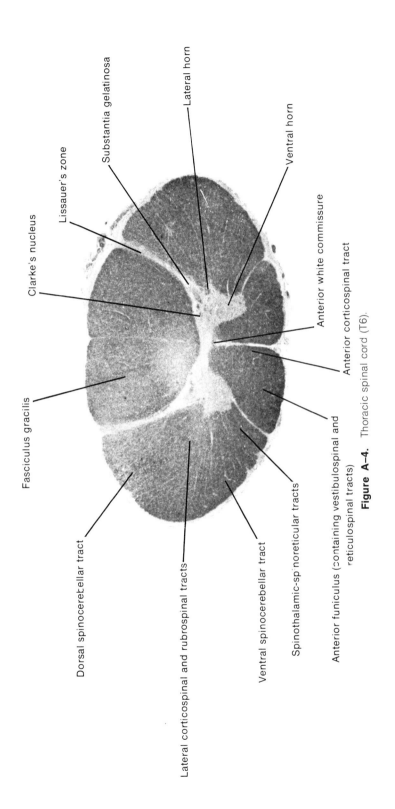

Figure A–4. Thoracic spinal cord (T6).

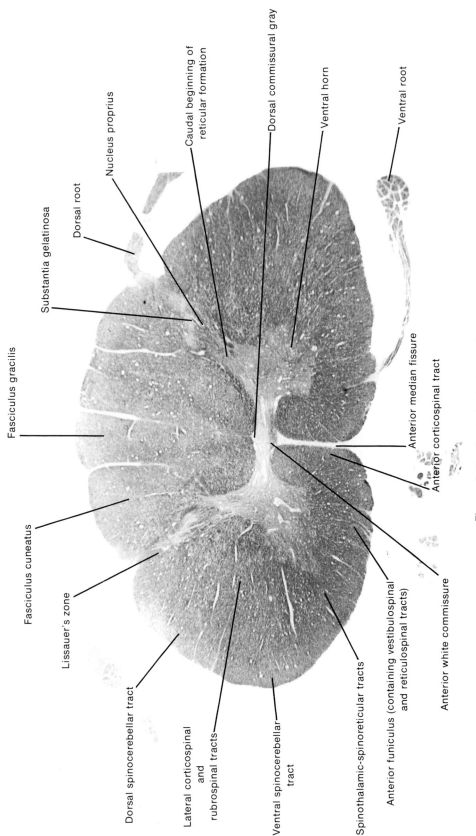

Figure A–5. Cervical spinal cord (C7).

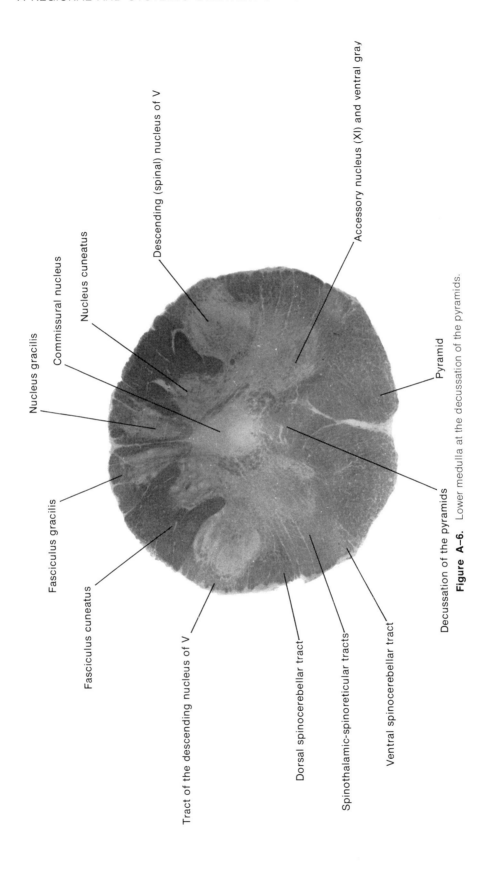

Figure A–6. Lower medulla at the decussation of the pyramids.

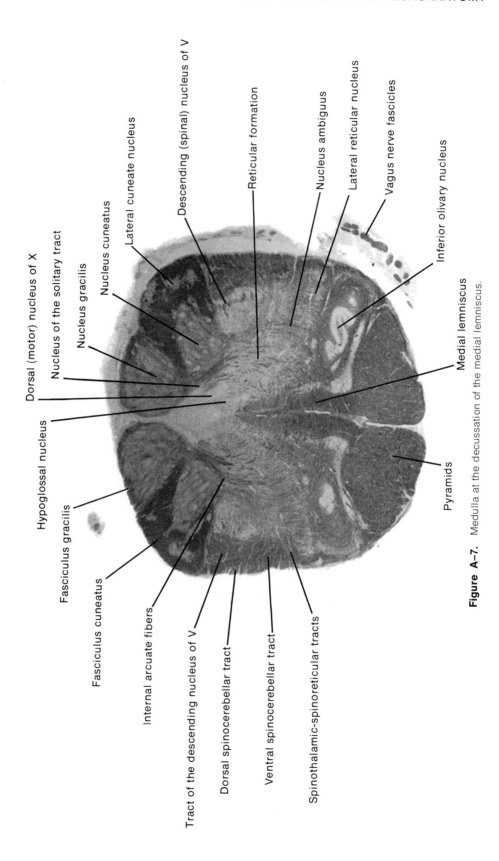

Figure A–7. Medulla at the decussation of the medial lemniscus.

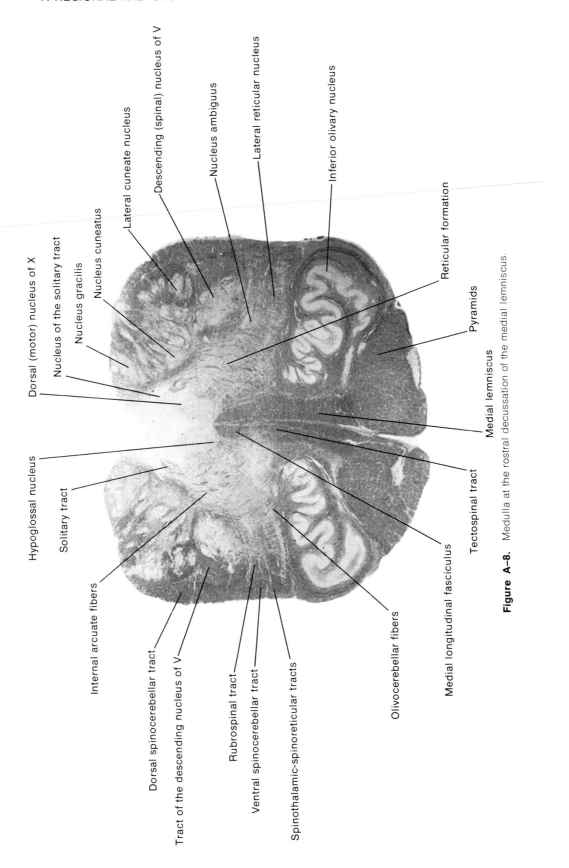

Figure A–8. Medulla at the rostral decussation of the medial lemniscus.

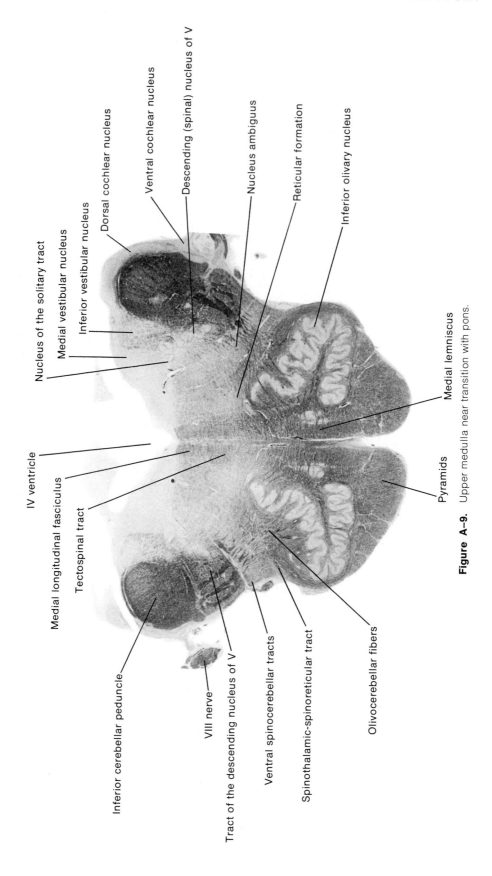

Figure A–9. Upper medulla near transition with pons.

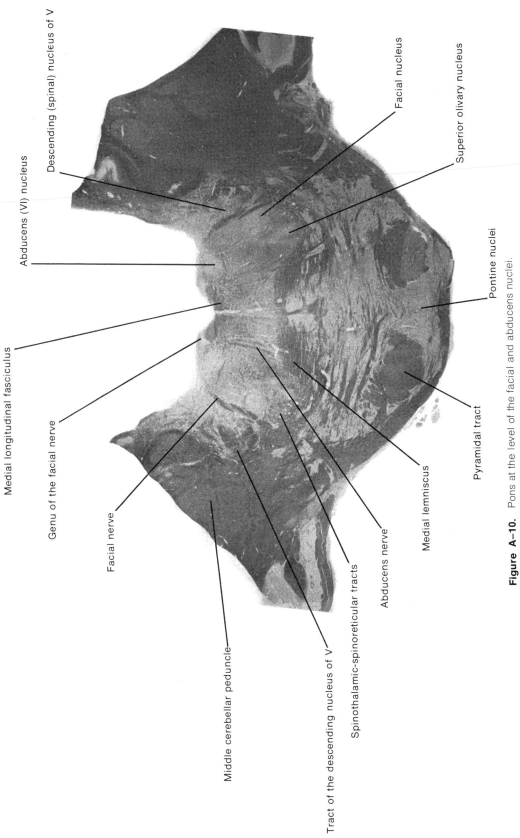

Figure A–10. Pons at the level of the facial and abducens nuclei.

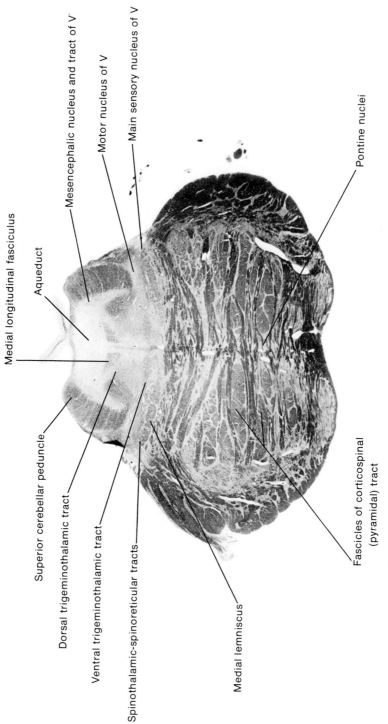

Medial longitudinal fasciculus

Aqueduct

Mesencephalic nucleus and tract of V

Motor nucleus of V

Main sensory nucleus of V

Pontine nuclei

Superior cerebellar peduncle

Dorsal trigeminothalamic tract

Ventral trigeminothalamic tract

Spinothalamic-spinoreticular tracts

Medial lemniscus

Fascicles of corticospinal (pyramidal) tract

Figure A–11. Pons at the level of the motor and main sensory trigeminal nuclei.

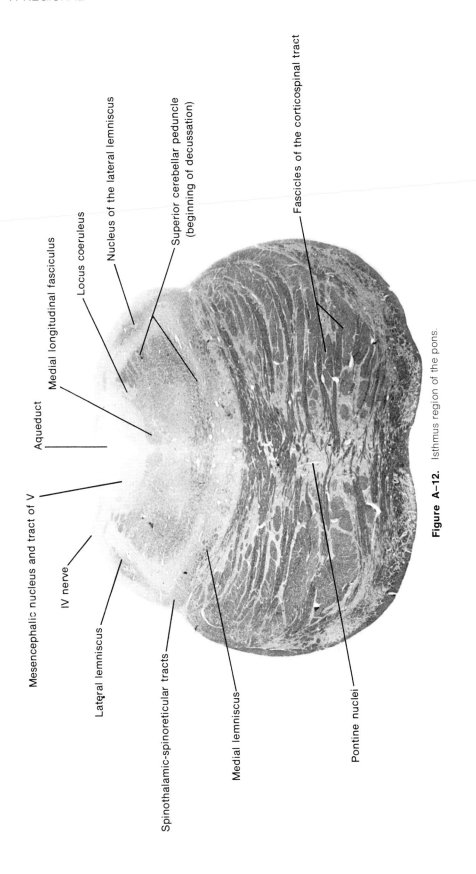

Figure A–12. Isthmus region of the pons.

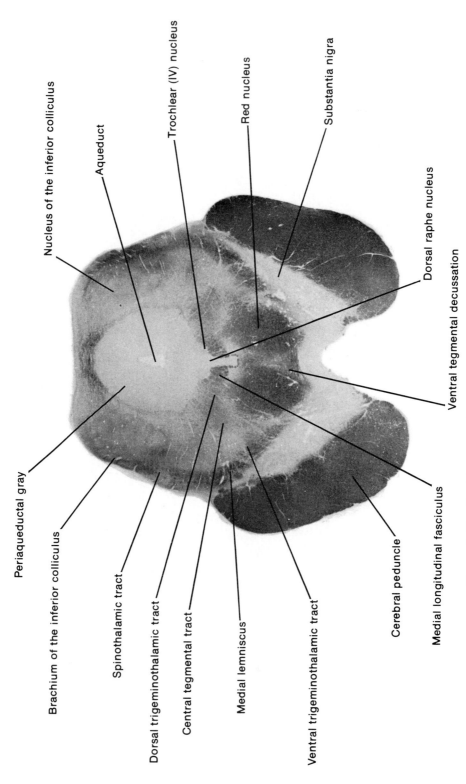

Figure A–13. Caudal mesencephalon at the level of the inferior colliculus.

Nucleus of the inferior colliculus

Aqueduct

Trochlear (IV) nucleus

Red nucleus

Substantia nigra

Dorsal raphe nucleus

Ventral tegmental decussation

Periaqueductal gray

Brachium of the inferior colliculus

Spinothalamic tract

Dorsal trigeminothalamic tract

Central tegmental tract

Medial lemniscus

Ventral trigeminothalamic tract

Cerebral peduncle

Medial longitudinal fasciculus

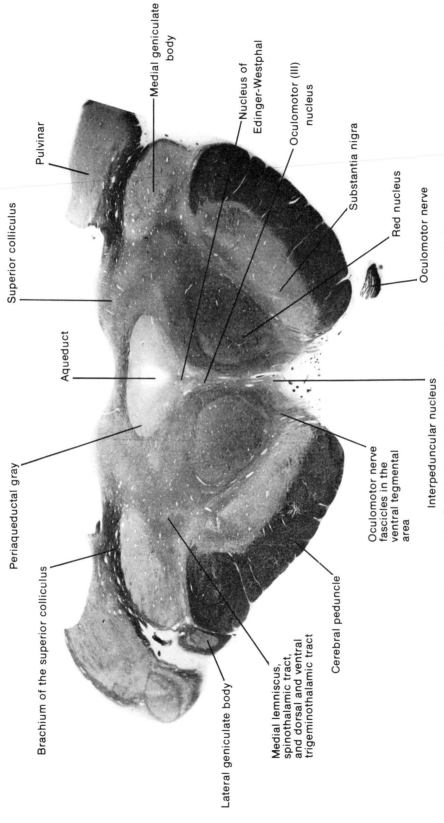

Figure A–14. Rostral mesencephalon at the level of the superior colliculus.

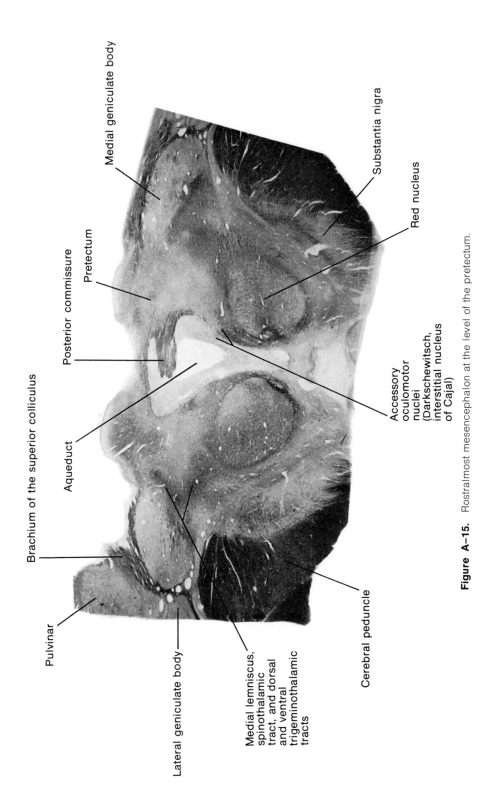

Figure A–15. Rostralmost mesencephalon at the level of the pretectum.

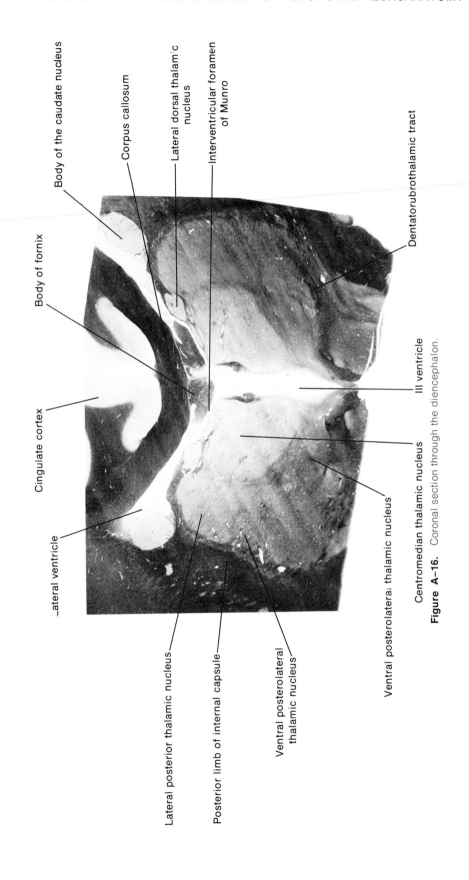

Figure A–16. Coronal section through the diencephalon.

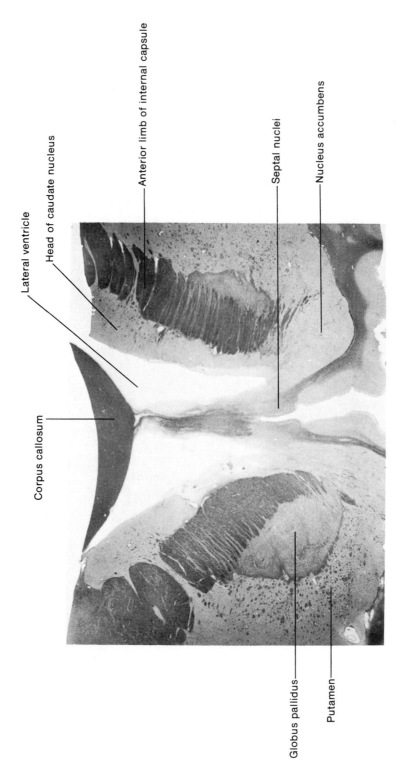

Figure A–17. Coronal section of basal ganglia rostral to the anterior commissure.

ANNOTATED BIBLIOGRAPHY

GENERAL AND INTRODUCTORY NEUROSCIENCES REFERENCES

Introductory References

1. Scientific American, September 1979, The Brain.

   The entire edition of Scientific American contains articles in brain sciences. An impressive group of scientists shares thoughts on the direction and future of neurosciences while presenting a solid core of information. This should be a starting point for the beginning student, but it is just as exciting reading for the professional neuroscientist. We particularly recommend the chapter on "The Organization of the Brain" by Nauta and Feirtog. Dr. Nauta's schematic model of the brain establishes the conceptual basis for neuroanatomy. Since one of the authors of the present chapter (D.L.F.) first learned neuroanatomy from Dr. Nauta at MIT, we are particularly fond of his approach. The more details and depth the reader adds to his or her own understanding of the brain, the more elegant Dr. Nauta's model seems. Read it, then reread it as your perspective changes.

2. Eccles JC.: The Understanding of the Brain, 2nd ed. New York, McGraw-Hill, 1973.

   Eccles presents a simple and elegant explanation of basic cellular neurophysiology, a field to which he has contributed so much. He then expands into motor control, learning and plasticity, speech and consciousness, and even a little philosophy. This neurophysiological introduction to the brain is a good starting point for the beginning student and informative reading for the more advanced student. He combines simplicity and complexity into a surprisingly power-packed paperback.

3. Bullock TH: Introduction to Nervous System, San Francisco, W. H. Freeman and Co., 1977.

   This book takes a unique approach to nervous systems. Cellular and molecular neurobiology are introduced, followed by more and more integrative approaches, often based on simple invertebrate nervous systems. The book presents concepts and basic principles of neurobiology in a superb fashion. The illustrations and diagrams are well done and extremely helpful in understanding the text. The book is a good introduction for the beginning student and is loaded with fascinating data and ideas often overlooked by medically oriented approaches to neurosciences. This book should be read as a prerequisite to studying the human nervous system. It provides the added benefit of an amazingly clear account of cellular neurophysiology, an area in which even the simplest of facts can be readily obscured or mired in a morass of complex graphs and incomprehensible symbols.

General Medical Neurobiology

1. Noback CR, Demarest RJ: The Human Nervous System: Basic Principles of Neurobiology, 2nd ed. New York, McGraw-Hill, 1975.

   This is one of the best systemically organized neurobiology textbooks available. The text reads clearly and the illustrations are excellent. While classical neuroanatomy is not as heavily emphasized as in many texts on the nervous system, functional systemic neuroanatomy is well presented. This book is our choice for a brief integrated neurosciences course with clinical correlations and a systemic slant.

2. Willis WD, Grossman RG: Medical Neurobiology, 2nd ed. St. Louis, C. V. Mosby Co., 1977.

   This text presents an integrated approach to neurobiology. After a brief regional neuroanatomical presentation, systemic neurosciences are emphasized. Numerous line diagrams are presented for aid in learning connections.

Introductory Texts to Selected Areas of Neurosciences

1. Shepherd GM: The Synaptic Organization of the Brain, 2nd ed. New York, Oxford University Press, 1979.

   Gordon Shepherd has bridged the gap between cellular neurobiology-transmitter events and neuroanatomical connections with a beautifully organized and lucidly written book. Following an introduction to neuronal structure, physiology, and transmission, Shepherd discusses the better-known neural regions for connectivity, such as peripheral ganglia, spinal cord, ventral horn, olfactory bulb, retina, cerebellum, thalamus, basal ganglia, olfactory cortex, hippocampus, and sensory and motor neocortex. For each area, he discusses the basic neuronal elements, synaptic connections, basic circuits, synaptic actions, neurotransmitters, and dendritic properties. The chapters are clear and build logically, are remarkably easy to read, are highly informative, and give an excellent hint of how the brain is actually "wired," through the anatomical, physiological, and chemical specificity of individual cell types in specific subportions of known structures. This book is a must for the student of neurosciences.

2. Jacobson M: Developmental Neurobiology, 2nd ed. New York, Plenum Press, 1978.

   This book presents a well-organized and scholarly account of developmental neurosciences. Both current research findings and classical descriptive work are merged into a single presentation. Cellular and molecular neurobiology are heavily emphasized, reflecting the research trends of the last decade. The book is relatively easy reading, with added depth that does not detract from the easier material. The advanced student will feel very comfortable reading it, while the beginning student will have to be selective. This is probably the best summary of developmental neurobiology available.

3. Kandel ER: Cellular Basis of Behavior. San Francisco, W. H. Freeman and Co., 1976.

   A well-written account of behavioral neurobiology characterizes the author's effort to explain behavior on a neuronal basis. This paperback discusses strategies in the study of behavior. It is excellent for beginning students and has numerous provocative ideas for more advanced students. It is oriented toward physiological psychology.

4. Worden FG, Swazey JP, Adelman G (eds): The Neurosciences: Paths of Discovery, Cambridge, MIT Press, 1975.

This unique book presents a highly personal glimpse of many great neuroscientists. The investigators were free to write about *how* they discovered, not just *what* they discovered. A great deal of highly personal feelings and hunches are discussed; the presentation lets the personality of the investigator come to the surface. The range of topics is highly diverse and presents both serious and humorous (The Gain in Brain Lies Mainly in the Stain, by Floyd Bloom) aspects. It is much more enjoyable to read the works of the respected investigators and proven contributors when they reveal a little of themselves, besides scientific data and interpretation. Once you start reading, it is difficult to put this book down.

Comprehensive General References

1. Quarton GC, Melnechuk T, Schmitt FO (eds): The Neurosciences: A Study Program. New York, Rockefeller University Press, 1967.
Schmitt FO, editor-in-chief: The Neurosciences: A Second Study Program. New York, Rockefeller University Press, 1970.
Schmitt FO, Worden FG, editors-in-chief: The Neurosciences: Third Study Program. Cambridge, MIT Press, 1974.
Schmitt FO, Worden FG, editors-in-chief: The Neurosciences: Fourth Study Program. Cambridge, MIT Press, 1979.

These large books are compendiums of information about virtually every aspect of the nervous system. The books have resulted from intensive Study Programs of the Neurosciences Research Program (based in Brookline, Massachusetts), which were held in Boulder, Colorado, in 1966, 1969, 1972, and 1977. The books are subdivided into sections investigating a specific theme ranging from molecular neurobiology to behavior. Individual chapters are written by well-known investigators in their field. The participating author list reads like a veritable "who's who in neurosciences," including the best known neurobiologists at the international level. Yet the chapters review large bodies of information, summarize past trends in research, bring out new ideas for the future, and speculate on where neurobiology is heading. Some of the information in the chapters is very straightforward and easy to understand, but a rapid development of ideas and directions can require a more extensive familiarity with the nervous system. These books are reasonable in price, broad in their scope, magnificent in the excellence of the authors and editors, and are, page-for-page, probably one of the great bargains available in the neurosciences literature.

2. Handbook of Physiology. Section I: The Nervous System, Volume I: Cellular Biology of Neurons, Parts 1 and 2. Brookhart JM, Mountcastle VB, Kandel ER, Geiger SR (eds): Am Physiol Soc., Bethesda, Md, 1977.

These two volumes represent the ultimate in detailed and comprehensive reviews on various aspects of cellular biology of neurons. Morphological, physiological, chemical, pharmacological, and behavioral topics are reviewed. The chapters present critical commentaries on research, usually reference many hundreds of original articles, and point out needed areas for further research. Many chapters require extensive background to understand. Yet some chapters (General Morphology of Neurons and Neuralgia, Chapter 2, by S.L. Palay and V. Chan-Palay) are so clearly written that they can be understood by a beginning student. Additional volumes will be published in the next few years.

3. Neurosciences Research Program (NRP) Bulletins.

These small bulletins are the results of NRP workshops, which bring a wide range of scientists together to discuss the future direction of a specific field. The monographs are intended for the more advanced student but can also provide some insights to the less advanced student. These are inexpensive and well worth obtaining as solid background material generated by respected neuroscientists.

4. Annual Review of Neurosciences, Cowan WM ed. Annual Reviews Inc., Palo Alto, Cal.

This series was recently begun (Vol. 1 in 1978) as a series of scholarly and detailed reviews in a broad range of topics in the neurosciences. The depth and breadth of coverage are impressive, as are the contributing authors. This is a good source to refer to for details in special areas that are not covered by traditional textbooks or reviews. But be prepared for high-power presentations of considerable length.

NEUROANATOMY REFERENCES

Major Textbooks

1. Brodal A: Neurological Anatomy, 3rd ed. New York, Oxford University Press, 3rd ed. 1981.

This neuroanatomy text is brilliantly written by a great researcher and neurologist. The chapters read remarkably smoothly despite great detail and many references. Dr. Brodal is not afraid to tackle outdated concepts such as pyramidal tract syndrome or extrapyramidal motor systems and presents compelling arguments for his point of view. The text is filled with excellent clinical examples. His coverage of motor systems and cranial nerves is unequaled elsewhere. The illustrations, while not numerous, are clear and concise. We recommend that an atlas or heavily illustrated text be used as a supplement by all but the seasoned neuroscientist. We view this text as the single finest neuroanatomy textbook written.

2. Carpenter MB: Human Neuroanatomy, 7th ed. Baltimore, Williams and Wilkins, 1977. Core Text of Neuroanatomy, 2nd ed. Baltimore, Williams and Wilkins, 1978.

The large text is a comprehensive text of human neuroanatomy covering regional neuroanatomy in detail and systemic neuroanatomy succinctly. References are provided in the text; illustrations are abundant, with particularly good pathway diagrams. This is a reference text or a neuroanatomy text for the hearty of spirit and memory. It is one of the finest neuroanatomy references available. The *Core Text* is a version of the large text pared down to permit its use as a course book. The emphasis is heavily on central connections and the discussion leaves out cellular neurobiology and peripheral nervous system material. The *Core Text* is highly recommended for studying an anatomical region or for learning basic pathways. A preliminary overview knowledge of systemic and/or regional neuroanatomy would aid in understanding the material.

3. Crosby EC, Humphrey T, Laver EW: Correlative Anatomy of the Nervous System. Macmillan, New York, 1962.

This text is a comprehensive summary of the anatomy of the nervous system as known in 1962. Detailed cytoarchitectural and pathway data are reviewed and many fiber systems are described in details not available elsewhere. The orientation is mainly toward regional anatomy. New data on transmitter and modulator systems have been uncovered since this was written, and new tracing techniques have altered or greatly expanded our knowledge of central connections. However, this book is still a standard reference for pre-1962 neuroanatomical knowledge.

4. Peele TL: The Neuroanatomic Basis for Clinical Neurology, 3rd ed. New York, McGraw-Hill, 1977.

The text of this book presents a highly detailed account of basic neuroanatomy. Myriads of connections and details are spelled out, making this an excellent reference. The student in a short course can have difficulty knowing where to place emphasis of study. Illustrations are somewhat sparse but are good. We recommend this text to students who already have a background in neurosciences or for use with both an atlas and an overview or review book.

5. Williams PL, Warwick R: Functional Neuroanatomy of Man. Philadelphia, W. B. Saunders Co., 1975.

This entire book is the Neurology section from British *Gray's Anatomy*. It is principally a neuroanatomy text and does not claim a multidisciplinary approach. The neuroanatomy is covered regionally and is beautifully done. The illustrations are superb and are often unequaled in any other source. Both central and peripheral nervous system anatomy is presented and sensory organs are also well covered. This is a neuroanatomy text well worth owning. A new edition (1981) of the entire Gray's Anatomy is now available, with a nicely updated section on Neurology. However, at present, you must buy the entire book to get the Neurology section.

Review Texts

1. Clark RG: Manter and Gatz's Essentials of Clinical Neuroanatomy and Neurophysiology, 5th ed. Philadelphia, F. A. Davis Co., 1975.

This little book is probably the only "quick reading" review paperback worth exploring. Ron Clark has done a laudable job of putting the 5th edition of this text in order. This is the medical student's

Bible for "how to squeak through neuroanatomy on the National Board exams." The anatomy is simple, regional as well as systemic in approach, and the book covers most of the basics. Clinical examples and correlations are presented in succinct and organized form. This is a good review book if you already have some background (introductory course), but would be difficult to use as a sole text.

Atlases

1. Netter FH: The CIBA Collection of Medical Illustrations, Vol I: Nervous System. Summit, NJ, CIBA, 1962.

This CIBA collection is a favorite of medical students and physicians because of the superb drawings of physician-medical artist, Frank Netter. Anatomical relationships of the nervous system, basic pathways of central tracts and peripheral and cranial nerves, and basic pathology (very simple) are nicely illustrated. The text and some of the anatomy are in need of updating in light of recent surges in research knowledge. However, many illustrations, such as those of the hypothalamic nuclei, are classics still shown in medical lectures throughout the world.

2. DeArmond SJ, Fusco MM, Dewey MM: Structure of the Human Brain: A Photographic Atlas, 2nd ed. New York, Oxford University Press, 1976.

In this atlas are seen good photographs and corresponding line drawings for spinal cord and brain stem cross sections, gross brain and brain stem, frontal sections, and horizontal sections in the CAT scan plane. The sagittal sections are of use mainly to more advanced students. This is a good, generally accurate atlas of the human CNS, useful for course work and references.

3. Rasmussen AT: Villager-Ludwig-Rasmussen Atlas of Cross Section Anatomy of the Brain, New York, McGraw-Hill, 1951.

This is an old but excellent atlas of the human brain. Plates are based upon Weigert fiber stains with labels pointing directly to the structures. This is a superb teaching atlas and a worthwhile atlas from which to learn basic regional neuroanatomy.

4. Ferner H, Staubesand J, Hild WJ (eds.): Sobotta/Figge Atlas of Human Anatomy. Vol 3: Central and Autonomic Nervous Systems, Sense Organs, Skin, Peripheral Nerves and Vessels, 9th Eng. ed. Baltimore, Urban and Schwarzenberg, 1977.

A volume of the classical Sobotta/Figge *Atlas of Human Anatomy*, this has a host of excellent atlas sections, illustrations, and schematic drawings of the human nervous system. The special sensory organs are particularly well covered.

5. Nieuwenhuys R, Voogd J, van Huijzen C: The Human Central Nervous System: A Synopsis and Atlas, New York, Springer-Verlag, 1979.

This atlas presents excellent line drawings, stained sections, and lucid explanations of the neuroanatomy. The brain stem sections are perhaps the best available. The accompanying text is quite detailed and well done. Unfortunately, the terminology and abbreviations are stodgy and are almost incomprehensible to anyone but a Latin scholar. We have found it well worth the effort to pencil in the English names and avoid the endless need for translation. If any book is worth the effort for such a task, this one is.

Special Anatomical Topics

1. Peters A, Palay SL, Webster H. de F: The Fine Structure of the Nervous System: The Neurons and Supporting Cells. Philadelphia, W. B. Saunders Co., 1976.

   This book is both an atlas and a scholarly, well-referenced text. It is the only definitive book on the ultrastructure of nervous tissue that actually presents details, explanations, current controversies, new methodological approaches, and good references between the same covers. It is an impressive work that takes cellular neurobiology to its finest morphological detail. It is recommended for the more advanced student, but anyone can learn from the beautiful electron micrographs. This is a work of art as well as a work of scientific content.

2. Hamilton WJ, Mossman HW: Hamilton, Boyd and Mossman's Human Embryology, 4th ed. Baltimore, Williams and Wilkins, 1972.

   Chapter 13 of this excellent classical embryology text presents one of the few detailed accounts of the morphological development of the nervous system currently available. The diagrams are particularly good.

NEUROPHYSIOLOGY REFERENCES

Introductory Texts

1. Schmidt RF: Fundamentals of Neurophysiology. New York, Springer-Verlag, 1975.

   This paperback on neurophysiology is a well-balanced introductory text. The diagrams are simple and to the point, the text is usually clear, and surprising detail is presented with minimal grief to the reader. This is a good starting source for those with a brief anatomical background or overview knowledge.

2. Ganong, WF: The Nervous System, 2nd ed. Los Altos, Cal, Lange Medical Publications, 1979.

   This is a very straightforward paperback "Lange Series" book on basic neurophysiology. It presents the core material simply and clearly. It is intended as an overview and introductory text for beginning students and does not get bogged down in controversies, numerous references, or extensive research background. This, of course, must be taken into account with any review book or chapter.

Major Textbooks

1. Mountcastle VB: Medical Physiology, 14th ed. St. Louis, C. V. Mosby Co., 1980.

   Medical Physiology is a scholarly and detailed physiology text with a strong emphasis on the nervous sytem. Expert contributors have reviewed wide areas of neurophysiological literature and discuss the research basis for current opinions and hypotheses. Unlike many neurophysiology texts, you are not asked to merely accept complicated hypotheses on faith or on the basis of strings of cited but undiscussed references. Virtually the entire first volume presents neurophysiology. Sensory and motor mechanisms and cellular neurophysiology receive emphasis while the autonomic nervous system and "higher functions" are a bit brief in comparison. This text should be a help to both the beginning student with enough time to explore a detailed text or to the advanced student seeking good summaries of related areas.

2. Eyzaguirre C, Fidone SJ: Physiology of the Nervous System: An Introductory Text, 2nd ed. Chicago, Year Book Medical Publishers, 1975.

   This text is an introductory book in plain English with a heavy emphasis on sensory and motor neurophysiology. For the most part, this book can be read and understood with a brief background such as the one supplied by Chapter 1 of the present book. This is a good "first source" for more detailed physiologic information than is normally given in an abbreviated course or chapter.

NEUROCHEMISTRY AND NEUROPHARMACOLOGY REFERENCES

1. Cooper JR, Bloom FE, Roth RH: The Biochemical Basis of Neuropharmacology, 3rd ed. New York, Oxford University Press, 1978.

   This brief text is perhaps the quickest and best introduction to neurotransmitter systems and associated neurochemistry currently available. After introductory chapters, each major transmitter is reviewed succinctly, including antomical, physiological, chemical, and pharmacological information. Appropriate clinical information is also correlated with the basic neurosciences. This is a good starting text for transmitters.

2. Goodman LS, Gilman A: The Pharmacological Basic of Therapeutics, 6th ed. New York, Macmillan, 1980.

   This book is a standard textbook used in many medical pharmacology courses in medical schools. Close to 30 chapters deal with drugs acting on the CNS, local anesthetics, and drugs acting at synaptic and neuroeffector junctional sites. The sections on autonomic neurotransmission and CNS drugs are particularly good. The discussion of drugs heavily emphasizes therapeutic uses, side effects, and history of the usage. References are extensive. We recommend this reference for obtaining information about specific nervous system drugs or transmitters but recommend an overview background for broad understanding.

3. Siegel GJ, Albers RW, Katzman R, Agranoff BW: Basic Neurochemistry, 2nd ed. Boston, Little, Brown and Co., 1976.

   Basic Neurochemistry is a detailed discussion of research findings in neurochemistry. At first glance it appears formidable; however, many chapters have simple introductions or discussions of findings. This is a good source book for students with a background in basic biochemistry or neurotransmitter systems.

NEUROPATHOLOGY REFERENCES

1. Escourolle R, Poirer J: Manual of Basic Neuropathology, 2nd ed. Philadelphia, W. B. Saunders Co., 1978.

   This paperback is a good, straightforward survey text of neuropathology intended to introduce students to the basics. The illustrations and diagrams are clear, and the text is succinct and easy to read. It is easily digestible in a short period of time and provides a real service for those wishing to read introductory information without getting bogged down in details.

2. Lewis AJ: Mechanisms of Neurological Disease. Boston, Little, Brown and Co., 1976.

   A scholarly approach to underlying mechanisms of neuropathology is seen in this textbook. An underlying basic sciences framework is provided in Part I. The chapters on gross brain anatomy and cellular neurophysiology are straightforward. The neuroanatomical chapters are compact and difficult to follow without a previous background. In Part III, an excellent summary is provided on numerous topics frequently slighted by other texts, such as cerebral edema, CNS dysfunction in homeostatic disorders, disorders of energy supply, birth injury, diseases of myelin, and mental retardation. The book represents a nice compromise between the highly cursory comments in many neurology texts and the endless details of most large neuropathology texts.

3. Blackwood W, Corsellis JAN: Greenfield's Neuropathology. London, Edward Arnold (Yearbook, Chicago), 1976.

   This text is a standard clinical reference in neuropathology. A comprehensive range of topics is presented by contributing neuropathologists. Both clinical and pathological details abound. A background in basic neurosciences and clinical neurology is helpful.

CLINICAL NEUROLOGY REFERENCES

Neurology Textbooks

1. Adams RD, Victor M: Principles of Neurology. New York, McGraw-Hill, 2nd Ed., 1981.

   This is a superb, well-organized, well-written textbook that our students prefer above all others. The first half of the book discusses "Cardinal Manifestations of Neurological Disease," emphasizing common symptoms. The student is immediately directed into "differential diagnostic" thinking. This coverage is certainly the best of its kind we have found. The last half of the book discusses the major neurological, muscular, and psychiatric disorders pertinent to a clinical neurologist. The entire book reads remarkably smoothly. An adequate basic sciences background is presented in the individual chapters to aid in understanding the diseases. For a non-neurologist, this is our first choice for a neurology text.

2. Baker AB, Baker LH: Clinical Neurology, Hagerstown, Md, Harper and Row, 1977.

   This three-volume set of neurology books is one of the best and most comprehensive available. Specific experts have contributed chapters on neurological techniques and neurological diseases that cover major aspects in depth with extensive references. Chapter 2 on Neuroradiology by Peterson and Kieffer has actually been published separately as a full textbook of neuroradiology. *Clinical Neurology* is updated yearly (a few new chapters at a time for a considerable yearly fee). This is a good source to use when you need details, references, and a discussion about current theories and approaches to the therapy and etiology of neurological disease.

3. Gilroy J, Meyer JS: Medical Neurology, 3rd ed. New York, Macmillan, 1979.

   This is a good standard textbook of neurology. The major diseases are well covered and the material is quite easy to read. Charts, tables, and illustrations are equally well done.

4. Isselbacher KJ, et al. (eds): Harrison's Principles of Internal Medicine, 9th ed. New York, McGraw-Hill, 1980.

   This classical textbook of medicine has a surprisingly good section on disorders of the nervous system. The major neurological diseases are covered by experts in a clear, succinct, and informative manner. This book is kept up to date with frequent revisions and is recommended as one of the first texts to consult for information about individual neurological disorders or general categories of neurological disorders.

5. Walshe F: Diseases of the Nervous System, 11th ed. London, Churchill Livingstone, 1973.

   Walshe presents a brief, well-written textbook of neurology written in a scholarly but pleasant British style. The introductory section on general principles of neurological diagnosis is particularly good for the beginning student. The descriptive account of the more common diseases of the nervous system is also excellent. This text is a pleasant change from some of the weightier, more stodgy neurology texts.

Neurological Examination References

1. Alpers BJ, Mancall EL: Essentials of the Neurological Examination, 2nd ed. Philadelphia, F. A. Davis, 1980.

   This is a straightforward, brief, and well-written introduction to the neurological examination. It explains how to test regions as well as systems, presents signs and their interpretation, and is highly recommended as a starting point for approaching the neurological examination.

2. DeMyer W: Technique of the Neurological Examination, 3rd ed. New York, McGraw-Hill, 1980.

   This programmed text reads in a smooth and comfortable style while teaching the student the practical and theoretical aspects of the neurological examination. It is both comprehensive and succinct. While neuroanatomy is not heavily emphasized in the text as an end in itself, it is heavily drawn upon. This is a pleasant and informative way to polish skills related to the neurological examination. The organization and cohesiveness of the text reflect on the excellence of Dr. DeMyer as a teacher as well as a clinical neurologist. We highly recommend it.

3. DeJong RN: The Neurological Examination, 4th ed. Hagerstown, Harper and Row, 1979.

This is a comprehensive textbook discussing the neurological examination in detail. The anatomical and physiological backgrounds necessary to understand clinical evaluations are presented, and signs, symptoms, and manifestations of neurological diseases and interpretation of findings are covered in a well-organized and understandable manner. It is a detailed book but an excellent reference.

Specialized References

1. Plum F, Posner JB: The Diagnosis of Stupor and Coma, 3rd ed. Philadelphia, F. A. Davis, 1980.

This book is volume 19 of the Contemporary Neurology Series. The series in general presents superb topical converage of areas of specific interest in neurology, such as clinical neuroendocrinology, mental retardation, disorders of the autonomic nervous system, clinical neurology of the vestibular system (excellent for therapists and others). Volume 19 is a new addition to a classical work on stupor, coma, and evaluation of the unconscious patient. This is the best coverage of coma and brain death currently available. The clinical emphasis is present throughout as with all Contemporary Neurology Series volumes, but the underlying basic sciences are brought into the discussion in a pleasing and valuable manner for the student.

CHAPTER 2

NEUROREHABILITATION EVALUATION CONCEPTS

Shereen D. Farber, MS, OTR, FAOTA

The purpose of this chapter is to review evaluation concepts and areas essential to neurorehabilitation. A comprehensive sampling of assessment tools is available in Hopkins and Smith (1978), including specific tests or evaluations, descriptions, and sources.

PRINCIPLES OF EVALUATION

Purposes

This is an age of accountability in which therapists are frequently expected to document the effectiveness of their treatment. Establishing a patient's behavioral baseline is necessary for critical review of treatment quality. The baseline should be quantified whenever possible to facilitate statistical comparison of baseline behavior with treatment-related behavior. In considering the example of a patient with spasticity, if a therapist uses only the term "spasticity" or "hypertonicity" to characterize baseline muscle tone, there will be inadequate data for quantification as tonal normalization occurs. A more specific approach is to measure initial muscle tone by electromyogram (EMG). Microvolt levels can then be compared and statistical significance may be determined.

It is frequently appropriate to *screen* a patient's performance in order to ascertain which areas need in-depth assessment. Screening is also helpful in selection of expedient evaluation tools. The initial interview with patient (or family) can be used as a screening tool to supply the therapist with vital information. It is also helpful in establishing rapport among therapist, patient, and family.

Reviewing a patient's medical record is another screening procedure. The medical record should be used to gather information before actual evaluation is conducted. The record should include medical precautions, history of illness, prognosis, family background, and reports from other disciplines. However, the therapist is urged to avoid prejudging a patient's performance based on recorded observation from other disciplines.

While allied health personnel do not actually diagnose patients' medical conditions, data from their evaluations may be utilized by physicians for diagnostic purposes. Many therapists are qualified to diagnose such conditions as developmental delay or sensory integrative dysfunction, and identify postural reflexive maturation and similar nonmedical indicators.

Evaluation procedures help identify a patient's needs so that treatment can be designed to address specific problems. The evaluation process should be ongoing to ensure the continued appropriateness of treatment. It is essential that clear, concise records be maintained during evaluation for purposes of analysis.

Guidelines for Analysis of an Evaluation Tool

Many medical supply houses are advertising new evaluation tools in neurorehabilitation. Because of the expense, one cannot order each new assessment battery for trial. The following questions can serve as guidelines to assist in discriminating purchasing.

1. Is the test or evaluation standardized? Therapists using an assessment as part of a research project would improve the research design by using an assessment tool that has been standardized. One must remember, however, that if the norms from a standardized evaluation are to be used, the evaluation must be given exactly as prescribed.

2. Is the test valid and reliable? Does the test measure what it is designed to and does it produce desired responses time after time? The manufacturer of a test should provide such data upon request.

3. As for test instructions, are the test administration and scoring instructions clear?

4. Are the age and diagnostic ranges applicable? Will the test be suitable for the patient population treated at a given clinic?

5. Is the test designed for group or individual administration? This factor would be of importance to therapists in situations in which there is a high ratio of patients to therapists. In such situations when an assessment can be conducted in groups, more of the patient population can be evaluated.

6. What about cost and reusability? The therapist must consider the initial expense of the evaluation tool as well as the price of replacement of answer sheets and other necessary equipment. If an answer sheet can be used for multiple trials, it will be less expensive.

7. What are the estimated administration and scoring times? The length of time it takes to administer, score, and interpret an evaluation may be critical to the therapist with a large case load. This information should also be available from the manufacturer.

8. Is there transcultural applicability? Does the test discriminate against members of a racial or ethnic group because of terminology or content?

EVALUATION AREAS

Autonomic Nervous System

It is critical to assess autonomic nervous system (ANS) function since this is intimately related to central nervous system (CNS) and peripheral nervous system function. Ongoing assessment in this area is recommended. Table 2–1 contains an ANS inventory useful in assessment of autonomic function.

The therapist must consider several concepts during the continuous monitoring of the ANS. When a patient is under chronic stress and is fatigued, it is easier to facilitate an undesirable sympathetic nervous system response. The patient's ANS cannot discriminate between real and apparent danger. For this reason, patients should be prepared for upcoming activities. If the sympathetic nervous system is stimulated, it will cause mass reactions throughout the body that will be difficult to reverse. The multisensory approach strives to promote homeostasis of the ANS; hence stimuli of high frequency are never suddenly applied without first preparing the patient.

TABLE 2–1 AUTONOMIC NERVOUS SYSTEM INVENTORY

Organ	Sympathetic Response	Parasympathetic Response	Method of Measurement
Eye	Pupil dilated	Pupil contracted	Direct observation.
Nose	Vasoconstriction of nasal glands	Thin, copious secretion from nasal glands	Direct observation.
Mouth (Salivary Glands)	Dry mouth and thick saliva	Increased parotid gland stimulation, thin watery saliva	Examine oral cavity. Have patient spit into a cup. Examine saliva.
Sweat glands	Copious sweating	No response	Can be measured by galvanic skin resistance test. With increase in skin moisture, a decrease in resistance occurs. One can palpate the patient's skin for wetness, although this is less precise.
Apocrine glands	Thick odoriferous secretion	None	Body odor change can be detected.
Gut	Decreased peristalsis and tone with increased sphincter tone (constipation)	Increased peristalsis and tone with decreased sphincter tone (defecation reflex).	Palpate abdomen, question patient regarding bowel habits.
Skin temperature and color	Less than 31–33°C when room is 26–27°C. Skin color pale. Blood vessels constricted.	More than 31–33°C when room is 26–27°C. Skin color pink. Blood vessels dilated.	Skin temperature can be measured by temperature tapes or by biofeedback units.
Piloerector muscles	Hair standing on end. Goose pimples.	None	Direct observation.
Muscle tone	Increased tone and strength	Decreasead tone and strength	Palpation of musculature; biofeedback (EMG) to measure tone and dynamometer to measure grip strength.
Mental activity	Increased activity, asynchronous cortical potentials, emotional excitement.	Decreased activity, synchronous cortical potentials. Relaxation.	Talk with patient. Ask questions. EEG can be used by qualified personnel.
Blood pressure	Most experts agree that blood pressure greater than 140/90 is hypertension at any age and bears watching.	Lower blood pressure than normal.	Measured by sphygmomanometer with arm held at the level of the aorta. Blood pressure values vary for age and sex, getting progressively higher with age. 118/73 is normal for a teenage male. 125/78 is mean value for a 25-year old male and 142/85 is mean value for a 60 to 65-year-old male.
Organ pulse	Sympathetic response is higher than normal	Parasympathetic response is lower than normal	Method of measurement is to palpate pulse at the wrist. Normal values vary with age (pulse rate/minute): Birth 122 2–5 114 range 5–9 103 range 9–12 89 range Adult 76 range
Respiration	Faster than normal; shallow pattern	Slower than normal	Count respiration cycles per minute. Normal values vary for each age: Birth 30 range 2–5 26 range 5–9 25 range 9–12 24 range Adult 17 range

The data in this table have been compiled from: Guyton, 1977; Peele, 1977; Adams and Victor, 1977; Altman and Dittmer, 1971; Sunderman and Boerner, 1949; Hurst, 1978.

Sensory Assessment

Motor milestones are readily available to therapists; however, knowledge of the relationship of these motor responses to sensory system development proves to be more difficult. The purpose of this section is to provide a sample of specific sensory tests in order to define and assess sensory system development. A gradual progression from generalized to more discrete responsiveness can be noted in each sensory system. For example, a light moving touch might initially facilitate a mass flexor pattern or an aversive response, but as the spinothalamic-spinoreticular system develops in response to therapy, a more discrete hand-to-face pattern should normally emerge. One must remember that damage to the nervous system may remove inhibition and discriminative ability, subsequently returning a sensory system to a more primitive level of function.

Table 2–2 contains a sensory system inventory that is designed for screening of sensory responsiveness. In patients with profound damage to the nervous system, cautious use of this inventory is advised. Overstimulation can result from successive application of stimuli representing many different systems. It may be necessary to screen one or two sensory systems per treatment session if the patient responds adversely to the multiple sensory system assessment. Specific directions and precautions for use of sensory stimuli are included in Chapter 3 under each respective system. The sensory system inventory is not intended to contain every sensory system test that should be assessed; instead, it provides examples and serves as a guideline for evaluation.

Developmental Appraisal

The therapist working in neurorehabilitation must have a thorough knowledge of the normal developmental progression and factors that can interrupt the acquisition of motor milestones. Each developmental pattern should be examined in terms of the component motions required to achieve a given pattern. For example, for a child to achieve the pivot prone pattern, he must be able to integrate the tonic labyrinthine in prone reflex and extend his neck, arms, back, hips, and knees against gravity. When a therapist studies a given developmental pattern in terms of its component parts, it is easier to plan remediation for deficits. Following an insult to the CNS in older children or adults, a developmental regression is likely to occur. Consideration of developmental proficiency is as important to an older patient as it is to a young child. In addition to testing motion components in a specific developmental pattern, the therapist must also assess the patient's ability to assume the posture, move within it, move to a more advanced pattern, and move back to a less advanced pattern. A comprehensive list of developmental tests and evaluations appears in Hopkins and Smith (1978).

Postural Tone Mechanisms and Reflex Integration

Many therapists make the mistake of attempting to assess the muscle tone of a patient having CNS damage without first understanding the mechanisms and characteristics of normal postural tone (see Chapter 1 for neurophysiological aspects of tone). Constant tonal change and fluctuation occurs during the execution of normal developmental patterns. Consider the tonic tonal increase of the weight-bearing extremity and the phasic tonal pattern of the swing-through extremity during gait. Normal muscle tone enables the individual to provide support against gravity. If the tone is in excess, mobility will be compromised and skilled movement will be difficult.

Muscles rarely work in isolation; reciprocal patterns of agonist and antagonist are seen that initially provide movement patterns. Co-innervation of agonist and antagonist facilitates stability and balanced tone around joints. Once stability is established, movement can be superimposed over a co-contraction (see Chapter 3 for a more detailed discussion of this topic).

When assessing tone, the therapist needs to develop a rating scale that will allow subsequent comparison with later

TABLE 2-2 SENSORY SYSTEM INVENTORY

Sensory System	Stimulus	Response	Possible Significance or Implications
Spinothalamic-spinoreticular system	°Maintained pressure: A. To perioral region	Head hyperextending away from stimulus	Aversive response. Use maintained pressure on abdomen, palms or soles of feet first. Retest.
	B. To other body surface areas, including abdomen, palms, soles of feet, or skin over specific muscles.	Generalized calming	Proceed with appropriate other sensory testing such as light moving touch.
		Specific calming of underlying muscle	Proceed to functional test of specific muscle function. (An example is to apply maintained pressure to the masseters, resulting in a relaxation of spasticity. Chewing function or jaw jerk should then be tested.
		Clawing of toes or reflexive grasp response	Hypersensitive skin in the palmar or plantar surface needing normalization.
	Light moving touch: A. To perioral midline	Total flexor pattern with the palmar surface out	More primitive response. Repeat light moving touch stimulus with rolling to assist pattern.
		Total flexor pattern with palms to face	More adaptive response. Proceed to activities using hand-mouth pattern.
	B. To T10 dermatome (adult)	Flexion of homolateral side leg	Proceed to activities using dorsiflexion and flexion of the leg (rolling, creeping, walking).
Vestibular system	Inversion	Reduction of hypertonicity, facilitation of midline trunk extensors, soleus, extensor carpi ulnaris and radialis, gastrocnemius, biceps femoris (long head), vasti, rectus femoris, triceps, gluteus maximus, deltoid. Good co-contraction pattern at the neck	Desired responses. Proceed to appropriate developmental pattern. Reinforce components of pattern with proprioceptive stimulation (see Chapter 3).
		Aversive response: flushed face, excessive sweating, other sympathic responses	Carotid sinus may not be properly functioning. Discontinue inversion.
		Hyperextension of neck (see Fig. 3–17)	Reflexive neck extension pattern instead of desired co-contraction pattern. Place visual stimulus on the floor to direct patient's visual responses.
	Anteroposterior motion in each developmental pattern		
	Slow, even movement →	Generalized relaxation →	Desired response, proceed to appropriate developmental or facilitation pattern.
	Fast, irregular motion →	Generalized increase in → tone	Desired response for patients with systemic hypotonia. Add proprioceptive stimuli to pattern when appropriate.
	Side-to-side movement in a slow even pattern	Weight shifting	Desired response. Add resistance to pattern if appropriate, then proceed to diagonal pattern.

Table continued on following page

TABLE 2–2 SENSORY SYSTEM INVENTORY *Continued*

Sensory System	Stimulus	Response	Possible Significance or Implications
	Diagonal rocking	Weight shifting	Desired response. Proceed to appropriate developmental pattern to reinforce movement (crawling, creeping, walking).
	Rotating: A. Rolling	Log-rolling response	Primitive reflex level. Need to do slow rolling pattern or other inhibitory handling to assist in integration of the primitive response. Follow with facilitation of segmental rolling.
		Segmental rolling response	Adaptive response. Proceed to next appropriate developmental pattern.
	B. Facilitory rotation in any developmental pattern	No change in muscle tone, no post-rotatory nystagmus	Patient may have sensory integrative dysfunction. Do comprehensive testing and carefully monitor vestibular input.
		Post-rotatory nystagmus and appropriate change in muscle tone	Adaptive response.
Olfactory	Banana/vanilla (see Chap. 3)	Reflex sucking	As an initial response, this would be considered an adaptive response. If the patient does not progress, the continued reflex sucking is no longer considered adaptive. More advanced behavior includes changes in facial expression, muscle tone, movement patterns, verbalization following stimulation.
	A variety of common odors	Patient is able to identify the odor	Advanced, adaptive response.
Gustatory	Sweet, sour, bitter, salt stimuli to appropriate tongue areas (see Chap. 3)	Change in facial expression; changes in muscle tone; reflex sucking; increased salivation; movement of tongue and lips; swallowing	Progressive adaptive responses.
Epicritic function	Quick stretch to a given muscle	Normal contraction of that muscle	Monosynaptic reflex (muscle stretch reflex) working properly.
		Hypertonicity of muscle stretched	Disinhibition of higher centers secondary to an upper motor neuron lesion.
	Vibrating tuning fork applied to bony prominences	Perception of vibration	Adaptive response; dorsal columns/medial lemniscus system intact.
	Vibration of a specific muscle with an electric vibrator	Appropriate contraction of muscle and relaxation of antagonist	Tonic vibratory response intact (see Chaps. 1 and 3).
	Placement of an object in hand for tactile discrimination without visual clues	Stereognosis	Adaptive response of epicritic system and development of association areas of brain.
		Astereognosis	Lesion in dorsal columns, medial lemniscus, or higher centers associated with stereognosis (see Chap. 1). Use stereognosis treatment procedures outlined in Chap. 3.

Table continued on opposite page

TABLE 2–2 SENSORY SYSTEM INVENTORY *Continued*

Sensory System	Stimulus	Response	Possible Significance or Implications
	Move patient's body part while asking him to identify direction of movement	Correct identification of movement direction	Adaptive response (kinesthetic sense)
	Move body part to a specific position then ask patient to identify position	Correct identification	Adaptive response (position sense)
Temperature	Cold or warm water in tubes applied to various skin surfaces	Lack of identification	Deficit in protopathic sensation. Instruct patient in compensation techniques until protopathic sense improves.
Auditory	Ring a bell 12 inches from patient's ear	Patient turns head to the sound or can identify stimulus	Adaptive response.
	Present a sequence of numbers	Patient cannot repeat sequence	Possible receptive problem or memory deficit. Assess further.
	Alternately stimulate each ear with tones of different pitches and volumes	Patient cannot hear many of the tones	Refer the patient to an audiologist for further evaluation.
Vision	In a dark room, press on patient's eyeballs (see Chap. 3); coma sequence	Patient changes facial expression, vocalizes, opens eyes, moves a body part	Adaptive response.
	In a dark room, move flashlight across visual fields	Patient does not track stimulus	Possible vestibular problem or cranial nerve lesion (see Chap. 1).
		Patient tracks stimulus in all directions, demonstrating conjugate eye movement	Adaptive response.

°It is recognized that maintained pressure is an epicritic stimulus. In this case, it is used to determine whether the patient is demonstrating tactile defensiveness.

measures. One such scale includes the following:

0 = Hypotonia: inability to resist gravity, lack of co-contraction at proximal joints; weakness.

1 – Decreased muscle tone: some co-contraction patterns starting to emerge; mild inability to resist gravity.

2 = Normalized muscle tone: co-contraction of proximal joints; balance between agonist and antagonists; ability to make a transition between mobility and stability as needed; ability to use muscles in groups or to isolate out a given muscle if necessary.

3 = Mild-to-moderate increased muscle tone: mild to moderate decrease in mobility; increased resistance to passive stretch; decreased balance between agonist and antagonist; reduced ability to separate out individual muscle action.

4 = Severe increase in muscle tone: severe decrease in mobility; joint contractures present; severe increased resistance to passive stretch; synergy patterns.

Another way to quantify muscle tone is use of EMG equipment.

Postural reflex integration is a critical aspect of the normal postural tone mechanism. Fiorentino (1973) and Crutchfield, Barnes, and Heriza (1978) have developed reflex testing procedures used frequently by therapists. A complete reflex assessment must be conducted to determine the status of primitive reflex integration and development of righting and equilibrium responses. The therapist must understand that a delay in primitive reflex integration will result in decreased segmentation of the trunk, decreased isolation of movement, decreased rotation component in any action, decreased responsiveness to postural change resulting in postural insecurity, decreased ability to develop antigravity muscles, increased synergy patterns (mass movement patterns), and increased dependence on environmental stimulation for changes in posture. One of the main goals of the multisensory theory of neurorehabilitation is to integrate primitive reflexes while facilitating higher-level responses (see Chapters 3 and 5 for additional information on postural reflexes). Reflexes are tested in all developmental patterns.

Occupational Performance History/Assessment and Environmental Assessment

In order to design treatment that is meaningful to the patient, the following information should be obtained: educational experience, work history, avocation interests, household responsibilities, and status of carrying out activities of daily living. In addition to this information, it is also helpful to discuss arrangements in or evaluate in person the patient's home so that necessary adaptation can be made to facilitate the patient's maximum independence. See Hopkins and Smith (1978) for specific evaluations in this area.

REFERENCES

Adams RD, Victor M: Principles of Neurology. New York, McGraw-Hill, 1977.

Altman PL, Dittmer DS (eds): Biology Data Book. Bethesda, MD, Federation of American Societies for Experimental Biology, 1971.

Crutchfield C, Barnes M, Heriza C: Neurophysiological Basis of Patient Treatment. Vol. 2, Reflex Testing. Morgantown, WV, Stokesville Publishing Co., 1978.

Fiorentino M: Reflex Testing Methods for Evaluating Central Nervous System Development, 2nd ed. Springfield, IL, Charles C Thomas, 1973.

Guyton AC: Basic Human Physiology: Normal Function and Mechanisms of Disease. Philadelphia, W. B. Saunders Co., 1977.

Hopkins HL, Smith HD (eds): Willard and Spackman's Occupational Therapy, 5th ed. Philadelphia, J. B. Lippincott Co., 1978.

Hurst JW (ed): The Heart, Arteries and Veins. New York, McGraw-Hill, 1978.

Peele TL: The Neuroanatomic Basis for Clinical Neurology, 3rd ed. New York, McGraw-Hill, 1977.

Sunderman FW, Boerner F: Normal Values in Clinical Medicine. Philadelphia, W. B. Saunders Co., 1949.

CHAPTER **3**

A MULTISENSORY
APPROACH TO
NEUROREHABILITATION

Shereen D. Farber, MS, OTR, FAOTA

HISTORICAL OVERVIEW

A variety of theories for sensorimotor integrative treatment have been developed in the works of Ayres, Bobath, Brunnstrom, Fay, Fuchs, Kabat, Knott, Rood, Voss, and others (Ayres, 1972; Huss, 1978; Pearson and Williams, 1972; Brunnstrom, 1970; Knott and Voss, 1968; and Trombly and Scott, 1977). Each of these investigators has developed a treatment rationale with techniques that should be studied in pure form and practiced under the supervision of competent therapists before their relative merits are judged.

In each system, this author finds many useful techniques and sound rationale. A solid foundation in central nervous system (CNS) structure and function is a primary prerequisite before one can adequately synthesize the components of any treatment system. Competency in neuroanatomy and neurophysiology prepares the serious student to compare and contrast existing treatment systems and to develop a personal treatment approach based on sound rationale and logical sequence of applying techniques. The multisensory approach to neurorehabilitation presented in this chapter is the product of this process.

Continuous review of neuroscience literature is essential in order to keep abreast of newer concepts. One efficient method of locating pertinent journal articles is to review *Current Contents,** a weekly publication that catalogues world-wide neuroscience literature by journal and subject heading. Many other efficient methods of literature search and synthesis can be developed. The reader is referred to the numerous texts available on Research Methodology.

*Published by the Institute for Scientific Information, 3501 Market St. University City Science Center Philadelphia PA 19104

RATIONALE FOR THE MULTISENSORY APPROACH TO NEUROREHABILITATION

Main Objectives

The main objectives of the multisensory approach include:
1. Development of homeostasis in the autonomic nervous system,
2. Facilitation of the normal developmental progression,
3. Enhancement of sensory integration,
4. Normalization of muscle tone
5. Integration of primitive reflexes and facilitation of higher level reflexes
6. Normalization of movement
7. Development of coordination
8. Normalization of affective state.

Description of Modalities

Modalities representing all sensory systems are used as stimuli to activate, inhibit, or facilitate motor responses. The sensory stimuli are carefully applied in a sequential order on the basis of their appearance developmentally. For example, touch is used early in treatment, followed by vestibular input, while vision and hearing, phylogenetically newer systems, are emphasized later in the treatment sequence. Exceptions may be made in the application sequence if a patient has a particular need for a given modality, such as proprioceptive input. Since the sequence of sensory treatment is based on the developmental succession of the sensory systems, Table 3–1 is included for reference.

TABLE 3–1 DEVELOPMENTAL STAGES OF THE SENSORY SYSTEMS

Sensory System* or Sensory Receptor	Developmental Stages and Characteristics
Auditory system	Internal ear begins development early. Cochlear ducts are coiled by 3rd fetal month. Newborn demonstrates imperfect responses to auditory stimulation due to gelatinous tissue filling middle ear and detritus (debris) in external auditory meatus. Acute hearing occurs a few weeks after birth (Arey, 1974). 6-month-old infant can localize sound (Lowrey, 1973).
Gustatory system	Tongue begins to develop by 4th fetal week (Moore, 1974); taste buds are developed by 8th fetal week. Reflex responses to taste are present in a premature infant of 7 months' gestation (Arey, 1974). At birth an infant's sense of taste probably cannot differentiate among sour, salt, and bitter stimuli (Lowrey, 1973). Newborns can differentiate good nutrient taste from foul taste (Steiner, 1974).
Neuromuscular Spindles and Golgi Tendon Organs (GTO)	These receptors begin differentiation at 3 months' fetal development (Arey, 1974). Large bag fibers in the spindle develop first; chain fibers are last intrafusal fibers to develop (Barker, 1974). Motor supply to capsule follows sensory innervation (Barker, 1974). By 15 weeks' fetal development, motor end plates are visible (Beckett and Bourne, 1972). By 24 to 31 weeks' gestation, some muscle spindles appear mature. There is a fetal response to stretching by midfetal life (Lowrey, 1973). Evidence suggests that morphological and functional development continues into postnatal period. In most muscles equal numbers of muscle spindles and GTOs exist (Myers, 1977).
Olfactory system	Olfactory structures begin to develop during 1st trimester (Moore, 1974). The olfactory nerve grows from the bulb toward the brain at 13 fetal weeks. From 2nd to 6th gestational month, nostrils are closed by epithelial plugs. Olfactory perception, although not well developed, is present by 8 months' gestation (Arey, 1974).

Table continued on following page

TABLE 3–1   DEVELOPMENTAL STAGES OF THE SENSORY SYSTEMS *Continued*

Sensory System* or Sensory Receptor	Developmental Stages and Characteristics
Temperature receptors	Development and function of these receptors is poorly understood (Hensel, 1973). Temperature differences are discriminated during early postnatal period (Arey, 1974). Facial skin has greatest thermal sensitivity (Darian-Smith, 1973).
Touch and tactile systems	First response to touch occurs in perioral area causing an avoidance reaction at 7½ fetal weeks. Fetal response to perioral stimulation includes responses in trunk and arms by 11–12 weeks (Hooker, 1977). When the lips of an 11-week fetus are touched, swallowing movements occur. Touch on the lips of a 22-week fetus causes pursing, and on the lips of a 29-week fetus causes sucking movements and sounds (Rose, 1973). All these touch responses imply that simple reflex arcs are differentiated for touch very early. Free nerve endings, the most common type of sensory receptor, invade epidermis by 3 fetal months. Merkel's discs are developed during 4th fetal month; simultaneously pacinian corpuscles begin to differentiate. Meissner's corpuscles begin to differentiate during 4th fetal month but are not complete until after birth (Arey, 1974). Protopathic (protective) touch develops much before epicritic tactile function (discriminative touch including stereognosis).
Vestibular system	This system, like touch responses, develops early. Vestibular ganglia differentiate during 6th fetal week and cristae and maculae differentiate during 7th fetal week (Arey, 1974; Klosovskii, 1963). By 3rd fetal month, the labyrinth has adult shape (Arey, 1974). Vestibular system is thought to function by about 14 weeks (Klosovskii, 1963). Ossification of periotic capsule occurs by 20 weeks (Arey, 1974; Lowrey, 1973). By 26th–29th fetal week, fetus assumes head-down position (Moore, 1974), which further reinforces input to vestibular system.
Visual system	Visual structures including the optic cup and stalk differentiate early, but system is imperfect at birth (Arey, 1974). Occipital lobe is immature anatomically and functionally at birth and neonate is hyperopic (Lowrey, 1973). Eye is ¾ its final diameter at birth (Arey, 1974). Several weeks postnatally, fixation occurs. During 8th postnatal month, infant can see details. Depth perception is achieved by 6 years (Lowrey, 1973). By 7 years of age, visual acuity ideally reaches 20/20.

*Sensory systems are listed in alphabetical order.

Summary of Table 3-1

Conception ⟶ Birth

System	1 mo	2 mo	3 mo	4 mo	5 mo	6 mo	7 mo	8 mo	9 mo	Birth	6 mo	8 mo	6 yr	7 yr
Auditory System		Cochlear ducts coiled							Debris in external auditory meatus; Acute hearing		Localize sound		Word associations	
Gustatory System	Tongue develops	Taste buds develop					Reflex response to taste		Differentiate good nutrient and foul tastes				Continued associations	
Neuromuscular Spindles			Receptors begin differentiation	Motor end plates form	Fetal response to stretching →		Some mature spindles →	Continuing development of muscle spindles						
Olfactory System		Olfactory structures develop	Nerve grows from bulb towards brain				Nostrils unplugged	Olfactory perception present (immature)		Continued associations →				
Temperature Sense									Temperature differences discriminated					
Touch and Tactile Systems	Perioral stimulus → avoidance response		• Trunk and arm motion • Reflex swallowing • Nerve endings invade epidermis	• Meissner's corpuscles begin • Merkel's discs • Pacinian corpuscles begin	Perioral stimulus → Lip pursing reflex		Perioral stimulus → sucking movements			Continuation of tactile (epicritic) sensation with development; Continuation of associations and integration				
Vestibular System	Vestibular ganglia cristae + maculae		Labyrinth assumes adult shape; Functional vestibular system		Ossification of periotic capsule		Fetus → assumes head-down position							
Visual System		Optic cup and stalk develop						Occipital lobe immature; Hyperopia	3/4 diameter eye fixation occurs			Details visible	Depth perception	20/20 vision

*Sensory systems are listed in alphabetical order.

Purpose of Sensory Stimulation

Sensory stimulation is designed to produce an *adaptive response* (Ayres, 1972; King, 1978; Lewontin, 1978), which is defined as behavior of a more advanced, organized, flexible, or productive nature than that which occurred before stimulation. The ability to produce adaptive responses ensures the individual a measure of independence from environmental change. This independence facilitates consistency in behavior. Stimuli used should be as natural or appropriate to the developmental experience as possible in order to productively shape adaptive response formation. Patients should not be bombarded with input because this might cause overstimulation and confusion.

To illustrate these concepts, some appropriate treatment modalities for a 2-month-old baby with hypertonia might include maintained touch (pressure); slow, even, rhythmical movement in the antero-posterior plane (rocking); and olfactory input using good nutrient odorants such as milk or bananas (Farber, 1978). All these modalities represent input to early developing sensory systems and are natural to the neonatal developmental experience.

An *inappropriate* sensory tool for a neonate, according to the multisensory approach, would be rotatory vestibular stimulation. Rotation is appropriate in the preschool and school-aged population (Stone and Church, 1975) but is unnatural to neonatal behavior. Maladaptive behavior could result from facilitory rotation applied to the neonate. Some rotation about the body axis is noted in the preambulatory population during the rolling pattern; however, rotation during early rolling is usually incomplete about the body axis and is not rapidly repetitive. For example, a young baby may roll from prone to supine but rarely completes the cycle back to prone.

Multisensory or Cross-Modal Stimuli

A multisensory stimulus is one that combines elements from more than one sensory system. For example, touching a patient while talking to him produces a multisensory input. Cross-modal stimuli are inputs designed to convey information acquired in one sensory modality to another (Gottfried, Rose, and Bridges, 1977). An example would be feeling an object without vision and then identifying the object from visual clues. Multisensory stimulation may produce cross-modal transfer in older patients with normal sensory integration (see stereognosis section of this chapter); however, neonates are easily overwhelmed by excessive simultaneous presentation of sensory stimuli. A 3-month-old infant demonstrates a variety of motor patterns, especially in the upper trunk region, before it can actually process sensory information (Rose, 1973).

Campbell and Wilson (1976) report that a multisensory approach should be considered for the neonate but that complex multisensory stimuli should be delayed until the infant reaches the developmental level at which some intersensory integration (cross-modal learning) occurs. This concept is applied to any patient population in which intersensory integration is in question. For example, Ritvo in his study of 1969 demonstrates that children with early infantile autism show significantly shorter duration of postrotatory nystagmus than normal controls when both are tested in a lighted room with their eyes open. When both groups are tested in a darkened room, again with eyes open, no significant differences are noted. Autistic children, therefore, demonstrated a more normal postrotatory response with visual input blocked. Thus one might speculate that adaptive responses would more readily occur following developmentally appropriate stimulation to one primary sensory system than following multisensory or cross-modal stimuli in patients with sensory integrative dysfunction. This concept needs to be tested in a variety of populations in which CNS function might be impaired. Since acquired CNS damage in an adult may reproduce immature CNS function, it is possible that this concept applies to adult brain injured patients.

Subcortical Activity

Use of subcortically monitored purposeful activity is central to the multisensory approach to neurorehabilitation. It requires less cortical concentration to keep a patient functioning on an automatic (or semiautomatic) than on a conscious basis (Moore, 1969). Carefully designed purposeful activity can be used as a means to reinforce any treatment objective while encouraging active patient participation. Table 3–2 illustrates cortical commands that are to be avoided when possible, contrasted with appropriate subcortical activity.

When designing relevant subcortical activity to reinforce treatment goals, the therapist must combine various types of information, including developmental ability; psychological, social, cognitive, motor and sensory integrative function; occupational performance history; and environmental factors (see Chapter 2). If the activity is not relevant, it will probably not be motivating to a patient and he may refuse to comply.

Cortical commands may be appropriate later in treatment after a patient consistently demonstrates adaptive responses and marked decrease in apraxia. If a cortical command is given, it should be brief. The therapist should allow a patient sufficient time to process the command without additional environmental interference. Excessive use of cortical commands should be avoided even with normal individuals because of the high degree of concentration demanded by cortically monitored activity.

Developmental Foundation

The multisensory approach uses as its developmental foundation many concepts gathered and synthesized by Rood (Stockmeyer, 1972). Motor development progresses from reciprocal innervation to co-innervation to heavy work movement and finally to skilled movement. *Reciprocal innervation* is defined as relaxation of the antagonist during contraction of the agonist. *Co-innervation* produces a simultaneous contraction of agonist and antagonist with the agonist being supreme (Crutchfield and Barnes, 1973; Basmajian, 1978). Co-contractions that result from co-innervation provide the body with stability. *Heavy work movement* is superimposed over the stable proximal joints, as during creeping. For *skilled movement* to occur, the individual's neuromuscular system must be able to combine automatically elements of reciprocal innervation, co-innervation, and heavy work movement as needed for a specific activity. Mobility and stability must also be balanced. Much repetition of an activity is needed before skilled movement develops. Table 3–3 represents an adaptation of the developmental sequence as described by Rood.

Consideration of muscle type and function is vital to understanding the developmental foundation. Rood (1962) has classified work into two subgroups, *light work*

TABLE 3–2 SUBCORTICAL ACTIVITY

Inappropriate Cortical Commands	Appropriate Subcortical Activity
1. "Close your lips and swallow. You are drooling."	1. Maintained pressure on lips and tongue reinforced by sucking on either banana- or vanilla-flavored ice Popsicle or a nipple or straw (see oral facilitation section in this chapter).
2. "Lift up your head."	2. Gain patient's attention with a visual stimulus. Move the object (stimulus) upward.
3. "Open your hand."	3. Invert patient to allow labyrinthine input to assist in hand opening (see section on vestibular stimulation in this chapter). Use joint compression of less than body weight placed into heel of hand. Place a hard object in patient's hand.
4. "Just relax."	4. Involve patient in even, rhythmical movement or supply even, rhythmical auditory input.

TABLE 3–3 NEUROPHYSIOLOGICAL SENSORIMOTOR APPROACH TO TREATMENT*

	Progression of Motor Development		
Reciprocal Innervation	Co-innervation	Heavy Work Movement Combined Mobility and Stability in Weight Bearing	Skill Combined Mobility and Stability in Nonweight Bearing
Mobility	Stability		

Withdrawal from stimulus
↓
Flexion pattern → Extension → Neck co-contraction → Head oriented to vertical → Speech articulation
toward stimulus   pattern   ↓   plane (rotation available)   eye control
↓
Roll   Prone on elbows
                                    ↓
                              Prone on extended   Weight shifting backward,   Unilateral upper extrem-
                              arms ——————————→ forward, side to side ——→ ity weight bearing and
                                                                           reaching
                              All fours ⇄   Weight shifting forward
                                  | and backward
                                  | ↓
                                  ↓   side to side ——————————→ Unilateral reaching
                              Bilateral lower   during creeping
                              extremity weight
                              bearing ———————→ Weight shifting in standing

                              Hold semisquat and ←——————————— Cruising
                              squat   ↓
                                      ——————→ Squat to stand ———————→ Walking
                                                                        ↓
                                                              Hands free for prehension

*Compiled by Becky Porter, MS, RPT, Indiana University Physical Therapy Program, 1978.

and *heavy work*. Muscles participating in heavy work are deep and positioned near a joint. They are one-joint muscles (uni-arthrodial), which lie in medial and proximal body regions. These vital muscles, which must be stimulated early in treatment, act as *stability* forces.

The heavy work muscles, primarily extensors and abductors, are under greater reflex control, i.e., from vestibular input, than light work musculature. Maintained stretch and heavy resistance will also activate these muscles. The distal segments are fixed during heavy work. Light work muscles are positioned in superficial lateral body regions or on distal body segments and function more voluntarily than reflexly. During light work, the distal segment is free and therefore moves through space (*mobility patterns*). The following are classified as light work muscles: two-joint extensors (multiarthrodial), flexors, and adductors. Low-threshold exteroceptive stimuli and light stretch are effective activators of light work musculature (Rood, 1962; Crutchfield and Barnes, 1973; Rood, 1978).

Children with neuromuscular dysfunction frequently manifest a pattern of active superficial lateral musculature without the stabilizing influence of the heavy work muscles. Before planning treatment, the therapist must analyze muscle function and stimulate a muscle so that it responds properly. Examples of this include using inversion and joint compression of more than body weight on heavy work muscles and using quick stretch, moving touch, and other low-threshold exteroceptive stimuli to activate light work musculature. These techniques are discussed later in this chapter.

The concepts of rostral to caudal adaptive motor responses, proximal to distal control, and gross to fine coordination are employed in the multisensory approach (Illingworth, 1975). For example, one would not attempt to develop fine coordination in the upper extremities of a patient who had not as yet developed proximal stability of the trunk and shoulder girdle.

The therapist must remember that no two individuals develop in exactly the same manner. Many normal children bypass complete stages of development. The developmental progression is therefore used as a guideline to determine the direction of a patient's treatment program. As a patient gains mastery in a developmental pattern, he is re-evaluated to determine if the next developmental pattern is appropriate for use in the treatment sequence. It is even conceivable that a therapist might attempt remediation of proximal instability within several developmental patterns during one treatment session.

If a patient is ready to progress to a specific pattern, such as the all fours position, but that pattern reinforces primitive reflexia and hypertonicity, components of the pattern may be used without actually using the specific pattern. In the creeping sequence, some of the movement patterns include swing-through, stance, movement over stance, weight shift and reciprocation. Reciprocal leg movements, for example, could be facilitated by using a tricycle.

TREATMENT SEQUENCE

Sensory Stimulation Concepts

When using various treatment modalities, one needs to recognize that a given modality may be used for different effects depending on how, when, and where it is applied. The amplitude and frequency of a stimulus and the site of stimulation may determine the outcome (Pederson and Ter Vrugt, 1973; Kornhuber, 1974; Sinclair, 1967). For example, light moving touch to the perioral area of a 7½-week human fetus causes an avoidance response of the head (Hooker, 1977). For a patient with a more mature nervous system, light moving touch applied in a slow stroking pattern in the direction of hair growth along the midline of the back for three to five minutes will usually produce calming (Farber, 1974; Frank, 1971). Stroking against the direction of hair growth may cause a tickle or pain response (Frank, 1971).

The touch example also illustrates that the developmental stage of the patient may determine how he responds to stimulation. A newborn baby is highly sensitive to a light moving touch owing in part to the fact that his skin is densely packed with receptors such as Meissner corpuscles

(Sinclair, 1967). The more end organs per unit area of skin, the more sensitive it will be. The number of Meissner corpuscles decreases with age (Sinclair, 1967), as does, consequently, the degree of sensitivity.

There are also sex differences for sensory thresholds. Women have lower thresholds for visual, auditory, and touch stimulation and for warmth and biological odors, while men have lower thresholds for vibration (Sinclair, 1967; Goleman, 1978; Koelega and Koster, 1974). Fear, anxiety, and previous experiences can change the way a patient responds to a given stimulus. Schneider (1974) reports that stressed individuals do not adapt to odor as rapidly as unstressed individuals; therefore, anxious patients may remain aware of environmental odors beyond the normal adaptation period.

The duration of a sensation does not necessarily correspond to the duration of the stimulus (Sinclair, 1967). There are times when the perception of the stimulus lasts beyond the application. Alternatively, there are occasions when perception of the stimulus decreases even while the stimulus is still being applied (adaptation). This adaptation varies with each modality (Sinclair, 1967).

When any sensory modality is used, care must be taken to avoid causing a pain response because pain can stimulate sympathetic nervous system tone. Any stimulus, even a normally non-nociceptive one, can cause pain if it is of sufficient intensity. The perceived quality of a stimulus often changes as the intensity increases (Sinclair, 1967).

One must also consider the concept of *rebound* (overcompensation) in relationship to the autonomic nervous system (ANS) when using sensory stimulation. For example, if one uses too many calming techniques on a patient, his body processes may speed up in an attempt to restore homeostasis (Gellhorn, 1967; Selbach, 1962) (see Chapter 1).

Inhibition Versus Facilitation

Table 3–4 describes basic characteristics of inhibitory versus facilitory stimuli. Knowledge of these characteristics is necessary for planning and implementing

TABLE 3–4 CHARACTERISTICS OF AN INHIBITORY COMPARED WITH THOSE OF A FACILITORY STIMULUS*

Inhibition	Facilitation
1. Rate of stimulation is generally slow, even, and rhythmical, perhaps affecting inhibitory regions of the reticular formation.	1. Rate of stimulation is generally fast, uneven, and intermittent.
2. Stimulus may be processed in peripheral and CNS regions. Both central and peripheral processing serve to direct excitation and produce localized responses.	2. Stimulus causes a condition of critical change in the body or specific body part stimulated. The spatial or temporal discharge pattern may change.
3. Following inhibitory input, either generalized or specific calming can be measured.	3. Following stimulation, a state of arousal can be measured in various body systems.

*Synthesized from Tamar, 1972; Andres and Von Düring, 1973; Farber, 1974; Noback, 1975; Guyton, 1977.

treatment sequences using sensory stimulation in order to meet specific needs of patients.

Assuming that the therapist understands the complexity of stimulation usage and has thoroughly assessed the patient's function as described in Chapter 2, he or she is then ready to plan and implement treatment. The following guidelines may be helpful in deciding whether to initiate treatment with inhibitory or facilitory activities.

Treatment Sequence Guidelines

The goal of the multisensory theory of neurorehabilitation is to promote homeostasis in the following areas: muscle tone, affective state, postural reflexes, ANS activity, and movement. Normalization of function involves therapeutic intervention beginning at the patient's baseline performance level and progressing in the appropriate direction toward homeostasis.

Under the following conditions, the treatment would begin with inhibition activities or patterns:
1. If the patient has hypertonicity;
2. If the patient is chronically or acutely dominated by sympathetic nervous system tone;
3. If spinal cord and brain stem postural reflexes dominate motor activity, indicating a reflexive maturational delay;
4. If activity or motion levels are excessive;
5. If behavioral state is excessively excitable;

6. If the patient demonstrates tactile hypersensitivity.

Systematic application of inhibitory activity begins with the use of modalities representing early developing sensory systems such as touch and progresses to include later developing sensory systems. The therapist must constantly evaluate the patient following application of the inhibitory input to assure the desired degree of response, whereupon the appropriate facilitation pattern or activity leading to the next developmental level is initiated. In some cases, one can inhibit certain behaviors at the same time as other behaviors are being facilitated. Facilitation *is always* followed by purposeful activity designed to promote the desired behavior (Table 3–5).

Under the following circumstances, the treatment sequence may start with facilitory activities or patterns:
1. If the patient demonstrates hypotonia;
2. If primitive reflexes have been integrated but midbrain and cortical (righting and equilibrium postural) reflexes have not as yet developed or need to be strengthened;
3. If the parasympathetic nervous system is dominating the patient's function or if the patient is calm, relaxed, and apparently ready to accept facilitation;
4. If activity or movement levels are depressed;
5. If the affective state is depressed, withdrawn, or flattened;
6. If the patient is hyporeactive to touch.

It is possible that a patient might dem-

TABLE 3–5 INHIBITION SEQUENCE

Treatment Sequence	Examples
Inhibition	Maintained touch, slow stroking, neutral warmth, slow rolling, slow rocking, etc.
↓	
Appropriate facilitation pattern	If patient cannot roll, for example, therapist would guide him through a rolling pattern, controlling at appropriate proximal joints.
↓	
Reinforcement at subcortical level	Involve patient in activities in which rolling is required, such as rolling inside a barrel or in inner tubes. Repetition will reinforce desired pattern and promote carry-over.

onstrate a mixed pattern of primitive reflexes with hypotonia. Under such conditions, the primitive reflexes must be inhibited or controlled first because normal movement patterns cannot occur until primitive reflexes are integrated. Facilitation patterns are also reinforced by purposeful activity at the subcortical level. Repetition of an activity at the subcortical level assists the patient to develop skilled movements.

A second critical decision must be made following the selection of the inhibition sequence or the facilitation sequence. The therapist must determine whether to use a given sensory modality in pure form or to use a stimulus combining components of several sensory systems. The author recommends initially applying a single sensory system modality in the early treatment sessions in order to evaluate adaptive responses. If the patient consistently demonstrates an improved behavioral response following the administration of a single sensory system stimulus, a second single sensory system stimulus from a different sensory system may be added to the program within the same treatment session. Multisensory stimuli should be initiated only after adaptive responses are consistently obtained following successive single sensory system stimulation. The therapist must constantly monitor the patient's responses, especially when complex multisensory stimuli are added to the sequence. If intersensory processing does not occur, and the patient fails to demonstrate an adaptive response, stimuli should again be simplified.

Ultimate progress toward more complex multisensory stimuli is necessary in order to promote firing of convergent or association neurons, which need input from more than one sensory modality in order to fire (see Chapter 1) (Shepherd, 1974). Additionally, a patient cannot always be in a sensory-controlled environment and must therefore develop intersensory processing if he is to cope adequately with the stresses in most environments.

The author views such *maladaptive behavior* as self-abusiveness or hallucinations as a probable result of inadequate sensory processing or a lack of interpretable sensory input. The brain requires constant input; when its input is not meaningful, for whatever reason, it creates its own stimuli in the form of hallucinations, for example (Hebb, 1963). Frequent findings in sensory deprivation studies include increases in hallucinations and other forms of maladaptive behavior (Freedman, Kaplan, and Sadock, 1975; Goldberger, 1970; Thomson, 1973; Zubek, 1969). To reduce such behavior, sensory input must be developmentally suitable; it must include use of the stimuli from the appropriate sensory system applied singly until adaptive responses occur. Active participation on the part of the patient seems to increase the likelihood of adaptive response formation. It is frequently helpful to use the type of maladaptive behavior as a guide in selecting proper stimulation. When a patient rocks himself, he may be indicating a need for more vestibular input.

Intersensory processing is a therapeutic goal, and remediation in this area is attempted by use of controlled application of stimuli from the early developing sensory systems. Once adaptive behavior consistently results, more complex sensory input is added to the program. Simply bombarding such patients with all types of stimuli does not assure that the input will be meaningful, especially if intersensory processing is inadequate. It is even conceivable that overstimulation designed to produce "reality orientation" may actually cause a rebound effect yielding more maladaptive behavior. Research designed to test the hypothesis that meaningful sensory input can reduce maladaptive behavior is needed.

The therapist must be aware of the total environment, with its human as well as nonhuman elements, when treating a patient in need of neurorehabilitation. All sensory input must be considered and controlled if possible during the early stages of therapy. If a patient needs an inhibitory treatment approach and is treated in a noisy, cluttered environment, it will be difficult to achieve the therapeutic goal. Even the therapist's body odor may have an effect on the patient (Farber, 1978).

Neurorehabilitation Equipment

The use of dynamic slings, splints, and positioning devices is preferred to the use of static equipment in the multisensory approach. Rationale and specific equipment will be discussed in depth in Chapter 7, on adaptive equipment.

Specific Therapeutic Modalities

The Touch System

As described in Table 3–1, simple reflex arcs differentiate early for touch, especially in the perioral region. Early touch responses are protective; a fetus moves his head away from the stimulus. Tactile discrimination (including stereognosis, two-point discrimination, position sense, and so forth) does not develop until much later after birth; therefore, activities designed to promote detailed tactile discrimination are incorporated into the treatment sequence following normalization of touch responses and improvement in movement patterns.

While the light moving touch system (the spinothalamic-spinoreticular system)

develops early and is subsequently a part of the early treatment sequence, initiating treatment with touch is often difficult. Members of our society are often reluctant to touch or be touched and many patients in need of touch are hypersensitive to it. In some cases, the patient may need to be calmed by other means before he can tolerate even inhibitory touch. Since touch input appears to enhance awareness or consciousness (Lassen et al, 1978), every effort is made to normalize touch responses as early as possible in the treatment sequence.

Inhibitory Touch. Inhibitory touch procedures are used to normalize hypersensitive skin, a condition that frequently results following central or peripheral nervous system damage (Sinclair, 1967).

MAINTAINED TOUCH OR PRESSURE. Maintained touch is an inhibitory technique useful in reducing body part disregard and in normalizing touch thresholds. This technique is effective perhaps because of pressure adaptation. When pressure is continuously applied, there is a decline in sensitivity; however, the adaptation may vary with the intensity of the stimulus and with the area of the body being stimulated (Geldard, 1972).

A recent study by Rogers et al (1980) provides possible neuroanatomical circuitry that explains the calming effect of maintained pressure in the perioral region. The pressure stimulus is afferent to the principal sensory trigeminal nucleus, which in turn communicates with the dorsal motor nucleus of the vagus. Thus a maintained pressure may facilitate an increase in parasympathetic tone.

Since the perioral area is quite sensitive and has a large cortical representation (Noback, 1975; Lassen, 1978; Guyton, 1977), maintained pressure in the perioral area is generally attempted first. The therapist should lightly place an index finger directly under the patient's nose. The finger should be in stationary contact with the skin rostral to the top lip while the remainder of the fingers should be kept out of the patient's visual field (Fig. 3–1). While keeping the finger above the top lip for a short time period, the therapist constantly monitors responses. Since each patient will respond differently, no precise period for maintaining the stimulus can be prescribed. This procedure may be repeat-

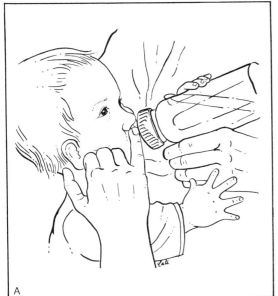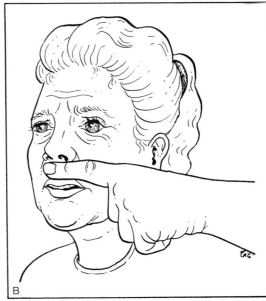

Figure 3–1.

ed as needed. If the patient pulls his head away from the therapist's finger or if other sympathetic nervous system responses become apparent (see Chapters 1 and 2), the patient may not be ready for input of any type to his face. In that case, maintained pressure to the palms, abdomen, or soles of the feet may be indicated.

When approaching a patient's face with an outstretched index finger, the therapist should move slowly and cautiously, being sure to avoid startling the patient and evoking undesirable responses. The patient can be actively involved in treatment by placing his own finger above his top lip. The therapist should briefly explain that

this technique is part of his therapy and may help him. One should generally avoid giving the patient detailed explanations regarding the purpose of treatment movements because this may cause the patient to attempt relaxation at a cortical level. It is interesting to note that many normal individuals who are upset often automatically place their own index fingers on their lips or mouth in an apparent attempt to regain emotional control.

Maintained pressure to the abdomen can also produce calming. The therapist places the palmar surface of the hand on the patient's abdomen (Fig. 3–2), utilizing light maintained pressure for a short

Figure 3–2.

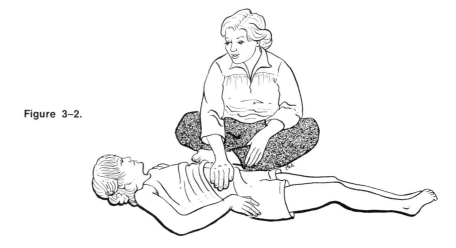

period of time. Before starting, the therapist should be sure that his or her hands are not cold because this could cause a facilitory response and disrupt rapport. Since each patient will respond differently, no precise period for maintaining the stimulus can be prescribed.

The use of maintained pressure into the soles of the feet or palms of the hands may decrease hypersensitivity of skin of the palmar and plantar surfaces in addition to producing some generalized calming. There are many ways to apply pressure to the palmar surfaces. Figure 3–3 demonstrates three equally effective methods. The first method involves placing the patient's palms together while he is in a sidelying, flexed position. The therapist can also apply maintained pressure to the soles of the feet while the patient is lying on his side. The second method involves having the patient place his palms on his abdomen. A third method involves having the therapist place his or her palms over the patient's. The therapist should never passively extend a patient's fisted, spastic hands in order to apply maintained pressure to the palms because this practice could facilitate the secondary endings of the muscle spindle and further facilitate flexion (Crutchfield and Barnes, 1973). Instead, one alternative would be to invert the patient, thereby facilitating wrist extension and open hand position due to labyrinthine excitation (see the vestibular input section of this chapter).

Figure 3–4 depicts two techniques for applying maintained pressure to the soles of the feet. The first method involves placing the patient's bare feet on a firm surface of neutral temperature. This can be done in a variety of positions, including sit-squat and sitting in a chair. In a second method, the patient's foot rests on the therapist's hand. If the therapist's hand is warm, this may further enhance inhibition (see the temperature section of this chapter). The therapist must be sure not to push up into the sole of the foot, especially over the region of the ball of the foot, as this might stretch the intrinsic muscles, facilitating a reflexive extension, positive supporting reaction (Fiorentino, 1973; Guyton, 1977).

When using maintained pressure on any part of the body, deciding how long and how often to apply the pressure is sometimes difficult. One is reminded that the goal is to achieve homeostasis of sensory responsiveness and not to render a hypersensitive patient comatose. When a patient can tolerate having an area touched that was previously hypersensitive and when generalized calming is evident, it is time to move on to other aspects of the program.

SLOW STROKING. This is an inhibitory procedure involving rhythmical moving touch instead of maintained touch. The patient is placed in prone position with his back exposed. Stroking must be done in the direction of the hair growth if it is to be calming (Frank, 1971). Before beginning the stroking for the first time, the therapist should examine the patient's back to make sure that there are not extensive hair whorls in the area. Patients having hair whorls are not good candidates for slow stroking because part of the stroke will be against the hair growth pattern. If the patient is hypersensitive on his back, maintained pressure can be used before stroking.

The alternate stroking is initiated by

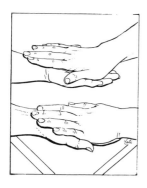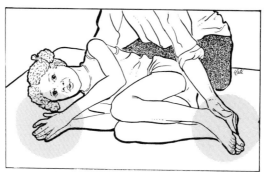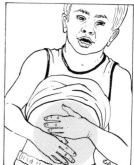

Figure 3–3.

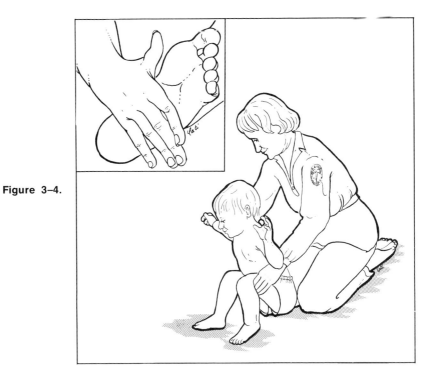

Figure 3–4.

placing one hand at the patient's occiput and stroking lightly in a caudal direction on the skin over the distribution of the posterior primary rami on either side of the vertebral column. As the first hand nears the coccyx, the other hand is placed up at the occiput. This ensures an even, rhythmical stroking pattern of continuous contact, which should be continued for no more than 3 to 5 minutes (Fig. 3–5) in

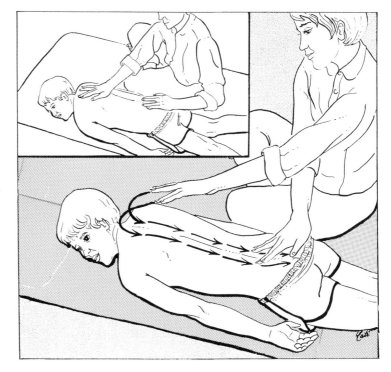

Figure 3–5.

order to avoid skin irritation and ANS rebound. Therapists applying the stroking might also experience a calming sensation because they are involved in an even, repetitive activity. Rood has had success in treatment of enuresis using slow stroking (Rood, 1978).

Facilitory Touch

BRIEF MOVING TOUCH. On the perioral midline, this modality will facilitate the flexor pattern seen in Figure 3–6. After maintained pressure to the upper lip is used for normalizing touch thresholds and to produce generalized calming, a movement stimulus is applied to the patient's face starting at the midline area directly under the nose and progressing caudally to the chin (Fig. 3–7). This stimulus generally must be reapplied several times before noticeable results occur; however, the therapist should apply each subsequent stimulus after a short rest. Constant stimulation can evoke primary afferent depolarization (PAD), a presynaptic inhibitory mechanism that prevents overstimulation (Schmidt, 1973; Rood, 1978). If the patient pulls his head away from the moving stimulus, he may not be sufficiently calmed or he may be demonstrating a remnant of the rooting response (see the feeding section of this chapter).

The flexor pattern (Fig. 3–6), evoked by the cumulative moving touch stimuli, is the first developmental pattern to appear.

Normal developmental oral stimulation causes a young infant to move his extremities toward the midline. Rood calls this pattern a "toward pattern" (Trombly and Scott, 1977) in which the upper extremities flex at the elbows and cross over the chest. The hands open with extended fingers, abducted thumb, and balanced tone at the wrist. A palm-out (aversive) response frequently occurs before the palm-to-face pattern. When used in therapy on a young child, perioral moving touch will also facilitate flexion of the lower extremities with knee flexion and dorsiflexion at the ankle. In contrast, perioral stimulation to an adult affects only the upper extremities. Thus moving touch at the level of the T10 dermatome (navel) is necessary to facilitate leg flexion on the same side (Fig. 3–8). The moving touch is applied within the dermatome in a midline to lateral direction on either side of the navel. Four to five repetitions of the stimulus may be necessary to evoke a response. Short rest periods between stimuli are again necessary to avoid causing a PAD.

The flexor pattern is frequently used in conjunction with the feeding and rolling patterns. Following the stimulation of the face (and abdomen), the patient may be rolled to assist the arm in coming diagonally up to the face or the leg in crossing over the body. An ice Popsicle flavored with banana oil can be placed in the pa-

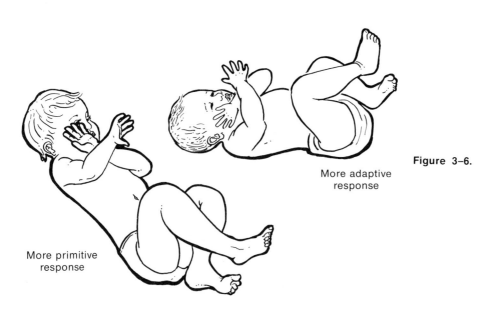

More primitive response

More adaptive response

Figure 3–6.

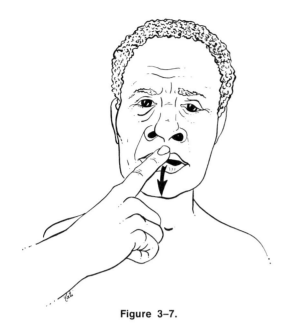

Figure 3–7.

feeding inhibits the aversive "moving away" response to oral stimulation. Patients who do not acquire sucking skills will maintain the aversive "moving away" pattern, which will interfere with the development of the flexor pattern used in feeding.

When the flexor pattern is used on a patient who has flaccid muscle tone, the upper extremity can be positioned in horizontal adduction with elbow flexion (so the hand rests on the opposite shoulder). The maintained and moving touch stimuli are applied and the patient is then rolled. This positioning causes the muscle spindles of the pectoralis major to adjust to the shortened range. The arm is allowed to move back to the patient's side prior to initiating rolling. The pectoralis is more sensitive to stretch; thus the flexion pattern is enhanced. In the horizontal adduction position, the triceps is placed on maintained stretch, which facilitates the secondary ending in the triceps muscle spindles causing excitation of the biceps (Rood, 1978). When the therapist is trying

tient's hand to encourage the hand-to-mouth and subsequent sucking pattern (Farber, 1978). Pressure on the tongue normally experienced during sucking and

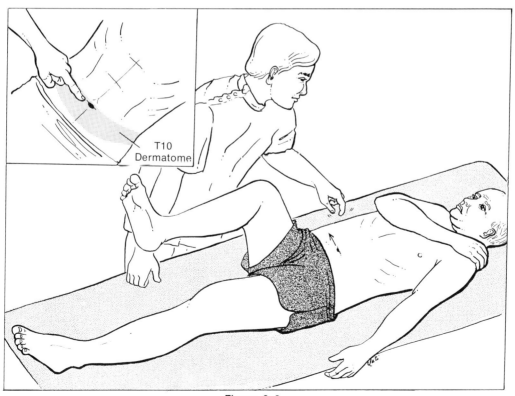

Figure 3–8.

to facilitate the flexion pattern in the early stages of a patient's treatment, passive abduction of the upper extremity should be avoided. This action might cause a traction response that would block the hand-to-mouth pattern normally facilitated in the flexor pattern (Rood, 1978; Bobath, 1978).

Once the perioral midline touch stimulus causes the desired response, the movement stimulus can be applied more laterally on the face (the corner of the lip or the cheek) still moving from rostral to caudal in direction. One must remember that as the touch stimulus moves away from the midline, it brings in more superficial musculature. It is important that the deep midline musculature be functioning before superficial muscles are brought into play. Stimulating the corner of the mouth causes a tilting of the head to the side stimulated as a result of the action of the sternocleidomastoid and trapezius muscles.

Once the patient achieves the flexor pattern, the second pattern, inverted suspension, is added to the treatment sequence. This pattern is discussed in depth in the section on vestibular stimulation. Development of these two early patterns provides a patient with the necessary components to progress through all developmental patterns. The flexor pattern brings in the components needed later for locomotion, including dorsiflexion and swing-through motion. Balanced tone at the wrist and ankle is also facilitated by the flexor pattern, and wrist extension is further reinforced in the inverted position. According to this author's experience, patients stimulated early in the treatment sequence for flexor and inverted patterns are least likely to develop wrist flexion deformities. Head and trunk balance are also enhanced by inversion. The feeding sequence described later in the chapter can be used in conjunction with both the flexor and inverted sequence.

BRUSHING. Brushing is a form of facilitory touch. A battery-powered camel's hair brush is used to stimulate the dermatomal area of a given muscle, thereby facilitating the underlying muscle. The fast repetitive stimulation supplied by the brush reportedly affects muscle spindles and sends impulses to the reticular formation (Rood, 1978). Brushing has a long latency period so that its maximum response follows stimulation by approximately 30 minutes, although an immediate response should occur within 30 seconds. Brushing may increase the excitability of stretch receptors in a given muscle (Harris, 1978). Therapists are urged not to use brushing unless they have studied both Rood's treatment rationale and technique and the neurophysiological effects of brushing. Although brushing was introduced as a therapeutic modality used in general muscle patterns, it is now used only to reduce disregard of body parts and to facilitate specific muscles that cannot be activated by other less powerful, developmentally appropriate methods.

Brushing of the face is avoided as it may interfere with the hand-to-mouth pattern. Midline areas are not brushed because many sensory fibers cross over in this region. Brushing the pinna of the ear is contraindicated; it stimulates a branch of the vagus (Trombly and Scott, 1977). Rood also uses brushing as part of the bowel and bladder training program she has developed. The reader is referred to her work for details on bladder and bowel training using brushing (Trombly and Scott, 1977).

Psychological Aspects of Touch. It is imperative that the therapist use a caring, empathetic, nontentative touch when handling patients (Huss, 1977). Insecurity and reluctance is easily communicated through touch, so that the patient will sense when a therapist lacks confidence. Self-assuredness and belief in a therapeutic modality can likewise be perceived by the patient. A patient's belief in the eventual success of therapy may in itself produce adaptive responses.

Vestibular Input

ADEQUATE STIMULI. The vestibular system is stimulated by movement in any plane, caloric stimulation, and gravitational pull (Tamar, 1972; Wirth, 1971). Visual stimulation (optokinetic input) and auditory input alter structures that are also influenced by the vestibular system. Therapists are mainly concerned with the effects of movement on the vestibular system and the subsequent effects on the whole body. Caloric stimulation is not recommended for therapeutic use because of its aversive and invasive nature.

Frequent acceleration and deceleration of the body causes the endolymph to move relative to the semicircular duct. The changes in pressure that this creates produce a facilitory response. In contrast, movement that is repetitive and maintained, with a uniform rate of speed, causes endolymph and the ducts to move together owing to inertia (Gardner, 1975). Movement of this second type will not promote the pressure changes of fluid relative to the ducts necessary for prolonged facilitation; thus a more inhibitory response may be produced (see Chapter 1).

GENERAL PRECAUTIONS. Before the types of vestibular input used in the multisensory approach are described, a general precaution regarding vestibular input is in order. Therapists in several disciplines have recently added vestibular stimulation to their therapeutic regimen. Unfortunately, misuse of this modality is common. This misuse involves but is not limited to rotatory stimulation of the neonate, inadequate monitoring during and following stimulation, improper rotatory patterns and velocities, and lack of understanding of neurophysiological rationale. As described in Chapter 1, the vestibular system has connections with many other structures within the CNS. Misapplication of technique can therefore have widespread deleterious effects.

VESTIBULAR INPUT USED IN THE MULTISENSORY APPROACH. Table 3–6 presents a summary of the various vestibular

or kinetic stimuli used in the multisensory approach listed in order of use.

Inversion. Inversion occurs early in development and is subsequently used early in the treatment sequence. As shown in Table 3–1, inversion occurs by the 26th to 29th fetal week. Moore (1974) suggests that this position results partially from the shape of the uterus and partially from the fact that the head is heavier than the feet. Moore's speculation, however, does not provide an adequate explanation for breech presentation.

This author hypothesizes that movement input is critical to the fetus. As the fetus increases in size, the available space for movement in utero decreases. It is possible that the inversion response of the fetus occurs partly as an attempt to maximize stimulation of the vestibular system. Perhaps a subtle vestibular malfunction may be responsible for the fetus not preparing itself for birth by inversion. This hypothesis might be tested by assessment of vestibular function of breech birth infants and comparison with that of infants with normal presentation.

The *tonic labyrinthine inverted reflex* was described by Tokizane in 1951 (cited by Payton, Hirt, Newton, 1977). Inversion activates the baroreceptors in the carotid sinus (Guyton, 1977) thus bringing into play the parasympathetic nervous system. Hypertonicity is thus reduced. The vestibular system is facilitated by inversion and Tokizane reports strong facilitory effects (+++) to the soleus and extensor carpi ulnaris and radialis; moderate facilitory effects (++) to the gastrocnemius,

TABLE 3–6 VESTIBULAR INPUT USED IN THE MULTISENSORY APPROACH

Stimulus Type	Examples
1. Inversion	1. Inversion of the total body over a ball (child) or leaning over while seated (adult), causing inversion of the upper trunk.
2. Anteroposterior movement	2. Rocking over ball or bolster in a horizontal plane; rocking in all fours position; gentle shaking or rocking.
3. Side-to-side movement	3. Rocking done in prone-on-elbows, all fours, kneel-standing, or standing position.
4. Diagonal rocking	4. Done in crawling, all fours, kneel-standing, and standing positions.
5. Linear Acceleration	5. Utilizing tricycles, scooter boards, ramps, and swings.
6. Rotation	6. Utilizing various types of equipment designed for rotation: merry-go-round, Sit and Spin,* Bárány chair (Bárány, 1907), net hammock (Ayres, 1972).

*Marx Toy Co.

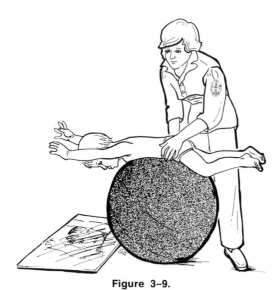

Figure 3–9.

mirror or appropriate toy is located on the mat surface, enabling the child to fix on the object. The child should actively extend his neck and maintain his head with his face parallel and not perpendicular to the floor (Fig. 3–9). The therapist should remember to avoid cortically directing the patient. Once some extensor tone results from facilitation of the vestibular system, the child's neck and deep midline back extensors can be vibrated to enhance extension. Wrist extensors can also be vibrated. When vibration is applied to a contracting agonist, the contraction is assisted and the patient's perception of contraction effort is reduced (McClosky, 1978). If the total inverted position is not possible, the patient can lean over a stool, the therapist's lap, or simply lean forward while seated in a chair (for the adult patient with a cerebrovascular accident (CVA), see Figure 3–10).

Rood has encouraged the development of many adaptations to the inverted position. For example, once some neck extensor tone is facilitated by the vestibular system, joint compression can be used at the neck to bring in co-contraction of neck musculature (see the section on joint compression in this chapter). In another adaptation, the therapist may want to "fold up" the patient's legs in order to concentrate on the upper extremity patterns (Fig. 3–11). Having the inverted patient work on a purposeful activity for brief periods of time reinforces the pattern and provides an infinite number of adaptations. For example, a child might be encouraged to

biceps femoris (long head), vasti, rectus femoris, triceps; and weaker facilitory effects (+) to the gluteus maximus and deltoid.

In the multisensory approach the inverted position is used in the treatment sequence following facilitation of the flexion pattern (see Table 3–3 and the section on touch in this chapter). The inverted sequence allows the infant to progress from the self-exploration seen during the flexor pattern (see Fig. 3–6) to exploration of the environment secondary to facilitated extensor tone (Fig. 3–9).

In the *procedure* for this stimulus, the child is positioned over a large ball with his head placed down near the mat. A

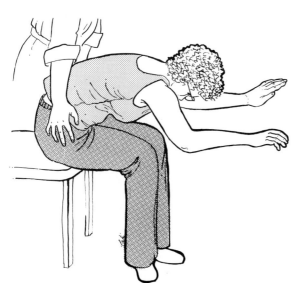

Figure 3–10.

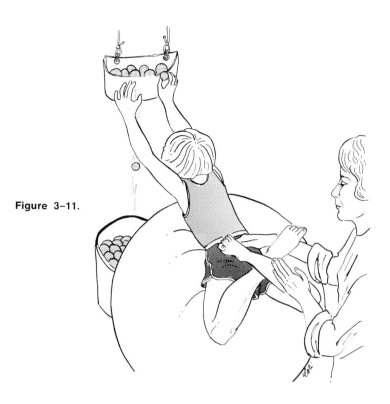

Figure 3–11.

drop objects into containers for balanced grasp and release patterns, or take a banana- or vanilla-flavored ice Popsicle to his mouth for sucking. The therapist can place the patient supine and can then pull the inferior angle of the scapula in a lateral direction to stretch the rhomboids (Fig. 3–12). This sequence can be added after

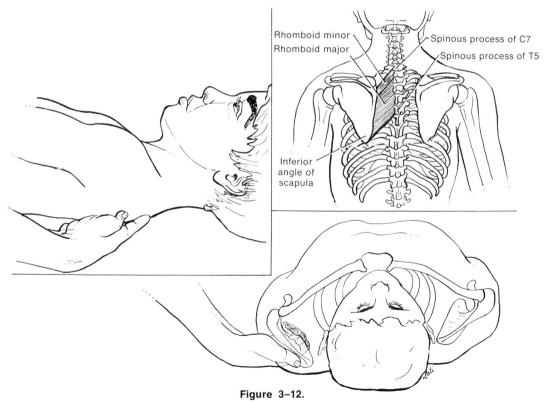

Rhomboid minor
Rhomboid major
Spinous process of C7
Spinous process of T5
Inferior angle of scapula

Figure 3–12.

135

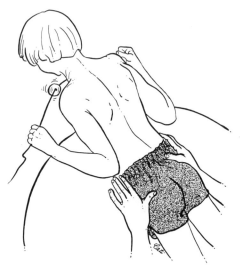

Figure 3–13.

some humeral flexion from inversion is achieved to enhance shoulder stability. The therapist should then design activities that will facilitate the upper extremity external rotation pattern (Fig. 3–13).

The *tonic labyrinthine inverted position* can be utilized in combination with a sit-squat pattern. The patient is placed in a sit-squat position with his weight centered over his heels. He then moves upward and forward while the therapist stabilizes him at the hips and trunk (Fig. 3–14). The sit-squat position is helpful in releasing spastic gastrocnemius muscles. The one-joint soleus muscle, when placed on maintained stretch during sit-squat, will fire its primary (Ia) and secondary (II) endings, promoting a co-contraction around the ankles (Rood, 1978; Crutchfield and Barnes, 1973). This modification of the inverted position can be done while the patient is positioned on a "shoe 2 × 4″ device" (see Fig. 7–39, Chapter 7) to avoid pressure into the balls of the feet.

If the patient demonstrates spastic hamstrings while inverted, pressure into the medial gluteal area will release the hamstrings (Fig. 3–15). Inversion can also be accomplished in supine position (Fig. 3–16). It is not possible to include every conceivable adaptation to the tonic labyrinthine inverted position. The therapist is urged to assess the patient's needs careful-

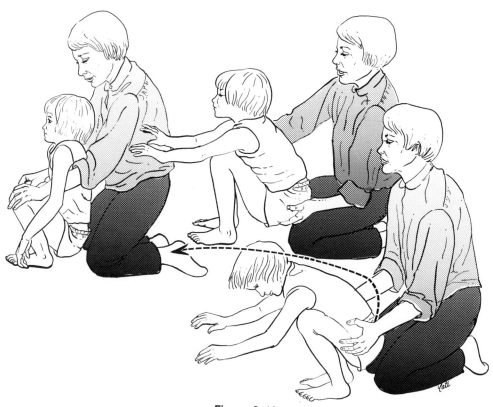

Figure 3–14.

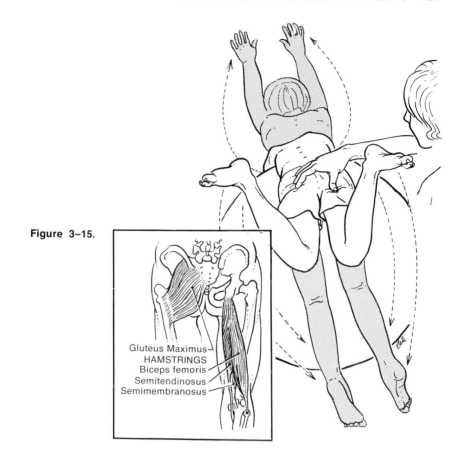

Figure 3–15.

Gluteus Maximus
HAMSTRINGS
Biceps femoris
Semitendinosus
Semimembranosus

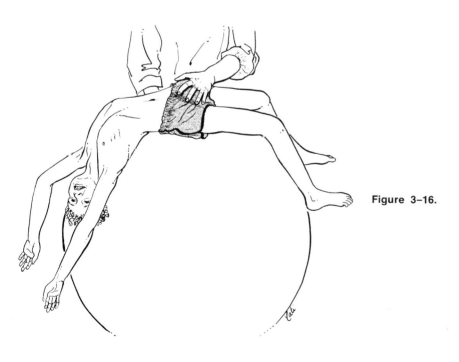

Figure 3–16.

ly and adapt this vital therapeutic sequence appropriately.

There are many *precautions* to heed when using inverted suspension. The patient must feel secure in inversion. If he is fearful, a sympathetic nervous system response could compete with the action of the baroreceptors of the carotid sinus. Also, the baroreceptors themselves may not be functioning properly. If this is the case, the patient will begin to manifest a variety of sympathetic responses. The patient should not remain in inverted suspension for extended time periods even if the baroreceptors of the carotid sinus are functioning properly because of possible adverse physiological effects such as venous pooling. The therapist must be sure that the patient assumes the proper head position during inversion. If the patient extends his neck so that his face is perpendicular to the mat instead of parallel to it, his symmetrical tonic neck reflex may actually be holding the neck in extension and not the desired co-contraction pattern of neck musculature (Fig. 3–17).

A toy or object of interest placed on the mat surface in the patient's visual field will encourage fixation on the object and direct head motion to some degree. The therapist must be sure to avoid placing pressure into the back (dorsal surface) of the head and to avoid stimulation of hair in this region because this could facilitate a reflexive extension instead of a co-contraction of neck musculature.

The therapist must be sure that the patient's hands are free and are not touching the ground during inversion. Fixing the distal segment (the hand) will hinder the desired movement pattern of the upper extremities. All therapists should work on a mat surface when inverting patients. The mat will assure some protection if the patient slips off the inverting equipment. Finally, the therapist is urged to monitor the patient's responses carefully and continually during the inverted suspension. One should never leave a patient unattended while inverted.

Anteroposterior Motion. Motion in this plane also occurs early in development and is therefore utilized along with inversion. Anteroposterior motion is used consistently throughout the developmental progression. In prone, the patient may be placed over a ball or a bolster. As with inversion, the patient must feel secure. For patients having problems with depth perception, the author has found a bolster to be less threatening than a large ball. The patient is rocked slowly back and forth (horizontally) in an even, rhythmical pattern if inhibitory responses are desired whereas a fast, uneven pattern with frequent starts and stops is used for facilitation. Following the use of anteroposterior motion in prone, a relevant occupational activity should be initiated, such as rocking the patient back and forth on a crawler or creeper as part of a game (see Chapter 7).

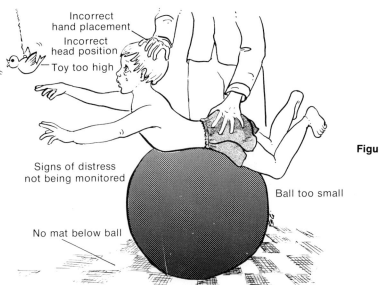

Incorrect hand placement
Incorrect head position
Toy too high
Signs of distress not being monitored
Ball too small
No mat below ball

Figure 3–17.

Gentle shaking or rocking is an adaptation of movement in the anteroposterior plane. The patient is placed in supine with his head ventroflexed in the midline. Ventroflexion of the neck will reduce the effect of the *tonic labyrinthine in supine reflex* on the body and should therefore be maintained throughout the rocking sequence. The therapist controls the patient by placing one hand under the patient's occiput and the other hand on the rostral surface of the head (Fig. 3–18); the head can also be held on the sides over the ears. Under no circumstances should any pressure be exerted on the dorsal surface of the head; this might strengthen the tonic labyrinthine in supine reflex. The therapist then gently pushes the patient's head into his body, compressing the neck in a rhythmical, even pattern for inhibition or in an irregular faster pattern for facilitation. As the therapist repetitively pushes the patient's head into his body, waves of motion spread down the entire body, possibly effecting a change in both mind and body states.

If the therapist is using gentle shaking or rocking with an adult, good body mechanics must be practiced. Trying to push an adult's head into his body can cause strain on the therapist's lower back unless the therapist leans into the patient while compressing the patient's neck.

The therapist must also be sure that the patient's head can tolerate the compression force. If there has been a section of bone removed from the patient's skull or if the patient has skin breakdown on the head, as frequently occurs in hydrocephaly, compression to the head may be contraindicated. If a patient has ventricular shunts, the therapist should discuss utilization of any vestibular stimulation with the physician to be sure that the intended technique is not contraindicated.

In the all fours position, movement in the anteroposterior plane occurs earlier than side-to-side or diagonal movement. A normal baby is often seen rocking himself before he initiates creeping (Stone and Church, 1975).

If a patient is ready to progress to the all fours position but primitive reflexes or hypertonicity interferes with the development of the pattern, the patient can be rocked slowly and evenly in the anteroposterior plane. Pads should be placed under the patient's knees to prevent inhibition of the quadriceps femoris from pressure on the patellar tendon. If the patient demonstrates spasticity in his hands, place them on a pair of cement smoothers or toy irons (Fig. 3–19 and Chapter 7). The pressure on the flexor insertions will assist in reducing spasticity and in avoiding stretch of flexors. Under no circumstances should fisted hands be spread open passively on the mat. Maintained stretch on flexors of the hands facilitates flexion (Crutchfield and Barnes, 1973).

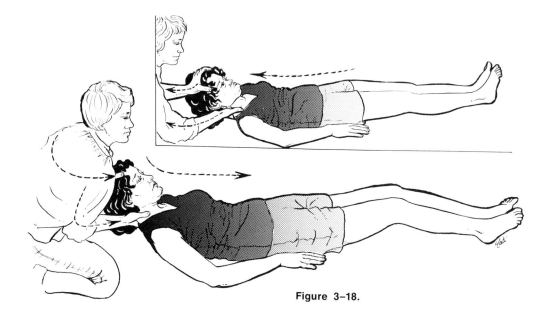

Figure 3–18.

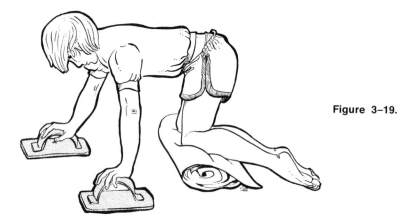

Figure 3–19.

One needs to be sure that the patient's back is as parallel to the ground as is possible. If his shoulders are higher than his hips as demonstrated in Figure 3–20, a symmetrical tonic neck reflex could be strengthened instead of inhibited. The longer a patient spends in a pathological reflex pattern, the more difficult it will be to integrate that reflex. As rocking on all fours is initiated, the therapist controls the patient by placing one hand on the rostral head surface and another hand on the buttocks (Fig. 3–21). If the patient demonstrates any abnormal increase in muscle tone during the even, slow anteroposterior rocking, perhaps the patient is not ready to utilize this sequence or is not properly positioned.

For facilitation in the all fours position, a rapid, uneven anteroposterior motion is used combined with frequent starts and stops. This activity would be appropriate for a baby with Down's syndrome who has developed enough extensor tone to assume the all fours pattern but who is not moving in the pattern. Play that promotes creeping would then follow the facilitation or inhibition sequence. Although it may seem humiliating for an adult to be placed into the all fours position, the author strongly recommends not bypassing this activity. If the patient is made to understand how the all fours position helps develop proximal stability at the hips and shoulders, cooperation is not usually a problem. Patients having decreased lower extremity sensation must be closely monitored during creeping so that they do not cause injury to their legs.

Inhibitory anteroposterior movement can be used in the kneel-stand and standing positions if the patient experiences hypertonicity and abnormal reflexes upon assuming these postures. The patient's knees or feet are fixed in one position (stance position) while the patient is rocked in the anteroposterior plane.

Side-to-side and Diagonal Movement. After adaptive responses occur following anteroposterior movement stimulation at a given developmental level, the therapist then adds side-to-side movement to the regimen at the same developmental level. This movement stimulus helps establish a weight-shifting pattern. Side-to-side movement stimulation can be easily achieved during prone-on-elbows, the all fours position, kneel-stand, and standing sequences.

When the patient is in the all fours position, preparation for side-to-side movement includes the use of the same positioning guidelines as are used during

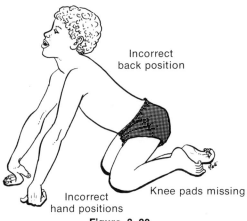

Incorrect
back position

Incorrect
hand positions

Knee pads missing

Figure 3–20.

Figure 3–21.

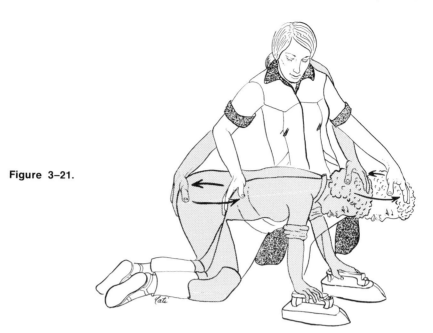

anteroposterior movement. Diagonal movement is added to the sequence after the patient begins to develop a weight-shifting pattern. One must remember to move the patient in both diagonal planes (Fig. 3–22). Whether the side-to-side and diagonal movement is done slowly, evenly, and rhythmically or done rapidly with frequent starts and stops depends on whether an inhibitory or facilitory effect is desired.

Linear Acceleration. Linear acceleration can be accomplished in a variety of methods. If done in a slow, even, continuous pattern, an inhibitory response will occur. Pulling a child in a wagon or pushing a baby in a carriage is an example of this concept. Crawlers (Chapter 7) can also be utilized for linear acceleration. For facilitory results, scooter boards with ramps can be used. In the scooter board activity, the vestibular system is stimulated by the linear acceleration and deceleration, resulting in a strengthening of neck and trunk extensors and thereby decreasing the effect of the tonic labyrinthine in prone reflex. Tricycles and bicycles can also be used for linear movement. Linear movement can be accomplished in all developmental patterns.

Rotatory Movement. As with anteroposterior, side-to-side, diagonal, and linear movement, rotatory stimulation can be done in all the developmental patterns. Rolling is the first rotatory pattern used in the multisensory approach. There are many ways to slowly and passively roll a patient in need of inhibition. A patient may be placed into a barrel and rolled. In *slow rolling,* an inhibitory technique, partial rotation about the body axis is utilized. The patient is positioned on his side. The therapist places one hand on the patient's rib cage and the other hand on the pa-

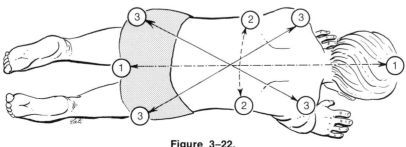

Figure 3–22.

tient's pelvis (Fig. 3–23). The patient is then rhythmically moved from sidelying toward prone and back to sidelying. Slow rolling should always be done to both sides and in a direction away from the therapist. If the patient is rolled toward the therapist, the patient's upper arm will contact the therapist in the region of the patient's biceps surface. This will facilitate flexion of that arm owing to the tapping-like motion on the biceps. Additionally, the patient may be visually stimulated while rolling toward the therapist.

After a passive rolling pattern of either an inhibitory or facilitory nature, active rolling is the goal. The patient may be encouraged to roll within a barrel. This type of activity assists in body side integration as the arms cross over each other while the patient makes the barrel roll.

A second activity that assists in body side integration is prone rotation on a scooter board. The patient is placed on the scooter board and encouraged to turn it around. As the patient improves in this activity, he will soon be crossing hand over hand while spinning (Fig. 3–24).

A net hammock, as described by Ayres (1972), can be used for spinning in supine, prone, or semisitting position. A variety of devices can be utilized for rotatory vestibular input in different developmental patterns.

As mentioned, misuse of vestibular

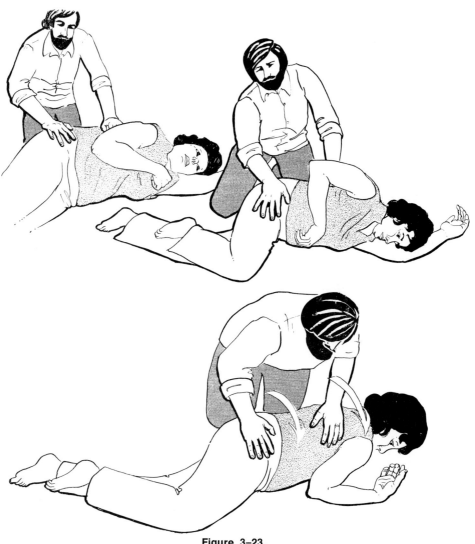

Figure 3–23.

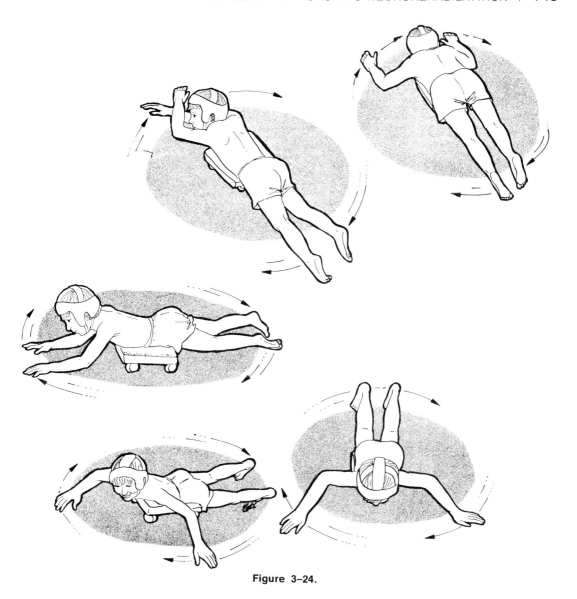

Figure 3–24.

input, specifically the rotatory type, is common. To prevent this, the following guidelines are offered:

1. Consult a physician before using vestibular input if the patient has some condition that might be aggravated by vestibular input, e.g., seizures, ventricular shunts, and so forth.

2. Inform all those who will be in contact with the patient that vestibular therapy has been initiated. Should any negative behavioral changes occur, such as increase in seizures or acting-out behavior, vestibular input can then be either suspended or decreased.

3. Always start movement slowly and progress toward facilitation when and if indicated.

4. Rotatory input should be used with visual input only after intersensory processing has been established.

5. Add only one new therapeutic activity to the regimen at a time. Determination of factors responsible for producing aversive effects is difficult when rotatory stimulation and other new activities are initiated within the same treatment session.

6. The patient must be carefully monitored during and following vestibular

input of any type. Use the ANS Inventory in Chapter 2 to be sure that the results of the input are the desired ones. Measure postrotatory nystagmus as well (Ayres, 1972).

7. As with all therapeutic modalities, reinforcement at the subcortical level is a necessity. Any time a reinforcing activity can be developed that is relevant to the patient's occupational interests and needs, the patient's active participation and motivation are likely to increase.

8. If a little of something is good, a lot of it may *not* be better. Be careful of overstimulation.

9. Many cerebral palsied children and adult patients with cerebrovascular accident have sensory integrational dysfunction; however, facilitory rotatory stimulation may increase their spasticity. Avoid use of facilitory rotation in patients with systemic hypertonia.

10. Avoid use of rotatory stimulation until the patient is developmentally ready.

Olfactory Input

GENERAL INFORMATION. Much research has been done describing the effects of olfactory input. The Monell Chemical Senses Center of The University of Pennsylvania has, as one of its main functions, research in the area of mechanisms of taste and smell (Monell Chemical Senses Center booklet, 1978). The therapist is advised to survey the olfactory literature before indiscriminately applying olfactory stimulation.

In earlier literature (Farber, 1974) it was reported that pleasant, good-nutrient odors were calming, whereas noxious odors were facilitory. This oversimplification can no longer be made. Farber (1978) reviewed the olfactory literature and reported that many factors influence responses to a given odorant, including age, sex, previous experience, and ANS status. Women have increased olfactory acuity during ovulation (Schneider, 1974).

Certain odors have been studied and generally produce consistent responses in populations tested. Odors of vanilla and banana facilitate sucking and licking motions (Steiner, 1974); those of anise, peppermint, and iodoform cause a decrease in sucking behavior (Cheal, 1974).

The multisensory approach uses olfaction in the feeding and coma treatment sequences described later in this chapter. Only natural odorants are used in the treatment, including odors to which a patient may have been previously exposed or odors common to a given developmental period; e.g., milk odor for a baby. The author advocates use of odorants previously tested on large sample populations instead of random selection of odorants. Odors that irritate the trigeminal nerve, such as those of vinegar and ammonia, are to be avoided (Farber, 1978). Cagan (1978) reports that there may be a relationship between parotid gland flow rate and irritation of the trigeminal nerve. Since salivary flow is an important influence on digestion, purposeful trigeminal irritation is generally considered a contraindication.

According to Cagan (1978), the human olfactory system is considered to have more sensitivity than the gustatory system. For this reason, in addition to the fact that the olfactory area of the brain (rhinencephalon) is one of the phylogenetically early-evolving brain structures (Carpenter, 1978) and is tied to survival behavior (feeding) via limbic connections, the author uses olfaction early in the treatment sequence. Also, there is evidence to suggest that primary olfactory neurons in adult mammals can regenerate following injury (Graziadei, 1975, 1977, 1978).

Engen and Ross (1973) report that subjects demonstrate a longer memory for odorants than for visual or auditory stimuli. While Cagan (1978) mentions that the significance of long-term olfactory memory in our daily lives is not understood, perhaps older, less vulnerable regions of the brain should be stimulated to assist newer damaged areas.

Therapists must be aware of *olfactory thresholds* and *effective odorant concentrations* when attempting to find an adequate olfactory stimulus. Engen (1970) and Patte et al (1975) discuss this area fully in their work. The following compound concentrations are a partial list calculated from Patte's work by Cagan (1978): Skatole (fecal) 5.0×10^{-12} M; butyric acid (rancid) 6.0×10^{-11} M; eugenol (spicy) 1.9×10^{-10} M; amyl acetate (fruity, banana, light) 3.0×10^{-10} M; methylsalicylate (cool, cooling) 3.7×10^{-10} M; benzaldehyde (almond-like) 1.0×10^{-9} M. Consulting a pharmacist is recommended in formulating proper concentration levels.

The therapist must also be aware of his or her own body odor. One way animals communicate is via body odors. Each human being has a unique set of odors, or pheromones, which cause behavioral changes in those around him (Cheal, 1974). Farber (1978) reports, for instance, that at the time of menses in female therapists treating children with emotional disturbances, measured increases in acting-out behaviors have been documented in these children. This area needs controlled studies before therapeutic conclusions can be drawn.

STIMULATION PROCEDURES. The actual procedure for providing olfactory input involves placing a cotton ball saturated with the appropriate concentration of odorant under a patient's nostrils. As he inhales through the nose, the bipolar olfactory neurons in the roof of the nose will be stimulated. The therapist must be careful to avoid touching the patient's face with the cotton ball as this might cause an aversive, protective response to the light touch of the cotton ball. Alternatively, olfactory input can be provided with a sniff bottle. A bottle is placed under the patient's nostrils so that he can sniff the substance during quiet breathing. The therapist should allow the odorant to remain long enough to stimulate but not so long as to cause adaptation (about 10 seconds). The patient should not be cortically directed to inhale.

Olfactometers are used in experimental laboratories to deliver a given amount of odorant, for a given time period, at a given concentration level (Moulton, Turk, and Johnston, 1975). While this precision is desirable, the cost of such equipment may be prohibitive for the average therapy department.

The therapist should have a good baseline behavioral assessment before initiating the therapeutic input. Once the odorant is introduced, the therapist must be alert to possible changes in level of consciousness, muscle tone, facial expression, verbalization, postural reflexes, feeding patterns, and affective state. Quantification of responses is necessary for purposes of accountability and proper modification of the treatment protocol. Biofeedback equipment can be used to monitor bodily responses, including the electromyograph (EMG), cardiac monitors, and so forth. Use of olfactory input can enhance a feeding sequence and is used in conjunction with various other treatment techniques designed to normalize the oral musculature discussed later in this chapter.

Gustatory Input

GENERAL INFORMATION. Gustatory input is frequently used as a part of the prefeeding sequence. The taste buds of the mouth are the primary receptors for gustatory sensation (Guyton, 1977; Coppe, 1978). The taste buds are located on the tongue, palate, oropharynx, mucosa of the lips and cheeks, and the floor of the mouth (Coppe, 1978; Geldard, 1972). A substance must be water-soluble to be an effective stimulus. Humans are capable of perceiving many different tastes, but these tastes are thought to be combinations of the four primary tastes: sour, sweet, bitter, salt (Tamar, 1972; Guyton, 1977; Cagan, 1978). "Umami" has been described as a fifth primary taste by the Japanese; the word means "delicious taste" (Cagan, 1978). There is much controversy as to the exact number of basic categories of taste.

Table 3–7 shows the areas of greatest acuity for each basic taste category.

It is known that the whole tongue surface is sensitive to all categories of taste but that the thresholds for specific substances are lower in the areas attributed to perception of that category. Humans are much more sensitive to bitter substances than to any others, perhaps as a result of

TABLE 3–7 TASTE CATEGORY SENSITIVITIES*

Basic Category of Taste	Location of Greatest Acuity
Sweet	Anterior dorsal tongue
Bitter	Posterior tongue margin and tongue tip
Salt	Anterior tongue margin
Sour	Lateral tongue edges

*Adapted from Cagan (1978).

survival mechanisms (Cagan, 1978, Guyton, 1977).

Several factors affect the sense of taste. Decreased sense of smell seems to affect taste, as anyone who has a cold can testify. Decreased sense of taste (and smell) can result from certain diseases, such as Sjögren's syndrome (Cagan, 1978). Taste preferences can change during certain conditions, such as the reported increase in preference for salt during hypertension (Schechter et al., 1974). Heavy smokers demonstrate a decrease in taste sensitivity as they age (Kaplan et al, 1965). Also, an altered ability to perceive sweetness may result from wearing dentures (Giddon et al, 1954). This may be due to the fact that the dentures block part of the palate.

STIMULATION PROCEDURES. Three implements are used to apply the gustatory input to the tongue, depending on the patient's ability to swallow. For patients who cannot as yet swallow, a dental tweezer (Fig. 3–25) is used to deposit minute amounts of the substance onto the tongue. For patients whose swallowing is intact, a cotton swab or a plastic eyedropper is used for application.

A small amount of the flavoring is placed in a medicine cup to avoid contamination of the larger bottle. The therapist dips the applicator into the cup and then deposits the substance in the appropriate area of the mouth. It is reintroduced at least one time. Before introduction of a second primary taste stimulus, a rinse with sterile water is utilized. If the patient is exposed to one taste stimulus for a prolonged, continuous period, a water rinse can assume a taste in and of itself (Bartoshuk, 1974).

Humans demonstrate a natural preference for sweet flavors at birth (Desor et al, 1973). When using *sweet stimuli*, high concentrations are required to reach a threshold response (in the range of 10^{-2}M or more) (Pfaffmann, 1959). Saccharin is used as the sweet stimulus by this author for two primary reasons: (1) It can evoke a sweet sensation at a very low level of concentration (sucrose-threshold concentration range 5 to 16 mM, saccharin-threshold concentration range 0.02 to 0.04 mM), and (2) some patients who require gustatory input may have a metabolic problem and cannot tolerate introduction of sucrose (sugar).

In patients with hypertension, salt substitute is used for the *salt stimulus*. The threshold range for sodium chloride is 1 to 80 mM (Pfaffmann, 1959). The therapist is advised to consult with a pharmacist or use a chemistry book in order to create a liquid with effective concentration levels.

Sour taste is stimulated by use of dilute acetic acid (vinegar). Threshold concentration range is 0.1 to 5.8 mM. *Bitter taste* is stimulated by quinine sulfate (threshold concentration range 0.0004 to 0.011 mM) or caffeine (threshold concentration range 0.3 to 1 mM (Pfaffmann, 1959). Bitter stimuli are presented last because they seem to trigger aversive reactions.

Much work needs to be done in the area of gustatory stimulation. One might question if the order of presentation is critical (i.e., sweet before bitter) or if the tempera-

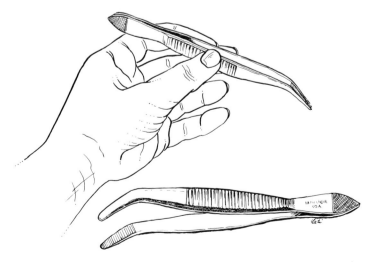

Figure 3–25.

ture of the substance might affect the perception. Some research has been done on measuring the taste responses to substances of different temperatures. In humans, the maximal sensitivity was to substances between 22° to 32° C with variation depending on stimuli tested (McBurney et al, 1973).

Temperature Input

GENERAL INFORMATION. Guyton (1977) has described three different nerve fibers possibly stimulated by temperature: cold-sensitive fiber; warm-sensitive fiber; and (3) pain-sensitive fiber. Extremes in temperature may affect the pain fibers. It is difficult to distinguish very hot from very cold. Sinclair (1967) provides the following temperature ranges* (adapted from Von Frey, 1904):

−10° to +10° = pain
+15° = burning cold
+16° to +30° = cool
+31° to +45° = warm (with tepid temperature in the lower end of this range)
+50° and higher = burning hot

Certain basic facts must be considered when using thermal stimulation. The critical difference between the thermal stimulus and the temperature of the body part on which it is to be used determines the degree of stimulation. If a patient has a skin temperature in the cool range (+16° to +30°), ice may not produce the desired facilitory result. Allowing the patient's skin to warm to the +31° to +45° range may enhance the effect of the ice. Individual variation is also important; women have a lower threshold for temperature changes than do men (Sinclair, 1967). Sinclair (1967) also reports that when large areas are stimulated, adaptation of thermal input is slow and incomplete. Guyton (1977) relates that summation of thermal signals occurs when large areas of the body are stimulated. The number of temperature endings in any small area of body surface is few; therefore, one may have difficulty judging gradations of temperature following stimulation of small areas. The hand, for example, adapts to all temperatures between +17° and +40° (Sin-

clair, 1967). If the hand is maintained at +18°, then +19° will seem warm in comparison. Patients respond faster to cold stimuli than to warm (Sinclair, 1967). Finally, warming and cooling the skin may affect adaptation of a pressure stimulus (Sinclair, 1967) and affect the action potential. Temperature is a protopathic modality that travels via the spinothalamic-spinoreticular system (see Chapter 1). Axons and collaterals from this system impinge upon the reticular formation.

INHIBITORY THERMAL INPUT. Neutral warmth is an inhibitory technique in which the +35° to +37° range of temperature is utilized. The patient may be wrapped in a thin thermal blanket in order to retain body heat. Adding additional heat is avoided. The total body or an individual part may be wrapped. Futuro-Thermolastic material* can be used to fashion mittens for spastic, fisted hands. Patients wearing such garments frequently demonstrate decreased hypertonicity following application of the garment. An alternative method of neutral warmth is to place the patient in tepid water or to have him take a tepid shower. The length of the time neutral warmth should be applied varies from patient to patient and depends on whether the whole body or just an individual limb is being stimulated. Total body wrapping takes about 15 to 20 minutes, whereas a 3-minute tepid shower has been effective. Neutral warmth can be initiated before the patient is brought to the therapy department, but care must be taken not to overstimulate the patient during transport. Skin receptors, especially pressure and vibration, have their lowest threshold in the +36° to +38° range (Geldard, 1972). Vibration might, therefore, have maximum effectivenss following neutral warmth.

Ice has been reported to be useful for inhibition of hypertonicity (Knott and Voss, 1968). Shaved ice on towels is applied to body parts, or patients are placed in ice baths for brief periods of time. There are certain critical rules to which one must adhere when using ice for inhibition: (1) The patient must be moved in meaningful patterns immediately following applica-

---

*Temperatures are in degrees C.

*Available from Jung Products, Inc., Cincinnati, OH 45227.)

tion of ice and closely monitored to prevent return of hypertonicity with pain (rebound). (2) The patient must be receptive to the use of ice. If the patient is fearful, inhibition may be blocked by increase of sympathetic tone. The reader is referred to the works of Knott and Voss (1968) for detailed explanation of use of ice for inhibition.

FACILITORY THERMAL INPUT. Ice is used in the multi-sensory treatment system as part of the feeding treatment sequence. The patient is either given an unsweetened ice Popsicle or one flavored with vanilla or banana extract. Small ice Popsicles are made by filling medium-sized plastic test tubes or similar containers with liquid and freezing them. The ice Popsicle is placed on the tongue with pressure. Maintained pressure applied by placing the fingers over the lips is used to encourage sucking (see the feeding section of this chapter). The most temperature-sensitive intraoral structures are the tongue tip and the hard palate; however, the highest thermal sensitivity in humans is in the perioral region and face (Darian-Smith, 1973). This region is more sensitive to temperature than any other body surface area. Because of this sensitivity, ice should be used around and in the mouth with extreme care. It could cause an aversive opening response at the lips. Ice should not be used on midline trunk areas or on the face above the mouth.

Ice can also be utilized with pressure for a few seconds to specific dermatomal areas in order to facilitate individual muscles. Abrupt temperature changes strongly stimulate thermoreceptors at initial contact. If the ice is maintained, adaptation will ensue (Guyton, 1977).

Thermal input probably chemically stimulates the temperature endings in the dermatomal area. Messages are then transmitted via the spinothalamic-spinoreticular system to the thalamus and then to the somatic sensory area I, and to the reticular formation (Guyton, 1977) (see Chapter 1).

As discussed previously, a therapist with very cold hands can unwittingly stimulate a patient. One whose hands are constantly cold can learn to warm them using biofeedback training (see Chapter 6).

Proprioceptive Input. The multisensory theory of neurorehabilitation considers stretch, traction, tapping, vibration, resistance, joint compression, stretch pressure, and stereognosis training to be important aspects of therapy. Much of proprioception travels in the dorsal columns and is considered an epicritic modality (see Chapter 1).

STRETCH AND TRACTION. Utilization of *stretch* is based on the two-neuron chain of muscle stretch reflex presented in Chapter 1. The purpose of using stretch as a modality is to modify the excitability of alpha (α) motor neurons, which in turn affect the stretched muscle (Harris, 1978). When a muscle is stretched, the muscle's sensory receptors (in the muscle spindles), send excitatory afferent messages to alpha motor neurons that innervate the stretched muscle, while inhibitory messages are sent to the alpha motor neurons of the antagonist (Harris, 1978). This is the principle of reciprocal innervation developed by Sherrington.

As mentioned previously in this chapter, the rate of stimulation determines the effect. In the case of stretch, the faster the stretch is applied, the more facilitory it will be (Harris, 1978). In the multi-sensory theory of neurorehabilitation, quick stretch is applied to extensor musculature after some tone has been facilitated via vestibular stimulation or to elongated muscles if modalities from earlier developing systems are not totally effective in increasing the muscle's tone to the appropriate level. The stretch stimulus may be applied diagonally to the joint over which the muscle is running. This diagonal application is based on the principle noted by Knott and Voss (1968) that diagonal stimulation is the most effective method to maximally stimulate elongated muscles.

The whole area of slow stretch, passive stretch, and maintained stretch is one of confusion and controversy in the therapeutic community. Harris (1978) describes a process of slowly stretching a muscle and maintaining the stretch over a prolonged period, thus causing adaptation of excitatory responses and producing an inhibitory response. Crutchfield and Barnes (1973) describe passive and maintained stretch as facility to II endings of the muscle spindle and subsequently facilitory to flexors (even if extensors are being stretched).

The following example is included to illustrate the use and sequence of quick stretch as a modality in the multisensory approach. A typical treatment order for a patient with a left cerebrovascular accident (right hemiplegia) includes normalization of touch responses, light moving touch to facial midline and T10 dermatome to facilate the phasic flexor response followed by rolling, olfactory and gustatory stimuli for the feeding sequence if appropriate, vestibular input in the semi-inverted position (patient leaning over in his chair). Once some extensor tone develops, a variety of proprioceptive techniques can be employed to enhance the response, including quick stretch, traction, resistance, vibration, tapping, and joint compression.

When quick stretch is applied, care must be taken to hold the patient's extremity properly to avoid inserting pressure into muscle groups one is trying to inhibit. For example, in quick stretch of the forearm extensors, the forearm should be held by the sides (bony prominences), while the dorsum of the hand is diagonally pushed down quickly into flexion; thus the extensors are facilitated (Fig. 3–26).

Quick stretch may also be used to facilitate flexor responses. Selective application of quick stretch to flexor muscles is recommended because many CNS-damaged patients demonstrate flexion contractions. If a patient already has hyper-responsiveness of flexors, internal rotators, adductors and pronators, the author recommends stimulating the antagonists of these muscles to reciprocally inhibit the hypertonicity in the flexors and avoiding stretch to the flexor group.

Passive range of motion exercises are avoided in the multisensory approach. Since passive stretch can fire II endings in the muscle spindle, thereby facilitating flexion, a more dynamic approach is used, including normalization of touch, facilitation of phasic flexor pattern, vestibular input to excite extensors, tapping, vibration, quick stretch, resistance, and joint compression all applied in function patterns. Even if passive range of motion is done very slowly, causing adaptation of excitatory responses and yielding inhibitory responses (Harris, 1978), this process does little to build up functional movement patterns.

Traction produces a separation of joint surfaces, thus facilitating joint receptors. Knott and Voss (1968) report that traction used in treatment seems to promote movement, whereas use of joint compression (approximation) facilitates joint stability. In keeping with use of natural stimuli, traction is used to simulate pulling movement.

RESISTANCE.   Resistance is a technique

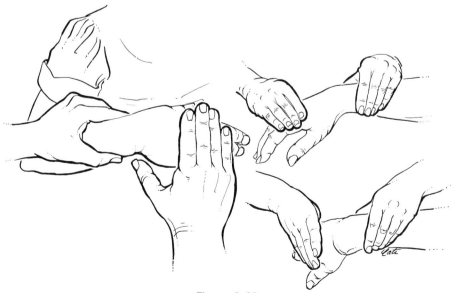

Figure 3–26.

frequently used following quick stretch to maximize the response. It must be applied correctly to avoid muscular fatigue. It requires maximum effort from the patient if strengthening is to occur (Hellenbrandt, 1951; Knuttgen, 1976). Determining the appropriate amount of resistance to apply during the therapeutic sequence is a skill that requires much practice and guidance from the experienced therapist.

In the area of resistance, the multisensory approach uses the proprioceptive neuromuscular facilitation (PNF) frame of reference developed by Knott and Voss (1968). Resistance is applied to isotonically contracting muscles that causes the patient to exert maximum effort while his body part is moved through a functional pattern. If skill and endurance are to develop, repetition of the resistance activity is a necessity (Knuttgen, 1976; Knott and Voss, 1968). Resistance should not be applied to uncoordinated movement patterns because it can reinforce the purposeless movement.

VIBRATION. Vibration, another modality that travels in the dorsal columns, is an effective way of artificially stimulating muscles. According to Sinclair (1967), vibration sense is actually derived from touch and can under certain circumstances suppress other sensations. Bishop (1974, 1975) has written an excellent series of articles on vibration in which the neurophysiology and therapeutic application of this modality are reviewed.

Amplitude and *frequency* are terms used in measuring vibration. Frequency refers to the cycles per second measured in hertz (Hz), while amplitude describes the amount of displacement or maximum deviation from zero measured in micrometers (μm). Figure 3–27 illustrates these two concepts. The *tonic vibratory response* (TVR), another term frequently used when discussing vibration, refers to the reflex effects resulting from high frequency vibration (100 to 300 Hz) of a muscle or tendon. This stimulates the Ia endings of the muscle spindle, producing a contraction. The Ia endings have been measured to discharge at the same rate as the frequency of vibration applied (Bishop, 1974). Pacinian corpuscles, a type of encapsulated nerve ending, have been described as receptors responsive to vibration (Sinclair, 1967). They send vibratory impulses to higher centers for development of conscious perception of vibration. Pacinian corpuscle stimulation does not produce a TVR; only stimulation of the muscular receptors can do so (McCloskey, 1978; Bishop, 1974).

Vibration of sufficient frequency to evoke a TVR in the muscle stimulated will also produce, via reciprocal inhibition, a depression in the motor neuronal activity of the antagonist (Goodwin et al, 1972; Bishop, 1974; Dimitrijevic, 1977). Therefore, by vibrating the antagonist of a spastic muscle, hypertonicity can temporarily be reduced in that spastic muscle.

Vibration, unlike brushing, has a short latency period and lasts only as long as it is applied (McCloskey, 1978; Bishop, 1974). It is subsequently enhanced when used in combination with other modalities, for instance vibration of a muscle when the patient is positioned in a reflex-inhibiting position (Hagbarth and Eklund, 1969), or vibration of a muscle followed by a resistance pattern.

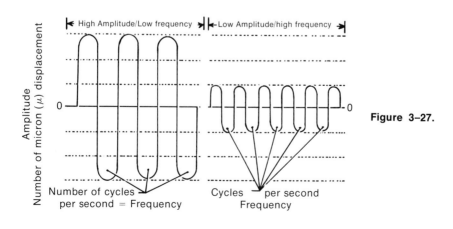

Figure 3–27.

It has been established that under certain circumstances, vibration of muscles and tendons can produce kinesthetic illusions (McCloskey, 1978; McCloskey, 1973; Goodwin, 1972). When using lower frequency, high amplitude vibration, patients report increased illusion of movement even though movement is not actually evoked (McCloskey, 1973). Movement illusions are more likely to occur when vibration is applied to a noncontracting muscle (McCloskey, 1973).

When utilizing vibration for facilitation purposes, the frequency should be between 100 and 200 Hz. There is a danger of vibration impulses spreading to adjoining muscles as the frequency increases. Effective amplitude is in the range of 150 μm. The vibrator is applied parallel to the extrafusal fibers or over tendons (in series with tendon force) (Bishop, 1974; Hagbarth and Eklund, 1969). Vibration can be applied to a contracting agonist to assist the contraction (McCloskey, 1978), to a flaccid muscle to decrease the threshold for excitation (Bishop, 1974, 1975), to the antagonist of a spastic muscle to reduce the hypertonicity in that muscle (Bishop, 1975), or to synergistic muscles by simultaneous application to enhance the synergy pattern (Bishop, 1975). Burke (1976) reports that vibration of a noncontracting muscle applied with passive movement maximizes the responsiveness. Vibration can be applied lightly or with pressure. It appears to this author that lightly applied vibration has a longer effect. More research is needed in this area.

Many factors can modify the patient's response to vibration. The TVR will be depressed in patients receiving barbiturates or other depressive drugs (DeGail et al, 1966). The initial length of the muscle can affect the TVR; as the initial length increases, the TVR increases. The patient's position may influence TVRs due to the interaction of the tonic neck and righting responses. In prone, flexor TVRs are increased, whereas in supine, extensor TVRs are enhanced (Bishop, 1974, 1975).

Some therapists use low-frequency vibration to normalize sensitivity of skin. The battery-operated vibrators that cycle between 60 and 90 Hz are most commonly used for this purpose. This author prefers maintained touch for skin normalization;

however, controlled studies are needed in this area.

Medaer and Kovacs (1978) report success in use of vibration for bladder emptying in patients having multiple sclerosis. They vibrated the area between the pubis and the umbilicus using 110 Hz frequency and 200 to 300 μm amplitude. Subjects in the study had decreased urinary frequency and residual urine. Some patients suffered from secondary diarrhea. Medaer and Kovacs attempted to vibrate patients with cord injury (paraplegics) using the same technique for bladder release without success.

There are many precautions that must be followed when using vibration as a therapeutic modality. The vibrator itself should not transfer impulses to the therapist's hands, as this can have an aversive effect (Sinclair, 1967). Since the vibrator generates heat, it should not be applied to any skin area for longer than 1 or 2 minutes (Bishop, 1975). Also, one should avoid startling the patient when turning on the vibrator. Vibration of the muscles of a patient having cerebellar disease can produce athetoid-like movements (Bishop, 1975). For obvious reasons, an electric vibrator should not be applied to a patient who is submerged in water. Vibration of facial skin is not recommended because of the risk of skin damage. Finally, a thorough knowledge of vibratory neurophysiological rationale, techniques, and precautions is a prerequisite before any therapist applies this modality to a patient. Bishop (1974, 1975) has her students experiment on themselves as part of the learning experience.

PRESSURE, TAPPING, STRETCH PRESSURES. Brief intermittent pressure into the belly of a muscle and tapping a muscle are both facilitory to the muscle (Hagbarth, 1952). These techniques are frequently used during active range of motion exercises. Since pressures to the belly of a muscle can facilitate the muscle, the therapist is reminded to handle the patient carefully to avoid inadvertently applying pressure into muscles that are to be inhibited. Knott and Voss (1968) use pressures or manual contacts as a facilitating mechanism as well as for sensory cues to assist a patient's anticipation of a movement pattern.

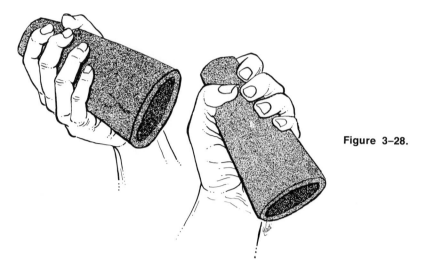

Figure 3–28.

Pressure at the point of insertion of a muscle appears to inhibit the muscle (Farber, 1974). Dayhoff (1975) investigated the use of hard cones placed in the hands of a limited sample of patients having severe flexion deformities secondary to CVA. The hard cones place pressure into the flexor insertions as well as supply a maintained pressure to the flexor surface (Fig. 3–28). Maintained pressure has been discussed previously in this chapter and is helpful in normalizing hypersensitive skin areas. Patients in Dayhoff's study demonstrated an increase in passive range of motion of extensors. Soft objects placed in the hands of brain-damaged patients seem to increase flexor tone, perhaps as a result of the primitive grasp response. Carefully controlled studies need to be conducted in this area.

The modality of *stretch pressure* combines use of pressure into a muscle belly with a stretching motion. Stretch pressure provides a mechanical deformation of the skin, causing tension within the cutaneous tissue and elongation of underlying muscle fibers and spindles that results in facilitation of the muscle (Geldard, 1972). The therapist's thumb and fingers are placed in a pad-to-pad position over the muscle belly, inserting pressure (Fig. 3–29). The therapist then stretches his or her fingers out over the muscle belly in the direction of the muscle fibers. Stretch pressures are used in active range of motion exercises, in the feeding sequence, and to stimulate any specific muscle after earlier-developing sensory stimuli have produced adaptive responses.

JOINT COMPRESSION. Rood (1978) and Knott and Voss (1968) use joint compression (or joint approximation) as part of their treatment approaches. The multisensory theory utilizes this modality as described by Rood (1978). Currently, an understanding of the function of joint receptors is, at best, incomplete. It is often difficult to analyze the joint and muscular components of a given nerve (McCloskey, 1978).

Several early studies have presented interesting findings. Boyd and Roberts (1953) describe joint receptors as responding to joint movement or local pressure applied to the joint capsule. Messages regarding joint position may also be transmitted by joint receptors with some angles being more excitatory, according to Andrew and Dodt (1953). Skoglund (1956) and Andrew (1954) report that some joint

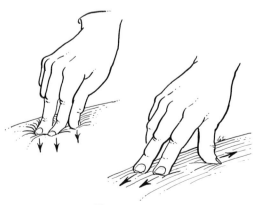

Figure 3–29.

receptors respond to tension applied to the ligament and may contribute to perception of joint position. Dee (1969) reports that increased pressure of the head of the femur in the acetabulum produces inhibitory reflex effects on hip joint musculature that last as long as the force is applied. There is a rebound facilitation in the muscles previously inhibited that lasts for a few seconds following removal of the force. Dee feels that Golgi tendon organs (GTOs) are stimulated during this action, which produces the reflex responses helpful in the prevention of dislocation and in load shift. Goldsheider, as described by McCloskey (1978), has reported that proximal joints have lower detection thresholds than distal joints.

The therapeutic use of joint compression involves two different methods of application. *Joint compression of body weight or less* by empirical measurements inhibits hypertonic muscles around a joint, thus temporarily assisting the balance of muscle tone at the joint. A compression force is applied to a joint with the force equal to or less than the weight of the body or body part over the joint. It is applied through the bone's longitudinal axis (Ayres, 1974). In the case of a patient with a "frozen shoulder" secondary to muscle tone imbalance, once thorough assessment is completed, the therapist might stabilize the patient's scapula while pushing the humerus up into the glenohumeral socket. Once the head of the humerus is compressed in the socket, the humerus can be moved in circles, thus increasing the range of motion (Fig. 3–30). Another instance of joint compression of body weight or less possibly proving helpful is its application at the wrist joint of a patient who has hypertonic flexors. The therapist places compression into the heel of the patient's hand while aligning the joint into a neutral position. Once again, it is essential to hold the patient's forearm by the bony prominences to avoid placing pressure into the flexors (Fig. 3–31). The joint compression will not be long-acting and needs to be reinforced by functional activity, promoting balance of tone around the joint. An example of such an activity is having a patient hit a 6- to 8-inch ball that has been pitched to him. The patient should use the heel of his hand to hit the ball. This

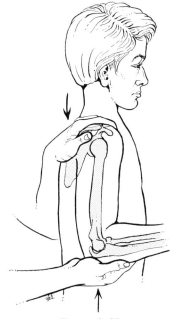

Figure 3–30.

promotes a repetition of the activity, which leads to the automatic performance of the act. The reader is reminded that the flexor pattern and inverted sequence are attempted before joint compression is, in order to produce a lasting balance of tone at the wrist.

Joint compression of more than body weight is the second method of therapeutic application. The force applied is more than the weight of the body or body part compressing a joint. A joint is compressed through the longitudinal axis of the bone as if it were supporting the body weight, and then an additional force is added. This

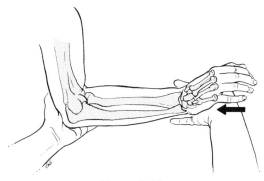

Figure 3–31.

technique has been empirically noted to facilitate a co-contraction at the joint being approximated (Farber, 1974). Two examples in the normal population are African women who carry objects on their heads and fashion models who improve their posture by walking with books on their heads. EMG studies are needed in this area to test whether more than body weight joint compression is actually producing the desired co-contraction. From the author's clinical experience, this modality appears to improve proximal stability when used at the shoulders, hips, and neck, especially when combined with other facilitory techniques and purposeful activity.

Some examples of how joint compression of more than body weight is used in the multisensory approach are given in the following discussion.

Head and Neck Pattern. A patient may be positioned in the sitting, or kneel-standing position or standing with his head in midline (Fig. 3–32). A compres-

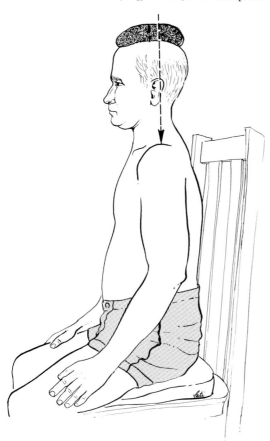

Figure 3–32.

sion force is applied to the rostral head surface either manually or by addition of a weighted object such as a sand bag. The head alignment must be maintained during this procedure. Following removal of the weight, a functional activity is utilized requiring the patient to maintain co-contraction of neck musculature. Joint compression can also be applied to the rostral surface of the head while the patient is in the inverted position. The force is applied for short intervals and then removed. It may be reapplied as needed.

Shoulder Patterns. Three examples of joint compression of more than body weight applied to the shoulder joints include prone-on-elbows position, all fours position, and sitting posture. The patient is placed in prone-on-elbows position on a mat with neck musculature co-contracting and arms maintained in approximately 90-degree elbow flexion. The elbows should be lined up under the shoulders or placed slightly laterally if the patient requires a wider base of support for improved head balance (Fig. 3–33). The therapist then manually applies a compression force to the shoulders. The force should be applied for about 10 to 15 seconds initially and then removed. Compression time varies with the patient's ability to co-contract. The objective of the compression is to facilitate a co-contraction and not to fatigue the patient's muscles. One must remember that when using joint compression at the shoulders, the force should equal the weight of the trunk over the arm(s) plus an additional weight graded to the patient's ability. Once some proximal stability occurs, it should be immediately reinforced in a functional activity such as playing in the prone-on-elbows position or belly crawling.

All Fours Pattern. As the patient prepares to assume the all fours position after mastering the prone-on-elbows and belly crawling patterns, joint compression of more than body weight can be employed to facilitate development of necessary proximal stability. The patient is placed on all fours with the neck musculature in a co-contraction pattern described previously. The therapist then manually applies the compression at the shoulders (and the hips) (Fig. 3–34). If the patient is not quite ready to maintain the all fours pattern, he

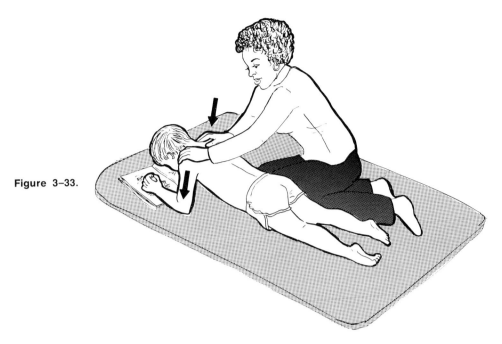

Figure 3–33.

can be positioned over a bolster to assist in supporting the weight of the trunk.

Joint compression can also be applied to the shoulders while the patient is *sitting*. The therapist positions the patient in a chair, on a mat, or on a bolster and then applies a downward force to the shoulders (Fig. 3–35). Dynamic chest straps made from dental dam can also be used for the same purpose (see Chapter 7, Fig. 7–29).

Hip joint compression of more than body weight may be applied in the all fours, kneel-standing, or standing postures. Compression in all fours has already been discussed. Joint compression in kneel-standing and in standing patterns is applied in the identical manner. The patient kneels or stands with the therapist positioned behind him if the patient is to move forward. The therapist places his or

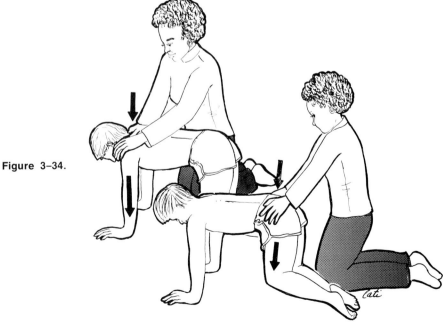

Figure 3–34.

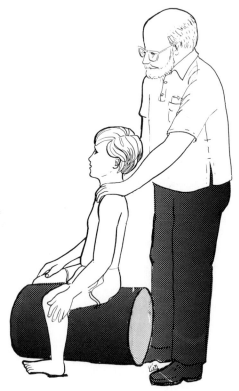

Figure 3–35.

her hands on the patient's hips. Compression is applied to the hip of the weight-bearing leg during the walking or knee-walking sequence (Fig. 3–36). The compression is removed as the patient prepares to use that leg for the swing-through pattern.

TACTILE DISCRIMINATION. *Stereognosis* is the ability to analyze tactile and kinesthetic data for the identification of an object. Locating and recognizing coins in one's pocket is an example of how stereognosis is used on a daily basis. Active manual manipulation of an object in order to obtain sensory information for object identification is also referred to as *haptic sensation* (Cashdan, 1968).

Stereognostic ability varies with the developmental age. Tyler (1972) and Jessen and Kaess (1973) report that there is a significant increase in ability to identify (through haptic sensation) objects correctly as the subject increases in age. Subjects under 2 years of age cannot be reliably tested for stereognosis (Tyler, 1972). Younger children (3 years) explore haptically before using vision for discrimina-

tion. As the child ages, visual exploration begins to dominate (6 to 7 years) and in the adult, visual discrimination is superior to haptic discrimination (Cashdan, 1968).

Roland and Larsen (1976) have localized lesions causing stereognosis dysfunction of the hand, mouth, and foot. Damage to the postcentral gyrus of the parietal lobe in the cortical region of the hand, mouth, and foot will result in *astereognosis* (absence of stereognosis) to the contralateral body side. Astereognosis commonly occurs in cerebral palsy and in cerebrovascular accident. Wilson and Wilson (1967) found no significant differences in stereognostic perception between spastic and athetoid subject groups.

Movement of the object on the contact surface will facilitate stereognostic perception, but active movement alone is insufficient to produce stereognosis in the absence of touch. Using two hands to identify an object and moving an object in the hand(s) of a patient who has a decrease of voluntary motion will also facilitate identification (Wolinski and Ayre, 1967).

Piaget and Inhelder (1956) describe image formation resulting from experience with an object in one modality (one-sensory system) followed by modification or correction of the image after exposure to other modalities (sensory systems). Gibson (1969) believes that during active exploration, the distinctive features of an object must be isolated by each sense modality independently. Cross-modal matching can only be successful after each sensory modality perceives the same distinctive features. There is good reason to believe that this progresses as association cortex matures.

Patients frequently lose both epicritic and protopathic sensation following a cerebrovascular accident; however, protopathic sensation often returns even though it may become hypersensitive (Sinclair, 1967). Epicritic sensation has a poorer prognosis for functional return. Several studies attempting to re-train patients in stereognostic perception have been conducted and researchers have reported improvement in patient function (Vinograd et al, 1962; Van Buskirk and Webster, 1955; Forster and Shields, 1959). The author's stereognostic treatment approach, explained in the following paragraphs, has

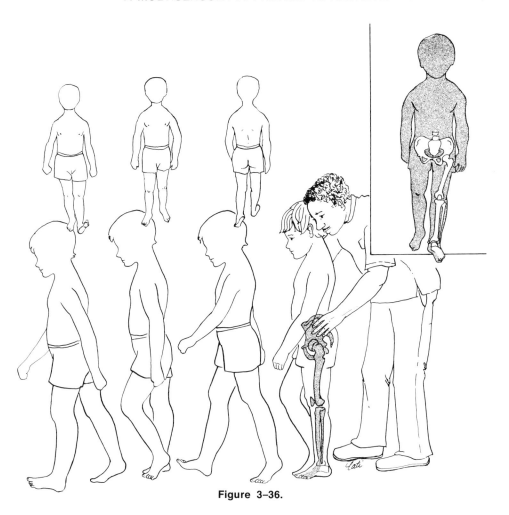

Figure 3–36.

been synthesized from these studies and from the survey of related literature presented in this section.

Stereognostic Therapeutic Approach. As it is with every treatment technique, a thorough baseline assessment is essential. Visual presentation of test objects is the first step of assessment to ensure that the patient is familiar with and can identify the object. If the patient is nonverbal, the therapist must determine if the patient can identify the object by yes and no questions.

During the *assessment*, common household objects including a key, dime, quarter, comb, rubber ball, small wooden cube, closed safety pin, tooth brush, pencil, and cotton ball are placed in the patient's more affected hand with the patient's vision occluded. If the patient cannot manipulate the item, the therapist does this for him.

The patient either verbally identifies the object or points to the correct object among a second set of identical objects. The other hand is also tested, with the therapist being sure to change the presentation order. Finally, the patient is asked to manipulate the object with both hands with vision occluded.

The *treatment* sequence for adults and children 2 to 3 years of age varies slightly. For adults and children over 3, the following order is used:

1. The patient visually examines an object that is rotated in all planes by the therapist.
2. The patient then handles the object with his less affected extremity while observing his hand.
3. The patient subsequently manipulates the object with both hands while observing his hands.

4. The object is then placed in the patient's more affected hand for manipulation with visual discrimination. The reader is reminded that other therapeutic techniques have been used initially to open the hand and normalize movement patterns before stereognostic perception is attempted. For steps 2, 3, and 4, a box lined with mirrors can be used. The patient manipulates the object in the mirror-lined box in order to increase the visual input (Vinograd, 1962; Forster and Shields, 1959).

5. Steps 2, 3, and 4 are then repeated without visual assistance.

6. Once the patient consistently identifies several objects, two objects can be placed in a can of sand or uncooked split peas or rice. The patient is then instructed to reach into the can and locate one specific object. If the additional sensory input of sand, rice, or split peas blocks object identification because of overstimulation, the objects can be placed in an empty bag. The patient is then asked to remove one specific object.

7. The patient is retested frequently for evaluation of program successfulness. If all objects are correctly identified, new objects can be added.

For children 2 to 3 years of age, step 1 of the previous sequence is done after steps 2, 3, and 4. The therapist is reminded to use objects familiar to children of this age group.

Auditory Input. The auditory system continues developing for two years postnatally, at which time the auditory cortex demonstrates many features of adult cortex (Baru and Karaseva, 1972). As such, it is one of the last sensory systems to develop and is therefore emphasized later in the treatment sequence.

As with any sensory system, continual stimulation of the auditory system can produce adaptation. Nordmark (1970) and Butler (1973) report that an even, constant auditory pulse train (serial pips of sound) will produce a cumulative inhibition of auditory responsiveness. Random pulse patterns can overcome the inhibition. In the auditory system, repetition of the stimulus does not result in complete disappearance of the sensation. Instead, a reduction in sensitivity will occur with a resultant increase in threshold. Three minutes of continuing auditory input produces neural adaptation (Elliot and Fraser, 1970). One to two minutes is required as a recovery period.

The ear may be permanently damaged by exposure to loud noises. Those subjected to constant loud noises may demonstrate audiological fatigue and gradual permanent hearing loss. Fatigue will more frequently occur at higher frequencies (4,000 to 6,000 Hz) (Elliot and Fraser, 1970).

INHIBITORY AUDITORY INPUT. Even, continuous auditory input (based on adaptation) is used as a method of calming patients in need of inhibition. The therapist should speak in a level, rhythmical monotone when communicating with the patient. Care must be taken to control other environmental stimulation during this process. Music with a repetitive rhythm may also provide some inhibition. Since many collateral fibers pass into the reticular formation from the auditory tracts and nuclei (Guyton, 1977), one might speculate that inhibitory auditory input affects other CNS thresholds. Constant monitoring of body processes, including muscle tone, attention span, and sensory responsiveness, is recommended. The length of time required to produce an inhibitory effect varies from patient to patient but seems to range between 3 and 8 minutes.

FACILITORY AUDITORY INPUT. A variety of facilitory auditory inputs are used in the multisensory approach, including random, rhythmical speech or music, auditory discrimination exercises, and cross-modal auditory, visual, tactile stimulus presentation. A critical change in stimulus application produces facilitory effects. If the therapist suddenly changes the *pitch* (the level in the musical scale), the *timbre* (harmonies), or the *loudness* of the sound (intensity measured in bels or decibels) (Gardner, 1975), a facilitory effect may be produced. The therapist should avoid startling the patient if possible.

Use of various sounds for discrimination help refine auditory adaptive responses. This aspect of treatment is frequently conducted or planned by an audiologist or speech pathologist. The patient is exposed to a variety of sounds. Initially an ability to match sounds is the objective, with treatment progressing to discrimination and identification of sound. For example, two identical sets of small cans are prepared by filling them with substances likely to produce distinctive sounds (gravel, split peas, coins, wood chips, rice). The patient is asked to match the sounds. Later in the treatment program, the patient is exposed to common sounds and asked to either name them or point to pictures representing those sounds. Objects that make noise when handled may also be used for tactile and auditory cross-modal learning.

It has been stressed that auditory input is not a major component of early treatment; however, it is critical that parents, family members, and health personnel talk to the patient outside of treatment sessions. With the hard of hearing, sound should not be indiscriminately increased in order to stimulate the patient — as exposure to loud noise can further damage hearing. Consultation with an audiologist is considered essential in order to determine effective stimulus levels.

Visual Input

VISUAL DEVELOPMENT. The eye is considered the most complex and developed sense organ (Geldard, 1972). Continual refinement of the visual system persists throughout the first 6 years of life (see Table 3–1). Bronson (1974) reports that 2-month-old infants use primarily peripheral instead of focal or central vision. By 3 months of age, infants are able to discriminate sad, happy, and surprised facial expressions (Young-Brown et al, 1977). This early discrimination may begin to shape social learning. Infants demonstrate interest in human faces even from birth, according to Goren, Sarty, and Wu (1975). Visual discrimination is measured by increases in the time spent looking at the novel stimulus.

Movement of the eyes is a critical aspect of visual development. Eye movements may serve to reduce distortion (Zinchenko and Vergiles, 1972; Zusne, 1970) and to integrate elementary perceptual components into more complex forms (Hebb, 1937, 1949, 1959). Early development of the vestibular system with its input to cranial nerves III, IV, and VI facilitates subcortical adjustments of eye movement

while cortical pathways, directed through synapses in the superior colliculus, direct voluntary eye movements (see Chapter 1). If vestibular dysfunction exists, inadequate stimulation of eye musculature may result in insufficient ocular motility.

While visual stimulation is not emphasized early in the multisensory approach, visual input is provided outside of initial treatment times to avoid the ill effects of visual deprivation. Zusne (1970) states that structural atrophy will occur in the visual system even after short periods of deprivation. File (1978) studied the effect of visual deprivation on rat exploration, discrimination, and habituation behavior. The findings of this study include an increase in random motor activity of experimental rats with a reduction in exploration and orientation compared to controls.

ADEQUATE STIMULI. Light is an adequate stimulus for vision. Geldard (1972) describes two light sources, incandescent bodies (hot sources) and luminescent bodies (cold sources). The visible spectrum of light waves ranges from 400 to 700 nanometers (nm) with a 1/10 second critical duration (Geldard, 1972). Pressure on the eyeballs is another adequate stimulus and produces dense, diffuse, luminous patterns called *phosphenes* (Geldard, 1972). Eyeball pressure is the first type of visual stimulation used during the coma sequence.

VISUAL ADAPTATION. Visual adaptation occurs as a method of bringing the retina into equilibrium with the environment. After prolonged exposure to a visual stimulus the retina becomes progressively less sensitive to it. Geldard (1972) reports that after being in the dark for 30 minutes, the retina becomes sensitive to a stimulus that is 1/100,000 of the intensity originally necessary to stimulate it. One is much more likely to evoke a visual adaptive response from a light stimulus if the patient has been in a darkened room for a time period preceding stimulation. Kitajima (1978) reports that repetitive flashes may fuse and have a cumulative inhibitory effect. Johnson and Brody (1977) suggest that visual habituation may be related to the type of play (play tempo) in a 1-year-old and may differ for boys and girls. Zusne (1970) describes stimulation of other sense modalities as being effective in reducing visual adaptation once it occurs.

CROSS-MODAL STIMULATION. The earliest age at which cross-modal learning occurs between visual and other sense modalities is currently being investigated. Tyrrell (1977) found that first grade children demonstrate transfer of dimensional information between two modalities. Visual-tactile cross-modal learning was present in preschool subjects. Blank and Klig (1970) also studied nursery school aged children and found that intradimensional transfers occur first (for example, keeping the same texture while changing the form). Carr, Bacharach, and Mehner (1977) analyzed the effect of telling 6-year-old subjects what they are about to see in order to determine if the auditory input assists the children in directing their attention. The study suggests that auditory preparation may provide a child with a "set" that is helpful in discrimination of detail.

McGurk, Turnure, and Creighton (1977) describe the sensory systems as functioning independently during the neonatal period. This finding supports the work of Piaget (1952), who believed that coordination between sensory systems does not occur until the second stage of sensorimotor development. We have, therefore, narrowed the age range for cross-modal learning from late infancy to early preschool age in children. One might speculate that the ability to convey information learned in one sensory modality to another modality occurs first in the earlier-developing sensory systems.

VISUAL STIMULATION PROCEDURES. For an *inhibitory visual effect*, a light stimulus is presented in an even, repetitive pattern, for instance, flashing a light at a set intensity and interval. Note: A pattern of 3 per second should be avoided for patients having petit mal seizures, or a seizure may be evoked. Cool colors may also provide some inhibition. The environment designed to calm the patient should *not* be cluttered, messy, or filled with different print patterns. Monochromatic cool color schemes seem to be effective in calming patients.

A variety of *visual stimulatory inputs* are used in the multisensory approach. For comatose patients who have demonstrated some responsiveness to sensory stimuli

from earlier-developing systems, pressure is applied to the eyeballs while the patient's eyes are closed. The therapist gently applies the pressure bilaterally for periods approximately 5 seconds in duration. The interval between application should be at least 20 to 30 seconds and should be irregular. Immediately following pressure stimulation, the therapist should observe for changes in state of consciousness. Use of a flashlight in a darkened room may promote eye tracking. Different objects such as plastic cookie cutters can be taped to the end of the flashlight to prevent visual adaptation. The use of Super–8 movies of family members has been an effective visual stimulus. In children over 6 years of age (developmentally), auditory preparation of visual stimuli is attempted. The patient is then asked to describe verbally the picture stimulus.

The Feeding Sequence

GENERAL INFORMATION. Since feeding is a survival behavior, normalization of feeding activity is critical to satisfactory developmental progression. A neonate uses his mouth for early interaction with the environment. Abnormality in oral function can subsequently interfere with that exploration, thus affecting all aspects of development.

Feeding is a function dominated by the parasympathetic nervous system. Consideration of this fact is vital to the treatment of patients who demonstrate oromotor pathology. If the environment is too stimulatory, a patient may be unable to maintain homeostasis of the ANS. When sympathetic tone dominates, production of adaptive feeding responses is difficult. This observation applies to both normal and abnormal populations. Many individuals eat "on the run" or in a noisy environment. Indigestion frequently results from parasympathetic suppression due to excessive sympathetic stimulation.

NORMAL DEVELOPMENT OF FEEDING BEHAVIOR. The therapist designing oromotor treatment must have a complete understanding of normal oral development and function. It is difficult to describe the precise movements involved in swallowing, sucking, and chewing because there are pattern variations from individual to individual.

Swallowing. Swallowing, which begins at 5 months' gestation, is the first oromotor behavior to occur (Humphrey, 1970). Walker (1978) states that when an individual swallows liquid his tongue proceeds anteriorly, stopping behind the incisors. A groove is then formed in the dorsal tongue surface. This groove is deeper in the posterior region and flattened near the tongue tip. The shape of the groove funnels liquid to the pharyngeal region.

As the liquid flows toward the pharynx, the teeth come together and the buccinators contract, exerting a lateral force (Garliner, 1976). Contraction of the mylohyoids raises the tongue to the palate, causing the tongue to apply pressure by bulging to the side and upward (Walker, 1978; Silverman and Elfant, 1979). Garliner (1976) reports that as the tongue moves up against the hard palate it tips in a 45-degree posterior angle. The posterior section of the tongue fits against the pharyngeal wall. The teeth and orbicularis oris supply a posterior force to prevent liquid leakage and forward tongue motion.

Once the swallowing action is initiated, motion is continuous. The opening in the nasopharynx closes to prevent regurgitation of liquid into the nasal cavity and to contribute to maintenance of oropharyngeal pressure. Elevation of the soft palate results from action of the palatoglossal sphincter.

The liquid or bolus then presses on the epiglottis, forcing it to fold over. Simultaneously, the glottis is shut off by muscular action. The cricopharyngeal sphincter relaxes as the bolus pushes its way past the retroverted epiglottis while moving toward the esophagus. The pharyngeal muscles contract reflexly (Walker, 1978).

The normal person swallows two times per minute when awake and once per minute during sleep (Garliner, 1976). A patient who has difficulty swallowing (dysphagia) and has an orofacial muscular imbalance will frequently drool. The normal infant drools during the first year of life (Knobloch and Pasamanick, 1974).

Sucking. Development of sucking follows swallowing. By 27 to 28 weeks after conception a fetus may suck on a nipple (Rose, 1973; Wolff, 1974), although mature sucking does not occur until 34 to 37 weeks (Bosma, 1974). The pattern of non-nutritive sucking — for instance, pacifier sucking — differs from nutritive sucking. Wolff (1968) characterizes non-nutritive sucking as rapid sucks with short bursts and pauses continuing over a long period. When fluid is introduced through a nipple, the duration of sucking bursts increases but the rate of sucking within a burst decreases to half of the non-nutritive rate (Lipsett, 1976). Burke (1977) suggests that nutritive sucking rate may be slower because the fluid necessitates swallowing, which in turn may play an organizational role in sucking. Another factor that affects the sucking rate is the fluid concentration. As the concentration of sucrose increases, the sucking rate decreases (Crook and Lipsett, 1976), perhaps as a result of the infant savoring the flavor.

Nose breathing is essential to normal nutritive sucking. Orofacial imbalance may contribute to malocclusion; a high arched palate may further complicate the picture by forcing the tongue into an abnormal position (Garliner, 1976) and thereby causing mouth breathing. While normal newborns do maintain lip closure during sucking, the corners of the mouth remain slightly open and the tongue protracts and retracts while attempting to remove liquid from the nipple. This early sucking pattern is also known as *suckling.* As sucking matures, jaw movement is reduced.

Basmajian (1978) states that the orbicularis oris is really two muscles, the orbicularis oris superior and inferior, and not just one sphincter-like muscle. This fact is not widely known among health care workers.

Chewing. The bite reflex, present from birth, normally integrates by 3 to 5 months. Integration of this reflex makes possible the emergence of individual jaw movements necessary for chewing. Failure to integrate the bite reflex results in an involuntary, forceful jaw-clamping movement whenever tongue or tooth surfaces are stimulated. Primitive chewing involves gross jaw movement with tongue elevation. It appears to be a transition from sucking to mature chewing (Knobloch and Pasamanick, 1974).

Mature chewing has several phases, according to Walker (1978), including maximum opening of the jaw, fast closing stroke, power stroke (in which food is sheared and crushed between the teeth), and opening stroke. Frequently food is primarily chewed on one side of the jaw, called the working side; the other jaw side is referred to as the balancing side. The tongue actively participates in the chewing process by pushing the food between the molars while the buccinators act as lateral retainers on the other side of the teeth (Walker, 1978). Hemiplegic patients with oromotor pathology frequently attempt to chew on the paralyzed side, according to Abd-el-Malek (1955), to enable the tonuge to continue pushing food between the molars. This action compels the balancing side to provide the bite force.

OROFACIAL MUSCLE SPINDLES. Some controversy exists in allied health science literature as to the existence of orofacial muscle spindles (Trombly and Scott, 1977, p. 78). Muscles of mastication and facial expression contain muscle spindles supplied with Ia afferent fibers by cells of the mesencephalic nucleus of V (see Chapter 1) (Lund et al, 1979). Muscle spindles are also present in all primate tongues but are morphologically less complex than spindles elsewhere in the body (Bowman, 1971; Fitzgerald and Sachithanandan, 1979). Existence of muscle spindles in orofacial musculature supports the use of stretch pressures as a facilitory modality because muscle spindle excitation could result. Electrical vibration of facial musculature is not used in the multisensory approach; it might produce aversive effects on delicate facial skin (Rood, 1978).

EVALUATION OF OROMOTOR FUNCTION

Breathing. Normal babies are obligate nose breathers, making sucking efficient. Muscle imbalance and palatal malformation may cause abnormal tongue placement and subsequent mouth breathing. Many brain-damaged patients demonstrate either mouth breathing or a combination of nose and mouth breathing. This breathing pattern may interfere with sucking. In addition, the normal neonatal respiration rate of 40 to 60 cycles per minute may increase and become shallow and irregular in the at-risk population.

Breathing assessment involves watching the patient at rest to determine baseline respiratory rate. The patient's lips are then held together for 5 to 10 seconds. A mirror may be placed under the nose to measure fogging resulting from nasal breathing. If the patient is a mouth breather, rest times between sucking bursts must be incorporated into the sucking treatment sequence to allow time for breathing.

Assessment of Position. One cannot expect to have normal oromotor function in a patient who is dominated by primitive reflexes causing poor body alignment. The ideal position for feeding includes hip flexion (at least 90 degrees or more), ankle dorsiflexion matching the degree of hip flexion, abduction of thighs, 90-degree knee flexion, trunk in midline, elbows flexed to 90 degrees (resting on a tray), and neck in midline with chin slightly ventroflexed. At no time should pressure be applied to the back of the head as mentioned earlier in the chapter. When feeding brain-damaged infants, the back of their heads should not rest against the feeder's arm because this will also apply pressure to the dorsal surface of the head or stimulate the hair in this region.

The therapist must continually evaluate the patient's posture during the treatment and feeding stages. If a patient hyperextends his neck, for example, swallowing skill will markedly decrease.

Internal Oral Function Assessment

The Tongue. Tongue position and function should be assessed while the patient is at rest, exercising, speaking, and feeding. At rest, the normal tongue lies symmetrically on the floor of the oral cavity with the tip behind the lower teeth. Gross pathological tongue movements that hinder feeding — for instance, the tongue thrust — can be easily observed by the therapist. Tongue thrusting is a rhythmic, forceful tongue protrusion that may occur when a patient is feeding or consciously attempting to move or speak. Cineradiographic studies or black light studies (Garliner, 1976) are helpful in providing more detailed assessment of tongue function during feeding. These studies are generally done in otolaryngology, dental clinics, or gastroenterology.

The examination of tongue movement patterns should include assessment of mid-dorsal tongue elevation (which occurs as part of sucking from birth), tongue lateralization (from about 4 to 6 months), and tongue tip elevation (from 10 to 12 months). These tongue movements should be observed during feeding or in response to cortical commands. The tongue should also be manually palpated to assess its tone. The tongue of a child with Down's syndrome is hypotonic and provides no resistance to palpation.

The Gag Reflex. This reflex persists throughout life; however, it should not disrupt normal feeding. In the normal infant, the reflex weakens as solid intake increases. Hyperactive gag responses, perhaps caused by lack of inhibition of brain stem nuclei from higher centers, are frequently observed in patients sustaining brain damage.

When testing the gag response, place an index finger on the anterior tongue midline with light pressure. Progress posteriorly, continuing to apply pressure to the tongue midline. The normal individual should be able to tolerate this stimulus applied to the first half or two thirds of the tongue before a gag response is evoked. Some patients are so hyper-reactive to the stimulus that they gag even as pressure is applied to the tongue tip. Hyporeactive gag responses (such as in pseudobulbar palsy) can also interfere with feeding, increasing the likelihood of choking. The head should be in midline when both gag and bite responses are tested.

The Bite Reflex should be tested by placing a small padded tongue blade or a rubber seizure stick on the patient's tongue, gum, and tooth surfaces. A sustained, reflexive clamping motion in response to stimulation after 3 to 5 months of age indicates a reflexive maturational delay.

Temperature and Taste Assessment. Older, cooperative patients can be tested for temperature and taste discrimination. Ability to differentiate between extremes in temperature may help protect a patient from severely burning the inside of his mouth. If it is determined that temperature discrimination is impaired, a patient must be taught to compensate for this skill by testing the food with a thermometer or on another part of the body that is intact for temperature discrimination, by observing the food substances for steam, or by asking someone else to test the food

temperature. Assessment of taste is less critical but may be helpful in providing information about cranial nerve function. Testing procedures have been discussed in the section on gustatory input.

Facial Sensitivity. The skin of brain-damaged patients frequently becomes hypersensitive (Sinclair, 1967). When this occurs, the muscles lying beneath the hyperresponsive skin fail to work properly. The therapist should observe the patient's response to facial stimulation of varying types, including maintained and light moving touch. If a patient moves his head back, away from the stimulus, and demonstrates other sympathetic responses, the stimulus is probably aversive. Normalization of facial skin is therefore indicated.

Light moving touch to a neonate is generally avoided, as mentioned earlier in the chapter. One exception is when testing the *rooting response.* This reflex, normally present at birth allows the neonate to locate the food source. By 3 to 5 months it disappears (Ingram, 1962). It may persist or reappear in patients with brain damage. When the perioral area is lightly stroked or naturally stimulated, the infant turns his head, mouth, and tongue to the stimulus and his mouth opens. If the response is hyperreactive or persists past 5 or 6 months, it can impede normal oromotor function. It should be noted that the rooting response includes a rotation of the neck along with flexion and extension (Barnes, Crutchfield, and Heriza, 1978) depending on the stimulus.

Sucking and Swallowing Assessment. When evaluating the sucking and swallowing of a premature infant or a neonate, place the baby supine with the head in the midline. Non-nutritive sucking is always assessed first for the safety of the baby. Either an index finger or a mechanical nipple that measures strength and frequency of suck should be placed in the baby's mouth with slight pressure on the tongue (Sameroff, 1965; Greenberg, 1978). The advantage of using an index finger is that the therapist can feel the tone and tongue pressure pattern; however, the mechanical nipple provides data useful for measurement.

Before a premature infant makes the transition from tube feeding and non-nutritive sucking to nutritive sucking and swallowing, use 10 cc of distilled sterile water for testing suck and swallowing patterns. This procedure is indicated only if the non-nutritive sucking pattern is coordinated. Water is preferable to milk or formula in the event of incoordinate swallow and aspiration. The therapist should remember that the premature infant or neonate will demonstrate some slight leakage from the corners of the mouth.

For assessment of sucking and swallowing in older children or adults, straws of varying diameters and squeeze bottles (see Fig. 7–49, Chapter 7) may be used. If excessive jaw movement is present during sucking and swallowing, the patient may have poorly developed musculature for jaw stability. Some patients tightly retract their lips over their teeth, making sucking almost impossible. This may be due to skin hypersensitivity over the perioral region and frequently responds to maintained pressure.

Jaw Stability Assessment. The temporalis, pterygoids, and masseters all participate in jaw stability, a necessary component of mature sucking and chewing. Patients lacking jaw stability frequently demonstrate a lack of temporalis muscle development; this creates a hollowed appearance to the temple regions of the head. Excessive jaw protrusion is common during sucking and chewing if the patient has poor jaw stability. The stability of these muscles can be tested by placing an index finger on the chin and quickly pulling down (the *jaw jerk reflex*). Patients having normal jaw stability musculature demonstrate slight resistance to the stimulus followed by a rapid return of the mandible to its resting position. Those lacking jaw stability may provide no resistance (hypotonia) or excessive resistance (hypertonia) to the stimulus. The mandible either remains depressed in hypotonia or shuts with a quick snapping motion and a possible bite reflex in hypertonia.

Ability to Handle Solids or Chewing Assessment. Normally, infants are maintained on formula or milk for the first two months owing to the fact that the tone of the inferior esophageal sphincter is not fully developed, causing frequent regurgitation of gastric contents (Lowrey, 1978). When assessing an infant's ability to handle semisolids, rice cereal is an ideal substance to use. Frequently, developmentally delayed infants demonstrate less difficulty eating semisolids than sucking and swallowing liquids. Choking in response to presentation of solids is quite common in young infants but gradually decreases until about 28 weeks. At this time, biting replaces mouthing as infant explorative play. By 36 weeks, infants bite off crackers using a primitive munching pattern (Knobloch and Pasamanick, 1974), in which the jaw moves up grossly and the tongue smashes the food against the roof of the mouth.

When testing chewing ability in older children and adults, a variety of food textures should be tried. Small amounts should be presented to the patient who has been properly positioned. The therapist observes the patient during chewing, noting tongue mobility, shearing and grinding of food, jaw movements, gag response, swallowing, and facial musculature balance.

It is essential that any therapist doing feeding training be well acquainted with the Heimlich maneuver in case a patient chokes during feeding evaluation or treatment (Heimlich, 1975). The principle of the maneuver involves pressing one's fist into the patient's epigastrium to produce an elevation of the diaphragm. This compresses the lungs, increasing the air pressure within the tracheobronchial tree. The food will be ejected by the pressure. For detailed procedures, the reader is referred to Heimlich (1975).

Patient-Family Interaction. It is important to observe the patient's interaction with family members during the feeding process. If either the patient or members of the family are stressed during the feeding process, effective feeding behavior could be disrupted. Sometimes, minor modifications in the feeding protocol can be suggested to alleviate stressful situations.

Assessment of Maladaptive Mouthing Behavior. As mentioned earlier, mouthing is a method of exploring the environment and persists throughout the first year of life. If mouthing continues to be the primary method of sensory exploration, it is considered maladaptive. Other types of maladaptive behaviors include rumination, continuous thumb, finger, or pacifier sucking, and smoking. Baseline frequency of maladaptive behavior should be noted before oromotor treatment or developmental stimulation is initiated. With intensive oral input such as maintained pressures to the lips and tongue, olfactory and gustatory input, and stimulation of appropriate gross motor developmental sequences, the author has observed marked decreases in oromotor maladaptive behaviors, especially rumination. Controlled studies are needed in this area.

The Treatment Sequence

Normalization of oromotor function should be initiated by *normalizing facial sensitivity*. This involves application of perioral maintained pressure (see Fig. 3–1). Pressures may also be applied to the cheeks and temples if necessary.

Once the patient is generally calmed, *maintained pressure* is applied to the dorsal surface of the *tongue* (Fig. 3–37). When applying tongue pressure, the therapist places an index finger or a rubber seizure stick on the dorsal tongue midline about one third of the way back. Pressure is maintained for 3 to 5 seconds while the therapist stabilizes the patient's head from the rostral surface. Initially, tongue pressure may elicit a gag or bite response or both immediately, but as it is repeated and

maintained, marked reduction in hypersensitivity ensues. As the patient increases tolerance for tongue pressures, the posterior tongue will elevate and a swallowing pattern will develop.

Decreased sucking behavior reduces the sensory stimulation of the hard and soft palatal regions of the mouth. The roof of the mouth can be stroked from anterior to posterior in order to simulate normal tongue action. In a neonate, the gum ridges can also be stroked.

A *hypoactive gag* may be present in patients with bulbar involvement. A rubber seizure stick is used to stretch the palatopharyngeal and palatoglossal arches (Fig. 3–38). Also, a small, soft toothbrush can be gently tapped on the tongue, inner cheek surfaces, and on the palatopharyngeal arches. Extreme care must be exercised with this procedure to avoid damaging intraoral tissues.

After the tongue sensitivity has been normalized, various developmentally appropriate *tongue motion patterns* should be facilitated. For patients with *tongue thrust*, three different procedures are used to actively encourage tongue retraction. The first pattern involves placing pressure under the chin to the tongue retraction musculature. The therapist may use a thumb under the chin midline while ap-

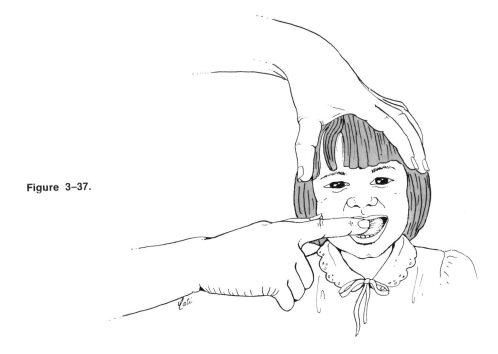

Figure 3–37.

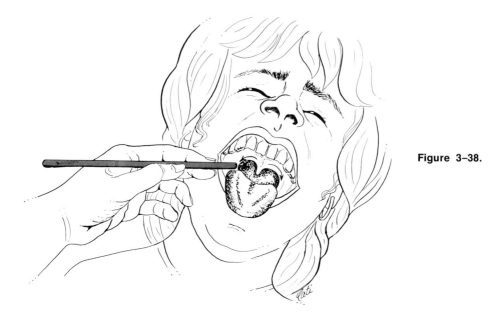

Figure 3–38.

plying maintained pressure on other appropriate orofacial surfaces (the cheeks, perioral area, or temples) with the remaining fingers (Fig. 3–39). The second tongue retrusion pattern involves manually vibrating the area under the tongue on either side of the frenulum. An index finger or rubber seizure stick is gently vibrated to stimulate tongue retrusion muscles (Fig.

3–40). Note: The sublingual area is sensitive. If the patient cries or is distressed, you are probably vibrating with too much pressure. In the third retrusion pattern, quick stretch is applied to the tongue by pulling the tongue out into protrusion, thus facilitating retrusion. The therapist grasps the patient's tongue between moist gauze pads and pulls the tongue out in

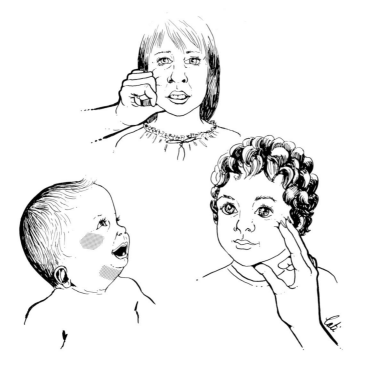

Figure 3–39.

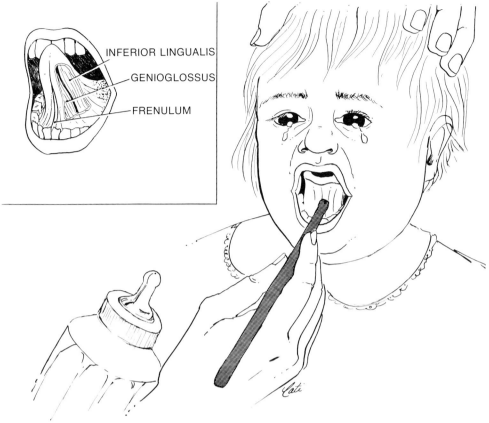

INFERIOR LINGUALIS

GENIOGLOSSUS

FRENULUM

Figure 3–40.

Figure 3–41.

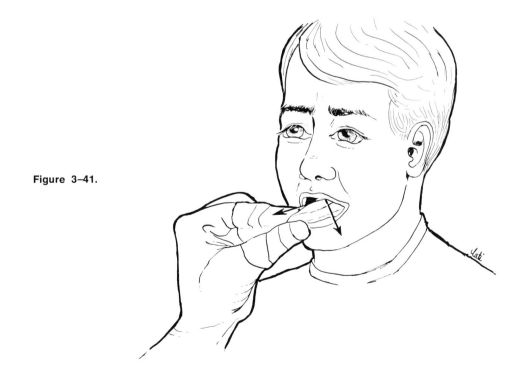

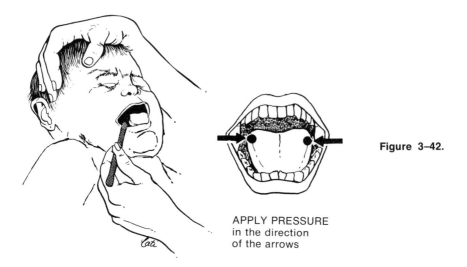

Figure 3–42.

APPLY PRESSURE
in the direction
of the arrows

diagonal protrusion movements (Fig. 3–41). This motion is followed by resistance to retraction by the therapist placing a finger on the tongue midline as it is retracting. It may be easier for the therapist to wrap his or her fingers with moist gauze strips.

Tongue lateralization is facilitated in children and adults who have normalized tongue retrusion and who are preparing for chewing. Pressure is applied against the sides of the tongue with an index finger or a rubber seizure stick so that the tongue is gently but quickly pushed toward the other side of the mouth (Fig. 3–42). Re-

peated bilateral application of pressure is recommended. The tongue should start resisting against the pressure as tongue lateralization develops.

Some patients demonstrate hyperretracted tongues. In such cases, pressure should be applied to the tip of the tongue (Fig. 3–43), pushing the tongue tip posteriorly. This facilitates protrusion. A light stroke to the roof of the mouth behind the front teeth may facilitate *tongue elevation*.

The patient must be able to maintain *jaw stability* before either sucking or chewing is efficient. The masseters, ptery-

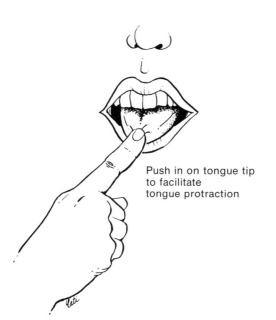

Push in on tongue tip
to facilitate
tongue protraction

Figure 3–43.

goids, and temporalis can be vibrated with the index finger in the direction of their fibers (Fig. 3–44). Since the skulls of neonates and young children differ from adults, the direction of muscle fibers varies slightly. Following manual vibration of jaw stability musculature, stretch pressures are applied to the same muscles in the direction of their fibers (see Fig. 3–29). If the jaw is too protracted, pull out quickly on the jaw; retraction will be facilitated owing to the fact that the digastrics and geniohyoid muscles are being quickstretched. Resist retraction to enhance the pattern. If the jaw is too retracted, *do not* stimulate the posterior fibers of the temporalis because this will increase retraction. Push in on the jaw to facilitate protraction. Apply resistance to protraction to enhance the pattern.

Maintained pressure over the orbicularis oris is effective in enhancing lip function for *sucking*. Manual vibration around the mouth should be followed by stretch pressures to the orbicularis oris (Fig. 3–45). The critical factor to remember when applying stretch pressures to the mouth is that the top lip must be stretched rostrolaterally while the bottom lip is stretched in a caudal and lateral direction. A piece of dental dam can be stretched over the lips to provide a stretch pressure. Following facilitation of suck, the patient can be given a banana- or vanilla-flavored ice Popsicle to suck. As sucking strength improves, use thicker liquids to increase the resistance to sucking.

Garliner (1976, p. 38) suggests the button pull exercise to increase lip strength. In this exercise, a plastic disc or button the size of a quarter is threaded on a string and then placed inside the mouth between the lips and the teeth. The patient then pulls on the string (Fig. 3–46).

Milk seems to thicken saliva possibly as a result of increase of mucus formation. If a baby is unable to suck milk or formula, a dietician can help in incorporating these

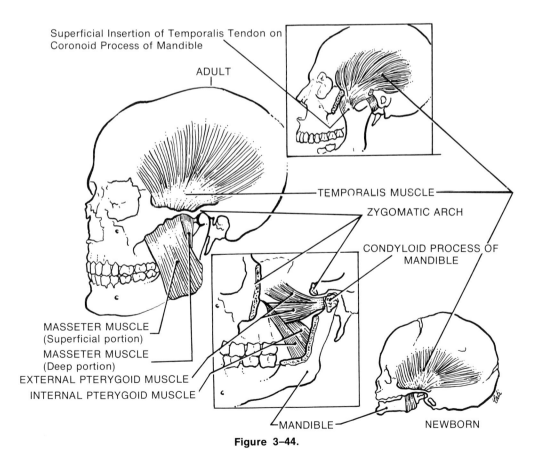

Superficial Insertion of Temporalis Tendon on Coronoid Process of Mandible

ADULT

TEMPORALIS MUSCLE

ZYGOMATIC ARCH

CONDYLOID PROCESS OF MANDIBLE

MASSETER MUSCLE (Superficial portion)

MASSETER MUSCLE (Deep portion)

EXTERNAL PTERYGOID MUSCLE

INTERNAL PTERYGOID MUSCLE

MANDIBLE

NEWBORN

Figure 3–44.

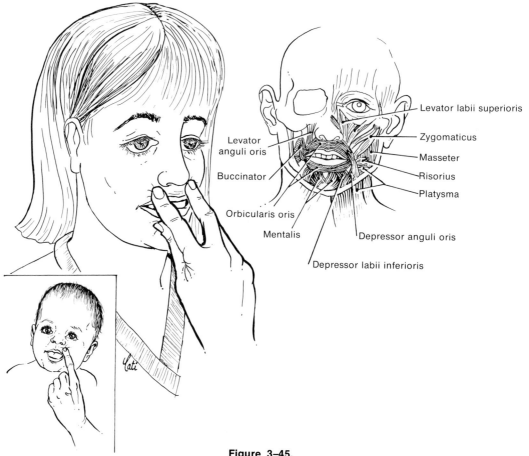

Figure 3–45.

foods into the diet. For sucking, the baby can then be given beef broth from which all fat has been removed. The animal juice helps to thin the mucus (Rood, 1978). Hot chicken soup has also been found to be effective in clearing mucus from nasal passages at a rate of 9.2 millimeters per minute compared with 8.4 for hot water and 4.5 for cold water (Saketkhoo et al, 1978). This is effective for patients in all age groups.

Facilitation of *swallowing* is done in conjunction with sucking patterns. The laryngopharyngeal musculature is digitally vibrated, starting under the chin and progressing down to the sternal notch. Stretch pressures are then applied to the same muscles in the direction of their fibers.

While jaw stability is facilitated, *chewing* musculature is automatically stimulated. Digital vibration and stretch pressures of the masseters can be applied after the food is deposited in the mouth to encourage chewing.

Feeding Patterns

Some patients may not be ready for oral feedings and are therefore maintained on tube feedings. Oral musculature used in feeding should be facilitated and then reinforced by non-nutritive sucking. Gustatory and olfactory stimulation can also be used.

Specific Feeding Techniques for Patients With a Tongue Thrust and Lack of Lateralization of the Tongue. Following application of the appropriate facilitation pattern mentioned previously, food should be deposited in the molar region of the mouth. Upon removing the spoon, place thumb under the patient's chin midline, avoiding the insertion area of the digastrics' anterior bellies, and apply maintained pressure to the perioral region. As the patient improves, food can be placed in a more frontal, midline position on the tongue.

Feeding Techniques for Patients Lacking Jaw Stability. Following facilitation

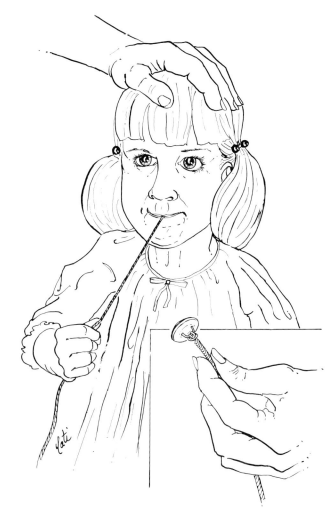

Figure 3–46.

of jaw stability musculature, food is placed in the mouth. The mandible is quickly pulled down to facilitate the temporalis. Maintained pressure is applied in the perioral region.

Specific Feeding Techniques for Patients With Hyperactive Bite Reflexes. Maintained pressure is applied to the tongue using a rubber seizure stick. The patient's head is maintained in an upright position with the chin tucked slightly. When the patient hyperextends his neck, the bite reaction may be exacerbated. If the patient should clamp down on the spoon, do not attempt to pry open his mouth. Instead, push up on the jaw to facilitate opening. Use a spoon with a small bowl in order to avoid stimulating the bite response. Rubber-coated spoons are available and help protect the patient's teeth. Avoid using plastic picnic tableware because it can splinter if the patient bites down on it. Once the bite response is

integrated, chewing can be facilitated by digitally vibrating the masseters and by gradually working toward solid textures.

Specific Feeding Techniques for Patients Who Do Not Suck and Swallow. After the sucking and swallowing patterns have been facilitated, special devices can be used to enhance sucking (see Fig. 7–49, Chapter 7).

The Coma Sequence

PURPOSE. The treatment sequence for comatose patients is included in this chapter because it represents an integration of multisensory treatment theory and pragmatics as applied to a specific situation. Much research needs to be done in the area of coma intervention in order to determine factors affecting consciousness. It is hoped that this presentation will provoke such action.

In order to understand the nature of

coma, one must have a thorough understanding of the functions of the reticular formation (see Chapter 1). One of its main functions is to preserve the state of arousal and attention through diffuse cortical stimulation (Peele, 1977; Noback, 1975; Gardner, 1975). In the normal individual, the brain continually processes sensory input. Even during sleep, which is an active process, higher centers are stimulated (Gardner, 1975; Plum and Posner, 1972). Injury to the reticular formation can produce a comatose state (Gardner, 1975; Peele, 1977; Plum and Posner, 1972).

Coma can produce a vicious circle of sensory deprivation. When a person incurs some damage to the CNS that renders him comatose, he is frequently hospitalized and treated in an intensive care unit (ICU). In this environment, most sensory input normally received by the individual before injury is markedly reduced. Tubes of various diameters are inserted in a variety of areas throughout the body. Medication, nutrients and liquids are introduced via these tubes. The sounds of monitors (often even, rhythmical, and repetitive) usually can be heard. Patients are moved once every two hours to prevent formation of decubitus ulcers. The lights frequently remain on 24 hours a day to enable staff to see their critically ill charges. Some individuals are hesistant to talk to the comatose patient. Thus, an already damaged system is further deprived of necessary sensory input. One might speculate that the threshold of the reticular neurons may rise first as a result of the damage, then rises further by sensory deprivation.

The purpose of the coma sequence in the multisensory treatment approach is to break this vicious circle and perhaps lower the threshold of reticular neurons. The same principles used in other aspects of treatment apply to the coma sequence. First a baseline assessment is initiated. These parameters are measured: level of responsiveness to each sensory system, postural reflexes, muscle tone, range of motion, verbalization, and cognitive functions (see Chapter 2 and Chapter 5, appendix 5–1). The order of application of sensory input may vary from patient to patient, depending on which CNS areas have been damaged and whether the patient has any intact sensory input systems that, when stimulated, produce consistent adaptive responses. If a given system produces more specific responses it can be used early in treatment; however, if all stimulation produces either no response or a generalized response, stimulation is applied according to the phylogenetic development of the sensory systems. Older systems are often less vulnerable to damage and are, therefore, used first.

TREATMENT CONCEPTS. Positioning the patient during the coma is critical in order to avoid deformity. Cones are used for spastic hands to keep them from becoming fisted. Footboards are avoided because they can actually reinforce plantar flexion in a patient with a positive supporting reaction. Special shoes are used to maintain ankles without causing pressure on the balls of the feet (see Chapter 7). If the patient is demonstrating extensor synergies (or decerebration), he can be positioned on his side with sandbags (Fig. 3–47), or a special device can be constructed to hold the patient in hip flexion.

For a patient who demonstrates no response to sensory stimulation (Stage 1) or generalized response (Stage 2), the early phases of treatment comprise use of touch and vestibular input presented several times daily for brief periods of time. Maintained touch is used to tone down hypertonicity followed by moving touch stimulation to the face to facilitate the hand-to-mouth pattern. Moving touch at the T10 dermatome is also used to facilitate lower extremity flexor pattern in adults, especially decerebrate patients. The therapist must constantly check the patient's responses following stimulation. There is a possibility that a stimulus might cause a brief arousal followed by a rebound into deeper coma. The therapist should also observe the various monitors to make sure that the sensory input is not threatening basal function stability. The patient's skin can be rubbed with a textured cloth such as terry cloth, beginning during this time.

Movement stimulation is initiated following use of touch modalities. Recommended methods of movement include moving the bed in several directions either by electrical or manual controls, moving the patient on a hospital cart (note: acceleration and deceleration are used *only* after medical clearance is obtained), movement of body parts, and rolling the patient.

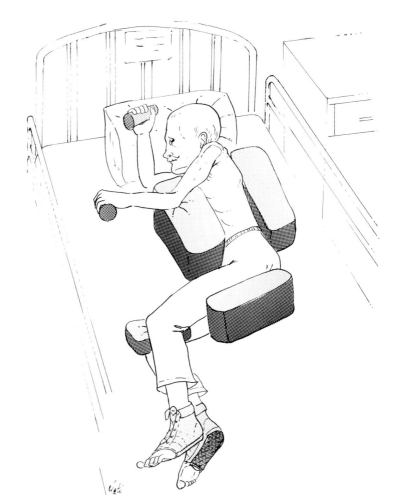

Figure 3–47.

Again, the patient's vital signs are closely observed.

Olfaction and gustatory input are also used in early treatment as part of the prefeeding program. The sensory stimuli are frequently paired and are presented in a treatment session in which the emphasis is on producing oral adaptive responses. Banana and vanilla odorants are usually presented to the patient first. Depending on the response, the treatment may progress to sucking reinforcement or to presentation of one or two additional odors with which the patient may have had some familiarity (hair spray, favorite foods, aftershave lotion, perfume). Gustatory input is provided by use of a dental tweezer or cotton swab to the appropriate intraoral structures as described in the gustatory section of this chapter. If a patient was known to have a particular taste preference, this substance is used during the stimulation process.

While auditory input is not the main thrust of the early treatment regimen, those caring for the patient should talk to him. This author identifies herself to the patient before initiating treatment and then informs the patient of what she will be doing. (On one occasion, a recovered patient later recounted several of the things this author had said to him while he was comatose.) A small radio can be used to provide auditory input. It should not be left on for long periods of time or adaptation may result. Tape recordings of family members talking to the patient have also been used.

As the patient moves from Stages 1 and 2 to Stage 3 (localization of response), more specific auditory input can be used, including playing tapes of sounds associated with various familiar objects and identifying them by name (for instance, during playing of tape of phone ringing, say "telephone").

Visual input during Stages 1 and 2 consists of placing pressure on the eyeballs, turning the light on and off, using a flashlight in a darkened room, and using bright-colored objects or a mirror. As the patient improves to Stage 3, more of a variety of visual stimuli can be introduced. Showing a Super–8 movie of family members may produce a sustained responsiveness.

During Stage 3, the goal of therapy is to combine the specific responses to each sensory stimulus into adaptive behavioral complexes. An example is to use a variety of related stimuli that could produce those basic skills necessary to promote feeding. The therapist might start with maintained pressure to the lips, then present a banana-flavored ice Popsicle for sucking reinforcement. The hand-to-mouth pattern might be facilitated by moving touch to the lips reinforced by a rolling pattern. It is likely that a patient will no longer be cared for in an ICU at this point.

Stage 4 indicates an improved level of consciousness with the patient fluctuating between various levels of confusion. The patient might try to pull out tubes (agitation), whereas during periods of less confusion, supervised activity such as simple self-care tasks can be initiated. Stage 5 is considered by this author to be the last stage of the coma sequence. The patient is consistently oriented and capable of self-care with minimal guidance.

REFERENCES

Abd-el-Malek S: The part played by the tongue in mastication and deglutition. J Anat 89:250–254, 1955.

Andres K, Von Düring M: Morphology of cutaneous receptors. In Ainsley Iggo (ed): Handbook of Sensory Physiology II. New York, Springer-Verlag, 1973.

Andrew BL, Dodt E: The development of sensory nerve endings at the knee joint of the cat. Acta Physiol Scand 28:287–296, 1953.

Andrew BL: The sensory innervation of the medial ligament of the knee joint. J. Physiol (London) 123:241–250, 1954.

Arey LB: Developmental Anatomy, 7th ed. Philadelphia, W. B. Saunders Co., 1974.

Ayres AJ: Sensory Integration and Learning Disorders. Los Angeles, Cal, Western Psychological Services, 1972.

Ayres AJ: Integration of information. In Henderson et al (eds): The Development of Sensory Integrative Theory and Practice. Dubuque, IA, Kendall-Hunt Publishing Co., 1974.

Banks RW et al: A study of mammalian intrafusal muscle fiber using a combined histochemical and ultrastructural technique. J Anat 123:783–796, 1977.

Bárány R: Newer methods of examination of the semicircular canals and their practical significance. Am Otol 16:755, 1907.

Barker D et al: The muscle spindle. Handbook of Sensory Physiology III/2. New York, Springer-Verlag, 1974.

Barnes MR, Crutchfield CA, Heriza CB: The Neurophysiological Basis of Patient Treatment. Vol II Reflexes in Motor Development. Morgantown, W Va, Stokesville Publishing Co., 1978.

Bartoshuk LM: NaCl thresholds in man: thresholds for water taste or NaCl taste? J Comp Physiol Psychol 87:310, 1974.

Baru AV, Karaseva TA: The Brain and Hearing Disturbances Associated with Local Brain Lesions. New York, Consultants Bureau, 1972.

Basmajian JV: Muscles Alive: Their Functions Revealed by Electromyography. Baltimore, Williams and Wilkins Co., 1978.

Beckett EB, Bourne GH: Histochemistry of developing skeletal and cardiac muscle. In GH Bourne (ed): The Structure and Function of Muscle, Vol 1, 2nd ed. New York, Academic Press, pp 150–180, 1972.

Bishop B: Vibratory stimulation. Part 1 Neurophysiology of motor responses evoked by vibratory stimulation. Phys Ther 54:1273–1281, 1974.

Bishop B: Vibratory stimulation. Part II Vibratory stimulation as an evaluation tool. Phys Ther 55:29–33, 1975.

Bishop B: Vibratory stimulation. Part III Possible applications of vibration in treatment of motor dysfunction. Phys Ther 55:139–143, 1975.

Blank M, Klig S: Dimensional learning across sensory modalities in nursery school children. J Exp Child Psychol 9:166–173, 1970.

Bobath B: Adult Hemiplegia: Evaluation and Treatment, 2nd ed. London, William Heinemann Medical Books Ltd., 1978.

Bosma JF: Examination of the mouth and pharynx of the infant. In C Heriza (ed): The Comprehensive Management of Infants at Risk for CNS Deficits. Chapel Hill, NC, Physical Therapy Division, School of Medicine, University of North Carolina, 1974.

Bowman JP: The Muscle Spindle and Neural Control of the Tongue. Springfield, IL, Charles C Thomas, 1971.

Boyd IA, Roberts TD: Proprioceptive discharges from stretch receptors in the knee joint of the cat. J Physiol (London) 122:38–58, 1953.

Bronson, G: The postnatal growth of visual capacity. Child Dev 45:873–890, 1974.

Brunnstrom S: Movement Therapy in Hemiplegia. New York, Harper and Row, 1970.

Burke D et al: The responses of human muscle spindle endings to vibration of noncontracting muscles. J Physiol (London) 261:673–693, 1976.

Burke D et al: The responses of human muscle spindle endings to vibration during isometric contraction. J Physiol (London) 261:695–711, 1976.

Burke PM: Swallowing and the organization of sucking in the human neonate. Child Dev 48:523–531, 1977.

Butler RA: The cumulative effects of differential stimulus repetition rates on the auditory evoked response in man. Electroenceph Clin Neurophysiol 35:337–345, 1973.

Cagan RH: Olfaction and gustation: Section B Functions and mechanisms. *In* JH Shaw et al (eds): Textbook of Oral Biology. Philadelphia, W. B. Saunders Co., 1978.

Campbell SK, Wilson JM: Planning infant learning programs. Phys Ther 56, 1976.

Carpenter MB: Core Text of Neuroanatomy, 2nd ed. Baltimore, Williams and Wilkins Co., 1978.

Carr TH, Bacharach VR, Mehner DS: Preparing children to look at pictures: advance descriptions direct attention and facilitate active processing. Child Dev 48:22–27, 1977.

Cashdan D: Visual and haptic form discrimination under conditions of successive stimulation. J Exp Psychol 76:215–218, 1968.

Cheal M: Social olfaction: a review of the ontogeny of olfactory influences on vertebrate behavior. Behav Biol 15:1–25, 1974.

Coppe MR: Olfaction and gustation: Section A, morphology of receptors. *In* JH Shaw et al (eds): Textbook of Oral Biology. Philadelphia, W. B. Saunders Co., 1978.

Crook CK, Lipsett LP: Neonatal nutritive sucking effects of taste stimulation upon sucking rhythm and heart rate. Child Dev 47:518–522, 1976.

Crutchfield C, Barnes M: Neurophysiological Basis of Patient Treatment. Vol I The Muscle Spindle, 2nd ed. Morgantown, W Va, Stokesville Publishing Co., 1973.

Darian-Smith I: The trigeminal system. *In* Ainsley Iggo (ed): Handbook of Sensory Physiology — Somatosensory System. New York, Springer-Verlag, p 278, 1973.

Dayhoff N: Re-thinking stroke: soft or hard devices to position hands? Am J Nurs 7:1142–1144, 1975.

Dee R: Structure and function of hip joint innervation. Ann Roy Col Surg Eng 45:357–374, 1969.

Desor JA, Maller O, Turner RE: Taste in acceptance of sugars in human infants. J Comp Physiol Psychol 84:496, 1973.

DeGail P, Lance JW, Neilson PD: Differential effects on tonic and phasic reflex mechanisms produced by vibration of muscles in man. J Neurol Neurosurg Psychiatry 29:1–11, 1966.

Dimitrijevic M et al: Reflex effects of vibration in patients with spinal cord lesions. Neurology 27:1078–1086, 1977.

Elliot DN, Fraser W: Fatigue and adaptation. *In* JV Tobias (ed): Foundations of Modern Auditory Theory, Vol 1. New York, Academic Press, 1970.

Engen T: Man's ability to perceive odors. Adv Chemorecept 1:361, 1970.

Engen T, Ross BM: Long-term memory of odors with and without verbal descriptions. J Exper Psychol 100:221, 1973.

Farber SD: Sensorimotor Evaluation and Treatment Procedures for Allied Health Personnel, 2nd ed. Indianapolis, Indiana University Foundation, 1974.

Farber SD: Olfaction in health and disease. Am J Occup Ther 32:155–160, 1978.

Fiorentino M: Reflex Testing Methods for Evaluating Central Nervous System Development, 2nd ed. Springfield, IL, Charles C Thomas, 1973.

Fitzgerald MJT, Sachithanandan SR: The structure and source of lingual proprioceptors in the monkey. J Anat 128:523–552, 1979.

Forster FM, Shields CD: Cortical sensory defects causing disability. Arch Phys Med 40, 1959.

Frank LK: Tactile communication. *In* CB Kopp (ed): Readings in Early Development for Occupational and Physical Therapy Students. Springfield, IL, Charles C Thomas, 1971.

Freeman MA, Wyke B: Articular contributions to limb muscle reflexes: I An electromyographic study of the ankle joint mechanoreceptors upon reflex activity in the gastrocnemius muscle of the cat. J Physiol (London) 171:20–21, 1964.

Freeman MA, Wyke B: Articular reflexes at the ankle joint: an electromyographic study of normal and abnormal influences of ankle joint mechanoreceptors upon reflex activity in the leg muscles. Br J Surg 54:990–1001, 1967.

Freedman AM, Kaplan HI, Sadock BJ (eds): Comprehensive Textbook of Psychiatry II. Baltimore, Williams and Wilkins Co., 1975.

Gardner E: Fundamentals of Neurology. Philadelphia, W. B. Saunders Co., 1975.

Garliner D: Myofunctional Therapy. Philadelphia, W. B. Saunders Co., 1976.

Geldard FA: The Human Senses, 2nd ed. New York, John Wiley and Sons, 1972.

Gellhorn E: Principles of Autonomic-Somatic Integration: Physiological Basis and Psychological and Clinical Implications. Minneapolis, University of Minnesota Press, 1967.

Gibson EJ: Principles of Perceptual Learning and Development. New York, Appleton-Century-Crofts, 1969.

Giddon DB et al: Relative abilities of natural and artificial dentition patients for judging the sweetness of solid foods. J Prosthet Dent 4:263, 1954.

Goldberger L: In the absence of stimuli. Science 168:709, 1970.

Goleman D: Special abilities of the sexes: do they begin in the brain? Psychology Today, November 1978.

Goodwin GM et al: The contribution of muscle afferents to kinaesthesia shown by vibration-induced illusions of movement and by the effects of paralysing joint afferents. Brain 95:705–748, 1972.

Goodwin GM et al: Cardiovascular and respiratory responses to changes in central commands during isometric exerise at constant muscle tension. J Physiol (London) 226:173–190, 1973.

Goren C, Sarty ME, Wu PYK: Visual following and pattern discrimination of face-like stimuli by newborn infants. Pediatrics 56:544–549, 1975.

Gottlieb GL, Agarwal GC: Response to sudden torques about the ankle in man: myotatic reflex. J Neurophysiol 42:91–106, 1979.

Gottfried AW, Rose SA, Bridges WH: Cross-modal transfer in human infants. Child Dev 48:118–123, 1977.

Graziadei PPC, Monti-Graziadei GA: The olfactory system: a model for the study of neurogenesis and axon regeneration in mammals. *In* CW Cotman (ed): Neuronal Plasticity. New York, Raven Press, 1978.

Graziadei PPC, Monti-Graziadei GA: Continuous nerve cell renewal in the olfactory system. *In* M Jacobson (ed): Handbook of Sensory Physiology IX. New York, Springer-Verlag, 1977.

Graziadei PPC: Neuronal plasticity in the vertebrate olfactory receptor organ. Tenth Int Cong Anat Tokyo, 1975, p 45.

Greenberg J: Sudden infant death. Science News 113, 1978.

Guyton AC: Basic Human Physiology: Normal Function and Mechanisms of Disease, 2nd ed. Philadelphia, W. B. Saunders Co., 1977.

Hagbarth KE, Eklund G: The muscle vibrator — a powerful tool in neurological therapeutic work. Scand J Rehab Med 1:26–34, 1969.

Hagbarth KE: Excitatory and inhibitory skin areas for flexor and extensor motor neurons. Acta Physiol Scand 26:1–58, 1952.

Harris FA: Facilitation techniques in therapeutic exercise. In JV Basmajian (ed): Therapeutic Exercise, 3rd ed. Baltimore, Williams and Wilkins Co., 1978.

Hebb DO: The innate organization of visual acuity: I. Perception of figures by rats reared in total darkness. J Genet Psychol 51:101–126, 1937.

Hebb DO: The Organization of Behavior. New York, John Wiley and Sons, 1949.

Hebb DO: A neuropsychological theory. In S Koch (ed): Psychology: A Study of a Science, Vol I. New York, McGraw-Hill, 1959.

Hebb DO: Semiautonomous process. American Psychologist 18, 1963.

Heimlich HJ: A lifesaving maneuver to prevent food choking. JAMA 234:398–401, 1975.

Hellenbrandt FA: Physiology. In TL DeLorme and AL Watkins (eds): Progressive Resistance Exercise. New York, Appleton-Century-Crofts, 1951.

Hensel H: Cutaneous thermoreceptors. In Ainsley Iggo (ed): Handbook of Sensory Physiology II. New York, Springer-Verlag, 1973, p 103.

Hooker D: Evidence of prenatal function of the central nervous system in man. In Payton et al (eds): Scientific Bases for Neurophysiologic Approaches to Therapeutic Exercise. Philadelphia, F. A. Davis Co., 1977.

Humphrey T: Reflex activity in the oral and facial area of the human fetus. In JF Bosma (ed): Second Symposium on Oral Sensation and Perception. Springfield, IL, Charles C Thomas, 1970.

Huss AJ: Touch with care or a caring touch? Am J Occup Ther 31:11–18, 1977.

Huss AJ: Sensorimotor approaches. In H Hopkins and H Smith (eds): Willard and Spackman's Occupational Therapy. Philadelphia, J. B. Lippincott Co., 1978.

Illingworth RS: The Development of the Infant and the Young Child — Normal and Abnormal, 6th ed. New York, Churchill Livingstone, 1975.

Ingram TTS: Clinical significance of infantile feeding reflexes. Dev Med Child Neurol 4:159, 1962.

Jessen BL, Kaess DW: Effects of training on intersensory communication by three to five year olds. J Genet Psychol 123:115–122, 1973.

Johnson D, Brody N: Visual habituation, sensorimotor development, and tempo of play in one year old infants. Child Dev 48:315–319, 1977.

Kaplan AR et al: Cumulative effect of age and smoking on taste sensitivity in males and females. J Gerontol 20:334, 1965.

King LJ: Toward a science of adaptive responses. Am J Occup Ther 32, 1978.

Kitajima S: The cumulative inhibitory effect of repetitively flashed stimuli on the recovery process of the human visual evoked potential to a test stimulus. Electroencephlogr Clin Neurophysiol 44:364–372, 1978.

Klosovskii BN: The Development of the Brain and its Disturbance by Harmful Factors. New York, Pergamon Press, Macmillan, 1963.

Knobloch H, Pasamanick B (eds): Gesell and Amatruda's Developmental Diagnosis, 3rd ed. Hagerstown, Harper and Row, 1974.

Knott M, Voss, D: Proprioceptive Neuromuscular Facilitation, 2nd ed. New York, Harper and Row, 1968.

Knuttgen HG: Development of strength and endurance. Neuromuscular Mechanisms for Therapeutic and Conditioning Exercise. Baltimore, University Park Press, 1976.

Koelega H, Koster E: Some experiments on sex differences in odor perception. Ann N Y Acad Sci 237:234–246, 1974.

Kornhuber HH: Vestibular system. Part 2: Psychophysics, applied aspects and general interpretations. Handbook of Sensory Physiology. New York, Springer-Verlag, 1974.

Lassen NA et al: Brain function and blood flow. Scientific American 239:62–71, 1978.

Lewontin RC: Adaptation. Scientific American 239:213–230, 1978.

Lipsett LP et al: The stability and interrelationships of newborn sucking and heart rate. Devel Psychobiol 9:305–310, 1976.

Lowrey GH: Growth and Development of Children, 6th ed. Chicago, Year Book Medical Publishers, Inc., 1973.

Lowrey GH: Growth and Development of Children, 7th ed. Chicago, Year Book Medical Publishers, Inc., 1978.

Lund JP et al: Activity of trigeminal alpha and gamma motoneurons and muscle afferents during performance of a biting task. J Neurophysiol 42:710–725, 1979.

Mathews PBC: Mammalian Muscle Receptors and Their Central Actions. Baltimore, Williams and Wilkins Co., 1972.

McBurney DH et al: Temperature dependence of human taste responses. Physiol Behav 11:89, 1973.

McCloskey DI: Kinesthetic sensibility. Physiol Rev 58:763–820, 1978.

McCloskey DI: Differences between the senses of movement and position shown by the effects of loading and vibration of muscles in man. Brain Res 61:119–131, 1973.

McGurk H, Turnure C, Creighton SJ: Auditory-visual coordination in neonates. Child Dev 48:138–143, 1977.

Medaer R, Kovacs L: Vibration-assisted bladder emptying in multiple sclerosis. Lancet 1:768–769, 1978.

Monell Chemical Senses Center, University of Pennsylvania, 3500 Market St, Philadelphia, PA 19104.

Moore JC: Neuroanatomy Simplified. Dubuque, Kendall-Hunt Publishing Co., 1969.

Moore KL: Before We Are Born: Basic Embryology and Birth Defects. Philadelphia, W. B. Saunders Co., 1974.

Moulton D, Turk A, Johnson W (eds): Methods in Olfactory Research. New York, Academic Press, 1975.

Myers GJ: Understanding the floppy baby. In RC Griggs, RT Moxley (eds): Advances in Neurology, Vol 17. New York, Raven Press, 1977.

Noback C: The Human Nervous System, 2nd ed. New York, McGraw-Hill Book Co., 1975.

Nordmark JO: Time and frequency analysis. In JV Tobias (ed): Foundations of Modern Auditory Theory, Vol 1. New York, Academic Press, 1970.

Patte F et al: Selected and standardized values of

suprathreshold odor intensities for 110 substances. Chem Sens Flav 1:283, 1975.

Pearson P, Williams C (eds): Physical Therapy Services in the Developmental Disabilities. Springfield, IL, Charles C Thomas, 1972.

Pederson DR, Ter Vrugt D: The influence of amplitude and frequency on the activity of two month old infants. Child Dev 44:122–128, 1973.

Pfaffmann C: The sense of taste. In J Field et al (eds): Handbook of Physiology, Neurophysiology, Vol 1. Washington DC, American Physiological Society, 1959, p 507.

Piaget J, Inhelder B: The Child's Conception of Space. London, Routledge and Kegan Paul, 1956.

Piaget J: The Origins of Intelligence in Children. New York, International Universities Press, 1952.

Plum F, Posner JB: Diagnosis of Stupor and Coma, 2nd ed. Philadelphia, F. A. Davis Co., 1972.

Ritvo ER et al.: Decreased postrotatory nystagmus in early infantile autism. Neurology 19:653–658, 1969.

Rogers RC et al: Afferent projections to the dorsal motor nucleus of the vagus. Brain Res Bull 5:365–373, 1980.

Roland PE: Astereognosis: tactile discrimination after localized hemispheric lesions in man. Arch Neurol 33:543–550, 1976.

Roland PE, Larsen B: Focal increase of cerebral blood flow during stereognostic testing in man. Arch Neurol 33:551–558, 1976.

Rood M: Unpublished class notes from Rood workshop. Indianapolis, Methodist Hospital, July 1978.

Rood M: The use of sensory receptors to activate, facilitate and inhibit motor response, automatic and somatic in developmental sequence. In C Sattely (ed): Approaches to the Treatment of Patients with Neuromuscular Dysfunction. Dubuque, Wm. C. Brown, 1962.

Rose S: The Conscious Brain. New York, Alfred A. Knopf, 1973.

Saketkhoo K et al: Effects of drinking hot water, cold water, and chicken soup on nasal mucus velocity and nasal airflow resistance. Chest 74:408–410, 1978.

Sameroff AJ: An apparatus for recording sucking and control-feeding in the first days of life. Psychon Sci 2:355–356, 1965.

Schechter PJ, Horwitz D, Henkin RI: Salt preference in patients with untreated and treated essential hypertension. Am J Med Sci 267:320, 1974.

Schmidt RF: Control of the access of afferent activity to somatosensory pathways. In Ainsley Iggo (ed): Handbook of Sensory Physiology — Somatosensory System. New York, Springer-Verlag, 1973, p 154.

Schneider RA: Newer insights into the role modification of olfaction in man through clinical studies. Ann N Y Acad Sci 237:217–223, 1974.

Selbach H: The principle of relaxation oscillation as a special instance of the law of initial value in cybernetic functions. Ann N Y Acad Sci 98:1221–1228, 1962.

Shepherd GM: The Synaptic Organization of the Brain — An Introduction. New York, Oxford University Press, 1974.

Silverman EH, Elfant IL: Dysphagia: an evaluation and treatment program for the adult. Am J Occup Ther 33:382–392, 1979.

Sinclair D: Cutaneous Sensation. London, Oxford University Press, 1967.

Skoglund S: Anatomical and physiological studies of knee joint innervation in the cat. Acta Physiol Scand 36(Suppl.):1–101, 1956.

Steiner JE: Innate discriminative human facial expressions to taste and smell stimulation. Ann N Y Acad Sci 237:229–233, 1974.

Stockmeyer S: A sensorimotor approach to treatment. In P Pearson and C Williams (eds): Physical Therapy Services in the Developmental Disabilities. Springfield, IL, Charles C Thomas, 1972.

Stone LJ, Church J: Childhood and Adolescence. New York, Random House, 1975.

Tamar H: Principles of Sensory Physiology. Springfield, IL, Charles C Thomas, 1972.

Thomson LR: Sensory deprivation: a personal experience. Am J Nurs 73:266, 1973.

Tokizane T et al: Electromyographic studies on tonic neck, lumbar and labyrinthine reflexes in normal persons. Jap J of Physio, 1951. As cited in Payton et al (eds): Scientific Bases for Neurophysiologic Approaches to Therapeutic Exercise. Philadelphia, F. A. Davis Co., 1977.

Trombly CA, Scott AD: Occupational Therapy for Physical Dysfunction. Baltimore, Williams and Wilkins Co., 1977.

Tyler NB: A stereognostic test for screening tactile sensation. Am J Occup Ther 26:256–260, 1972.

Tyrrell DJ: Dimensional effect in cross-modal transfer of discrimination learning in children. Child Dev 48:625–629, 1977.

Van Buskirk C, Webster D: Prognostic value of sensory deficit in rehabilitation of hemiplegics. Neurology 5:407, 1955.

Vinograd A, Taylor E, Grossman S: Sensory retraining of the hemiplegic hand. Am J Occup Ther 16:246–250, 1962.

Walker A: Functional anatomy of oral tissues: mastication and deglutition. In JH Shaw et al (eds): Textbook of Oral Biology, Philadelphia, W. B. Saunders Co., 1978.

Wilson, BC, Wilson JJ: Sensory and perceptual functions in the cerebral palsied: II. Stereognosis. J Nerv Ment Dis 145:61–68, 1967.

Wirth G: Interdependent influence on movement sensation by auditory and vestibular stimulation. Z Laryngol Rhinol Otol 50:60–67, 1971.

Wolff PH: The serial organization of sucking in the young infant. Pediatrics 42:943–956, 1968.

Wolff PH: Abnormalities in the sequential organization of non-nutrient sucking. In C Heriza (ed): The Comprehensive Management of Infants at Risk for CNS Deficits. Physical Therapy Dvision, School of Medicine, University of North Carolina, Chapel Hill, 1974.

Wolinski GF, Ayre E: Contribution to the history of psychology V: Translation of stereognostic perception by E Claparede. Percept Mot Skills 24:35–41, 1967.

Zinchenko VP, Vergiles N Yu: Formation of Visual Images. New York, Consultants Bureau, 1972.

Zubek JP (ed): Sensory Deprivation: Fifteen Years of Research. New York, Appleton-Century-Crofts, 1969.

Zusne L: Visual Perception of Form. New York, Academic Press, 1970.

CHAPTER **4**

NEONATOLOGY

Shereen D. Farber, MS, OTR, FAOTA
and
Sammy Williams, MS, RPT

In this chapter the application of the multisensory approach to the neonate will be discussed. In order to encourage the development of effective neonatal programs, resources and guidelines are suggested for allied health professionals working in existing programs and those interested in developing new ones.

Neonatology is defined as the "art and science of diagnosis and treatment of disorders of the newborn infant" (Schaffer and Avery, 1977). Three per cent of all live-born infants require admission to a neonatal intensive care unit (NICU) because of life-threatening conditions (Evans and Glass, 1978). Determination of the incidence of permanent disability among these infants is difficult owing to the various definitions of disability and the time periods over which these infants are evaluated for disability. Calame and co-workers reported in 1976 that among 111 high-risk

newborns followed to 3 years of age, 71 per cent were normal, while 29 per cent exhibited neurological sequelae and developmental abnormalities. This incidence of neurological sequelae and developmental abnormalities was about four times greater than in the normal infant population.

Thompson and Reynolds (1977) discussed the results of neonatal intensive care and long-term prognosis for high-risk infants with respect to specific birth weights and diagnoses. They concluded that while a percentage of survivors may be permanently disabled, there is an increased number who demonstrate improved physical and developmental status as compared to infants born prior to the advent of neonatal intensive care. For example, although the number of low birth weight survivors has increased as a result of intensive care, the reported incidence of

178

cerebral palsy has decreased (Franco and Andrews, 1977).

Rationale for Intervention

The problems of the intellectually and neurologically impaired infant are compounded early (Bobath, 1967; Campbell, 1974; Brazelton, 1977). To prevent the exacerbation of already existing handicaps, appropriate social and sensorimotor intervention programs should be initiated as soon as the medical condition of the infant allows. *Guideline 1: The therapist initiates timely neurorehabilitative evaluation and treatment procedures only when the neonate is medically stable and survival seems assured.*

Suggested Qualifications for Allied Health Professionals Treating the Neonate

Presently, a variety of allied health professionals function in NICUs. Because of the narrow range of occupational behavior in the neonate, there is a potential for overlap of roles among these professionals. Each professional's role in this situation should be determined by his or her qualifications, postgraduate training and experience, expertise, and interest rather than by undergraduate degree alone. Coordination of team members' roles is essential to avoid redundancy that would add to the high cost of caring for a neonate in the NICU.

Allied health professionals preparing to work in neonatology should acquire:

1. Knowledge of normal and abnormal child development beginning in the prenatal period.
2. Concepts of neuromuscular maturation.
3. Knowledge of the perinatal literature in the areas of:
    a. Medical conditions peculiar to the neonate
    b. Outcomes or results of neonatal intensive care
    c. Research studies of neonatal sensorimotor intervention

References in each of these areas may be found in the bibliography at the end of the chapter.

Occupational Behavior of the Neonate

Chapters 2 and 3 have stressed the importance of examining the occupational behavior of a patient in order to assure relevance of treatment. This is of special significance in the neonatal population because failure to consider occupational behavior may result in a treatment plan that is too stimulatory, that may interfere with adaptive behavior formation, and that could threaten the infant's survival.

A period of rapid growth occurs during the neonatal stage (Stone and Church, 1979). The newborn infant appears to conserve his energy for growth processes and demonstrates a narrow spectrum of occupational behavior, including ingestion and digestion of nutritive substances, elimination of metabolic waste products, crying, sleeping, and brief periods of alertness. The majority of neonatal behavior is influenced by the parasympathetic nervous system. A therapist working with the brain-damaged neonate may spend most of the initial treatment time using inhibitory activity. The rationale for this practice is that in upper motor neuron damage, disinhibition frequently occurs (see Chapter 1). The neonate may become hyperresponsive to his environment; in this state, sleep and feeding behavior may be interrupted. *Guideline 2: The therapist provides input to normalize infant responses and enhance appropriate occupational behavior.* The authors choose to label treatment concepts presented in this chapter "infant normalization procedures" instead of infant stimulation. Campbell and Wilson (1976) alternatively describe an approach to neonates as "infant learning programs."

The Typical Neonatal Intensive Care Unit

The NICU is a highly technical unit requiring enough space to house the specially trained personnel and bulky equipment necessary to provide care for critically ill infants. Important pieces of equipment include open radiant heaters, respirators, monitoring devices, phototherapy lamps, and portable radiograph and electrocardiograph machines (Evans and Glass, 1977).

Besides neonatologists and nursing staff, other medical specialists such as the pediatric surgeons, cardiologists, neurologists, radiologists, and ophthalmologists may be involved in the primary treatment of infants in the NICU. Dieticians, laboratory personnel, psychologists, medical social workers, and physical and occupational therapists arc among allied health professionals who may be consulted according to the therapeutic needs of each infant.

Prolonged hospitalization of critically ill infants promotes strong attachment between unit personnel and the infants housed there. Because of this strong attachment and the comparatively high mortality rate of critically ill newborns, the emotional atmosphere of the unit is intense and often highly charged. *Guideline 3: Therapists wishing to become involved in the treatment of NICU infants are advised to remember that the primary medical and nursing staff members have arduously fought to promote these babies' survival. They are rightfully protective of their charges. Therefore, **Guideline 4:** The NICU therapist should intimately involve the primary medical and nursing staff in all aspects of therapeutic intervention, including screening of appropriate candidates and selection of suitable techniques and procedures.* As a result of continual contact with a given infant, primary medical and nursing staff members can provide valuable guidance and insight.

INTERVENTION STUDIES WITH HIGH-RISK INFANTS AND IMPLICATIONS FOR RESEARCH

In the past 15 years, several investigators have conducted experimental programs designed to prevent the developmental disabilities often associated with prematurity and low birth weight. The studies reviewed in the following paragraphs are those aimed at determining the effects of a variety of sensorimotor interventions on the behavior and development of high-risk infants.

Cornell and Gottfried (1976) reviewed the various aspects of intervention studies in a comprehensive article. Two rationales

for the studies reviewed by Cornell and Gottfried were: (1) premature (and low birth weight) infants are at high risk for developmental disabilities and (2) sensory deprivation occurs in the high-risk nursery as a result of inadequate environmental stimulation. The characteristics of the interventions were considered in terms of sensory modalities stimulated, use of singular or multisensory stimulation, and intensity, frequency, and length of stimulation.

Sensory modalities stimulated were proprioceptive, tactile, auditory, and visual. The investigators attempted to stimulate either one modality or a combination of these modalities by means of: rocking and handling; recorded voices and mothers' heartbeats; and mobiles and other visual stimuli placed in the nursery area.

The intensity, frequency, and length of stimulation varied from study to study. Cornell and Gottfried stated that the differing dimensions of stimulation among the studies reviewed appeared to indicate among the researchers a lack of agreement or knowledge or both with respect to appropriate types and levels of stimulation for the premature infant.

In the studies reviewed by Cornell and Gottfried (1976) the most common measure used to evaluate effects of stimulation on physical development was weight gain, while performance on a standardized battery of tasks such as the Neonatal Behavioral Assessment (Brazelton, 1973) was used to evaluate the effects of stimulation on behavioral development. The most inconsistent finding was weight gain while the most consistent trend was a positive effect on motor development, a subset of behavioral development.

Additional intervention studies similar in design, rationale, use of assessment measures, and findings to the experimental programs evaluated by Cornell and Gottfried include White and Labarba, 1976; Rice, 1977; Korner, Kraemer, Haffner, et al, 1975; Korner and Thoman, 1972; Kramer and Pierpont, 1976.

Following a review of the literature, many questions need further exploration: 1. What is the ideal environment for the high-risk infant? 2. Does a given type of environment promote sensory deprivation or sensory bombardment for the high-risk infant? 3. What are appropriate types, levels, and sequences of stimulation for high-risk infants? 4. What is the normal developmental progression for high-risk newborns (prematures, small for gestational age infants, infants of diabetic mothers, post-term infants)? It is critical that these questions be addressed to assist professionals in determining the result of therapeutic intervention and to inspire more effective treatment.

NEONATAL APPLICATION OF THE MULTISENSORY APPROACH TO NEUROREHABILITATION

Assessment

The medical record and parental interview are used to obtain the following information about a neonate:

1. History of the pregnancy: any known complications
2. Perinatal history
   a. Gestational age
   b. Type of labor and complications, if present
   c. Type of delivery
      APGAR scores (3 minute, 5 minute)
   d. Birth weight
   e. Occipital Frontal Circumference (OFC)
   f. Height
   g. Physical condition during the first 2 weeks of life
      (1) Acidosis
      (2) Infection
      (3) Respiratory distress
      (4) Presence of congenital anomalies
      (5) Reports of other consultants
      (6) Other
   h. Involvement of parents in neonatal care since birth
3. Physical examination at the time of initial therapy assessment
   a. Height
   b. Weight
   c. OFC
   d. Vital signs
   e. Average sleep behavior, feeding behavior
4. General precautions that may affect evaluation and treatment procedures

The Problem-Oriented Perinatal Risk Assessment System (Hobel, 1973) can be used as another means of gathering information about the neonate, and the Denver Developmental Screening Test (DDST) (Frankenburg et al, 1970) is often used as a screening tool by those in many different disciplines.

Once the general information is obtained, a more comprehensive assessment is performed. The following assessment tools should be reviewed by the NICU therapist to determine which tool best meets the needs of the program (service- or research-oriented) or of a specific neonate:

1. The Brazelton Neonatal Behavioral Assessment Scale (Brazelton, 1973)
2. The Graham-Rosenblith Behavior Test for Neonates (Rosenblith and Anderson-Huntington, 1974)
3. The Bayley Scales of infant development (Bayley, 1972)
4. A graphic method for the evaluation of motor development in infants (Zdánska-Brincken and Wolánski, 1969)
5. Gesell Developmental Schedules (Knobloch and Pasamanick, 1974)
6. The Milani-Comparetti Developmental Examination (Milani-Comparetti and Gidoni, 1967)
7. Ordinal scales of infant psychological development (Užgiris and Hunt, 1975)
8. Graham's behavioral differences between normal and traumatized newborns (Graham, 1956)
9. Reflex evaluation (Barnes, Crutchfield and Heriza, 1978)
10. Neonatal signs as predictors of cerebral palsy (Nelson and Ellenberg, 1979)
11. Feeding assessment (Chapter 3 of this text)
12. ANS assessment (see Chapter 2)
13. Sensory assessment (see Chapter 2)

After initial evaluation data is gathered, any neonate who demonstrates the following conditions is considered at risk for brain damage and is therefore a candidate for an infant normalization program.*

---

*This list was compiled from the following references: Nelson and Ellenberg, 1979; Naeye, 1979; Hobel, 1973; Jeffcoate, Humphrey, and Lloyd, 1979.

1. Abnormal muscle tone
2. Abnormal reflex development
3. Abnormal sleep-wake cycles
4. Abnormal skull size or OFC larger or smaller than normal by two to three standard deviations
5. Anoxia, hypoxia, or multiple apneic episodes
6. Asymmetrical neurological findings
7. Extended respiratory assistance
8. Extreme irritability or abnormal cry
9. Feeding dysfunction: weak or absent sucking, weight loss greater than 10 per cent from birth weight, retarded growth
10. Five-minute APGAR score less than 5 or significant drop noted between 3- and 5-minute APGAR scores
11. Jerky or myoclonic movement patterns
12. Meconium staining
13. Nonmetabolic seizure activity
14. Nystagmus
15. Severe birth trauma
16. Severe infection

Summary of Assessment Concepts. It is frequently a difficult task to assess a neonate. Assessments must be planned around the infant's feeding and care schedule. Because some assessments require large amounts of time to administer, it is often necessary to conduct these tests over several days to avoid overstimulating and fatiguing the neonate.

Even after medical stability is reached, the infant may remain connected to various monitors and have an assortment of tubes attached to diverse body parts. Additionally, uncorrected congenital malformations such as cleft palate and conditions requiring tracheotomies and gastrostomies complicate positioning and handling of the neonate. Certain areas cannot be assessed until the neonate reaches a particular gestational age. For example, muscle tone is best tested after 28 weeks; before that time passive hypotonia is observed (Lubchenco, 1976). It is also impossible to differentiate strength and muscle tone in the neonatal population (Myers, 1977). Although reflex sucking and swallowing have been observed as early as 20 weeks, nutritive sucking cannot be adequately tested until 34 weeks' gestation (Lubchenco, 1976).

Assessment of reflex development presents another dilemma. If a given reflex is not present at the time of testing, one may wonder if it has already been integrated or if it has yet to appear. *Guideline 5: As a result, one must examine the total pattern of postural reflex development instead of just looking at one isolated reflex in order to determine reflexive maturation.*

Treatment Concepts

The multisensory theory of neurorehabilitation has specific application to many populations. Analysis of the specific data, problems, and needs of a given population allows one to discriminately select appropriate treatment rationales and techniques described in Chapter 3 and other sources and apply them correctly. Perhaps *neurohabilitation* is a more expedient term to use in relation to the neonate, since we are working with a developing nervous system and trying to prevent secondary problems. The neonate has a high degree of CNS plasticity (Lund, 1978; Cotman, 1978), making it critical for therapeutic intervention to be appropriate to the infant's developmental needs. Inappropriate therapy may have prolonged deleterious effects.

Some typical treatment goals for the NICU infant include:
1. Normalization of the autonomic nervous system, including feeding and sleeping behavior.
2. Integration of postural reflexes
3. Enhancement of sensory integration
4. Enhancement of the developmental progression
5. Facilitation of social interaction (parent-infant bonding)

Additional goals may be utilized for an infant depending on the nature of his problem.

In the area of *autonomic nervous system normalization,* a variety of calming techniques have been successfully employed that are natural to the neonatal developmental experience. Rocking an infant is almost a universal calming technique employed by parents transculturally. Rocking chairs are or should be standard equipment in the NICU. When a premature infant is removed from an isolette or warmer for rocking, the parent must be taught to wrap the infant carefully to prevent temperature loss. Body fat develops during the last gestational month; therefore, the premature infant is "poorly insulated." Voluntary muscle contraction generates very little heat production in the newborn (Lubchenco, 1976). As mentioned in Chapter 3, anteroposterior rocking is used early in the treatment sequence. The baby's ventral surface is turned toward the ventral surface of the caregiver. However, a particular baby may not calm down until he is positioned so that the rocking produces a side-to-side pattern. Therefore, the use of hard and fast rules for application of rocking is not advocated. *Guideline 6: Parents and caregivers must be trained to observe infant responses following use of techniques so that the behavioral response of the neonate is used to verify the appropriateness of the intervention.*

Normal newborns spend approximately 75 per cent of their time sleeping (Lubchenco, 1976). *Guideline 7: One should not wake an infant in order to apply "sensory stimulation" just because it is the scheduled therapy time.* Sleep is a survival behavior and unless it has been determined by evaluation of sleep patterns that excessive sleep is interfering with feeding, one should allow the baby to sleep undisturbed.

When promoting normal feeding behavior in the neonate, perioral maintained touch, maintained tongue pressure, olfactory input (vanilla and banana), digital vibration of appropriate muscles, and stretch pressures are commonly used. Chapter 3 describes these procedures in depth. A prefeeding program is used with infants under 33 to 34 weeks' gestational age. Non-nutritive sucking is facilitated and then reinforced by use of a premature infant nipple pacifier. Also during this period, the neonate's hard palate and gums are stroked to simulate the motion of the tongue during sucking. Before a neonate is started on formula, 10 cc of sterile, distilled water is used as a test for "nutritive" suck-swallow coordination. If a coordinate pattern is observed, the infant may be tried on the formula or breast as recommended by the physician and the dietician.

Integration of postural reflexes may be promoted by proper handling and positioning. In cases of severe brain damage, a baby may be observed to be dominated by primitive reflexes or abnormal postural and movement patterns or by both reflexes and patterns. The longer an infant remains in a primitive reflex pattern, the harder it will be to reduce the reflex's influence. Secondary handicaps such as scoliosis, loss of joint mobility, asymmetrical head shape, and poverty of motor patterns may occur.

For the therapist wishing to *enhance sensory integration,* detailed knowledge of developing sensory systems and perceptions is required. Chapters 3 and 5 contain helpful information in this area. The state of the art is still not advanced enough to be able to describe unequivocally when one should use a given sensory modality or when multisensory stimuli are necessary. The therapist must utilize the neonate's response as the guideline to treatment. If adaptive responses are obtained (such as improvements in feeding, sleeping, and motor development) therapeutic intervention has been appropriate.

Appropriate developmental patterns are encouraged as sensory integration occurs. Handling and positioning activities that occur naturally in the normal infant environment will provide the neonate or special care infant with the opportunity to acquire those components of movement that are necessary for later skill development. These activities might include varying the infant's position throughout the day to promote the development of head and trunk righting, and movement in space appropriate to the developmental level of the infant, such as that movement which occurs as the newborn infant's mother carries, dresses, and rocks him.

Health personnel play an important role in providing support and training for parents of high-risk infants. Parental training should begin early and progress slowly and gradually while the infant is still hospitalized to prevent bombardment at the already emotional time of discharge (Yu, 1977). If parents of atypical infants can be instructed *early* to reach out to their infants and to encourage feedback from them, a cycle of communication develops that facilitates parent-infant bonding. There is a growing body of evidence that points to poor bonding as a major contributing factor in such problems as child abuse and other psychological, emotional, and developmental disturbances (Solomons, 1979; Jolly, 1978; Taft, 1978).

FOLLOW-UP PROCEDURES

When an infant is discharged from the NICU to go home or to a hospital nearer to his home, his parents are usually asked to bring the infant back to an "alumni clinic" at various time intervals for evaluation of medical and developmental status. This provides the opportunity to initiate, update, or discontinue neurorehabilitation programs according to the specific needs of the infant. *Guideline 8: The problems of each infant dictate the intensity of follow-up required.* For example, an infant without apparent handicap may return to the clinic on a yearly basis for screening, while the child with a diagnosed disability will return more often for program revision. *Guidline 9: If an infant and his family require intensive follow-up and training, referral to a local agency is desirable to allow more frequent contact between the family and health personnel involved in their program.*

Parent Support Groups. As parents learn to understand and deal with their own infants, they will be better able to provide support for other parents in the same situation through organized parent groups. These parent groups are excellent sources for encouragement and support for families after discharge from the NICU, as are the alumni follow-up clinics. Parent groups have been formed to assist other parents whose infants have died in sudden infant death syndrome or from complications of their conditions. Referral of a troubled parent to such a group may be vital.

REFERENCES

Avery CB (ed): Neonatology: Pathophysiology and Management of the Newborn. Philadelphia, J. B. Lippincott Co., 1975.

Barnes MR, Crutchfield CA, Heriza CB: The Neurophysiological Basis of Patient Treatment. Vol II. Reflexes in Motor Development. Morgantown, WVa, Stokesville Publishing Co., 1978.

Bayley N: The Bayley Scales of Infant Development. New York, Psychological Corp., 1972.

Bobath B: The very early treatment of cerebral palsy. Dev Med Child Neurol 9:373–390, 1967.

Brazelton TB: Neonatal behavioral assessment scale. Spastics International Medical Publications Monograph No. 50. London, Heinemann, 1973.

Brazelton TB: Newborn learning and the effect of appropriate stimulation. *In* L Gluck (ed): Intrauterine Asphyxia and the Developing Fetal Brain. Chicago, Year Book Medical Publishers, Inc., 1977.

Burpee B: Effect of oral stimulation in premature infants. *In* CB Heriza (ed): The Proceedings of the Comprehensive Management of Infants at Risk for CNS Defects. Chapel Hill, University of North Carolina, 1974.

Calame A et al: Psychological and neurodevelopmental outcome of high-risk newborn infants. Helv Paediat Acta 31:287–297, 1976.

Campbell SK: Facilitation of cognitive and motor development in infants with central nervous dysfunction. Phys Ther 54:346–353, 1974.

Campbell SK, Wilson J: Planning infant learning programs. Phys Ther 56:1347–1357, 1976.

Carter RE, Campbell SK: Early neuromuscular development of the premature infant. Phys Ther 55:1332–1341, 1975.

Connolly K (ed): Mechanisms of Motor Skill Development. New York, Academic Press, 1970.

Cornell EH, Gottfried AW: Intervention with premature human infants. Child Dev 47:32–39, 1976.

Cotman CW (ed): Neuronal Plasticity. New York, Raven Press, 1978.

Dunn D, Lewis AT: Some important aspects of neonatal nursing and family involvement. Pediatr Clin North Am 20:481–498, 1973.

Evans HE, Glass L: The neonatal intensive-care unit. Pediatr Annals 7:232–239, 1978.

Franco S, Andrews BF: Reduction of cerebral palsy by neonatal intensive care. Pediatr Clin North Am 24:639–649, 1977.

Frankenburg WK, Dodds JB, Fandal AW: Denver Developmental Screening Test Manual. Denver, University of Colorado Medical Center, 1970.

Graham FK: Behavioral differences between normal and traumatized newborns. I The test procedures. Psychol Monogr 70:1–16, 1956.

Hobel CJ, Hyvarinen MA, Okada DM, et al: Prenatal and intrapartum high-risk screening. I Prediction of the high risk neonate. Am J Obstet Gynecol 117:1–9, 1973.

Hoskins TA, Squires JE: Developmental assessment: a test for gross motor and reflex development. Phys Ther 53:117–126, 1973.

Illingsworth RS: The Development of the Infant and Young Child, Normal and Abnormal, 6th ed. Edinburgh, Churchill Livingstone, 1975.

Jeffcoate JA, Humphrey ME, Lloyd JK: Disturbance in parent child relationship following pre-term delivery. Dev Med Child Neurol 21:344–352, 1979.

Jolly H: The importance of bonding for newborn baby, mother . . . and father. Nurs Mirror 147:19–21, 1978.

Knobloch H, Pasamanick B (eds): Gesell and Amatruda's Developmental Diagnosis, 3rd ed. Hagerstown, Harper and Row, 1974.

Korner A, Kraemer H, Haffner M, et al: Effects of waterbed flotation on premature infants: a pilot study. Pediatrics 56:361–367, 1975.

Korner AF, Thoman EB: The relative efficacy of contact and vestibular proprioceptive stimulation in soothing infants. Child Dev 43:443–453, 1972.

Korones SB: High-risk Newborn Infants: The Basis of Intensive Nursing Care. St. Louis, C. V. Mosby Co., 1978.

Kramer LI, Pierpont ME: Rocking waterbeds and auditory stimuli to enhance growth of preterm infants. J Pediatr 88:297–299, 1976.

Lubchenco LO: The High Risk Infant. Philadelphia, W. B. Saunders Co., 1976.

Lund RD: Development and Plasticity of the Brain: An Introduction. New York, Oxford University Press, 1978.

McGraw MB: The Neuromuscular Maturation of the Human Infant. New York, Hafner Publishing Co., 1963.

Milani-Comparetti A, Gidoni EA: Routine developmental examination in normal and retarded children. Dev Med Child Neurol 9:631–638, 1967.

Moore KL: Before We Are Born: Basic Embryology and Birth Defects. Philadelphia, W. B. Saunders Co., 1974.

Myers GJ: Understanding the floppy baby. In RC Griggs and RT Moxley (eds): Advances in Neurology, Vol 17. New York, Raven Press, 1977.

Naeye RL: Underlying disorders responsible for the neonatal deaths associated with low apgar scores. Biol Neonate 35:150–155, 1979.

Nelson KB, Ellenberg JH: Neonatal signs as predictors of cerebral palsy. Pediatrics 64:225–232, 1979.

Paine RS: Early recognition of neuromotor disability in infants of low birthweight. Dev Med Child Neurol 11:455–459, 1969.

Prechtl HFR, Fargel JW, Weinmann HM, Bakker HH: Postures, motility and respiration of low-risk preterm infants. Dev Med Child Neurol 21:3–27, 1979.

Rice RD: Neurophysiological development in premature infants following stimulation. Dev Psychobiol 13:69–76, 1977.

Robinson RT (ed): Brain and Early Behavior. New York, Academic Press, 1969.

Rosenblith JF, Anderson-Huntington R: Behavioral examination of the neonate. In CB Heriza (ed): Comprehensive Management of Infants at Risk for CNS Deficits. Chapel Hill, University of North Carolina, 1974.

Saint-Anne, Dargassies S: Neurological maturation of the premature infant of 28–41 weeks gestational age. In F Falkner (ed): Human Development. Philadelphia, W. B. Saunders Co., 1966.

Scarr-Salapatek S, Williams ML: The effects of early stimulation on low-birth weight infants. Child Dev 44:94–101, 1973.

Schaffer AJ, Avery ME: Diseases of the Newborn, 4th ed. Philadelphia, W. B. Saunders Co., 1977.

Solomons G: Child abuse and developmental disabilities. Dev Med Child Neurol 21:101–108, 1979.

Stone LJ, Church J: Childhood and Adolescence, 4th ed. New York, Random House, 1979.

Taft LT: Child development: prenatal to early childhood. J Sch Health 48:281–287, 1978.

Thompson T, Reynolds J: The results of intensive care therapy for newborns,. J Perinat Med 5:59–75, 1977.

Tjossem TD (ed): Intervention Strategies for High Risk Infants and Young Children. Baltimore, University Park Press, 1976.

Uzgiris IC, Hunt J: Assessment in Infancy: Ordinal Scales of Psychological Development. Chicago, University of Illinois Press, 1975.

White JL, Labarba R: Effects of tactile and kinesthetic stimuli on neonatal development in premature infants. Dev Psychobiol 9(6):569–577, 1976.

Yu V: Caring for parents of high-risk infants. Med J Aust 2:534–537, 1977.

Zdańska-Brincken M, Wolański N: A graphic method for the evaluation of motor development in infants. Dev Med Child Neurol 11:228–241, 1969.

CHAPTER 5

SENSORIMOTOR INTEGRATION THEORY AND THE MULTISENSORY APPROACH

Zona R. Weeks, MS, OTR

The purpose of this chapter is to provide a foundation for understanding the relationship between sensory integrative dysfunction and sensorimotor integrative therapy. The multisensory approach to sensorimotor integrative therapy is discussed in the context of several areas of practice: brain damage and minimal brain dysfunction, learning disabilities, emotional disturbances, mental retardation and cerebrovascular accident (CVA). Neurophysiological information and treatment principles presented earlier in the book apply to the multisensory treatment approach advocated in this chapter. Literature research findings are presented that demonstrate the application of neurophysiological information to the multisensory approach and that indicate areas for further development. Thus, concepts of development and treatment that have appeared earlier in the book are synthesized.

Terminology

The term *sensory integration* has been widely used to explain the process that occurs within the CNS when sensations from one or more types of sensory receptors are received. In brief, sensory integration means that sensations are coordinated, filtered, and interpreted in relationship to the individual's needs to perceive and act in response to the human and nonhuman environment.

Sensorimotor refers to the interrelationship between the sensory and motor systems of the body. The systems are highly interdependent, with sensory input affecting voluntary and involuntary motor output, and with movement causing increased sensory input. Sensorimotor treatment techniques are used to enhance CNS inte-

gration. *Sensorimotor* and *sensory integration* can in many instances be combined into one term, *sensorimotor integration*, because the sensory and motor systems are so closely interrelated neurophysiologically that it is difficult to speak of one without the other in human performance. Therefore, the term *sensorimotor integration* will be used in discussions of the multisensory treatment approach, except in discussion of underlying sensory integrative processing or of tests and approaches labeled *sensory integration* by their developers. The author believes that the term sensorimotor integration seems to fit the process of treatment, in that the sensory input usually results in a motor response followed by sensory feedback and motor modification. Others, including Ayres (1972), prefer to use the term sensory integrative therapy; they emphasize that the internal organization and integration in the CNS is the most important factor, and motor output is merely a visible means of inferring some change in sensory integration.

Behavior and Sensorimotor Integration

Behavior may be thought of partially in terms of input and responses. Input refers to stimuli reaching the individual through the various sensory channels: visual, auditory, tactile, proprioceptive, olfactory, gustatory, pain, and temperature. Input leads to responses or reactions, some of which are purely mental operations or other unseen CNS occurrences, while others are visible in behavior. Responses may be classified as gross and fine motor (including both voluntary and reflexive responses) and cognitive (including problem-solving and other thought processes with or without language, and social or psychological reactions). Behavior thus develops through a sequence of stimuli and responses, which, in turn, act as stimuli. If the neuromotor process is defective or if the natural environment does not provide sufficient and appropriate stimulation, experiences must be artificially provided to assist the desired development.

The multisensory approach as it applies to sensorimotor integrative therapy refers to the knowledgeable use of sensory stimuli to bring about improvement in an array of behavioral manifestations caused by inability of the CNS to properly filter, organize, and process incoming sensory data.

The Effect of Sensory Integrative Dysfunction

Various disorders resulting from problems in sensory reception, transmission and integration, or resulting from inadequate environmental stimulation, appear to respond to similar sensorimotor integrative therapy. Among these disorders are learning disabilities, severe or minimal brain dysfunction (MBD), emotional disturbances, and mental retardation.

Inaccurate sensory input due to abnormalities in peripheral sensory reception or transmission can interfere with sensory integration. Disordered central or peripheral neurological functioning frequently leads to difficulties in effective motor responses because of the reliance on sensory data for planning and carrying out movements. The severe CNS damage that results in motor functioning problems in persons with diagnoses of cerebral palsy, cerebral vascular accidents, and related conditions can lead to sensory integrative difficulties. Individuals with CNS degenerative diseases, tumors, traumatic brain injuries, and related disorders are also potential prime candidates for sensory integrative problems.

Recovery through sensorimotor treatment may be hampered if sensory input and integration needed for motor control are not adequate. Deviations in CNS functioning may also be manifested in a number of cognitive problems, as well as in such problems as lack of ability to attend, and abnormal activity level (Clements, 1973).

Perception refers to the ability to acquire knowledge through the senses and implies recognition of sensory input by the CNS. Awareness of the proper meaning of sensory input is necessary to develop concepts about one's environment and to make adaptive responses to it. The term *perceptual-motor dysfunction* concerns the inability to accurately perceive and interpret sensory stimuli, as well as the individual's frequently ineffective motor responses to these stimuli. Movement based on erroneous perceptions is likely to be poorly carried out. Inaccurate visual perception or deficient awareness of limb positions, for example, may lead to ineffective muscle movement. "Perceptual-motor dysfunction" is in current use by educators and others as an all-encompassing term, whereas sensory integrationists consider the perceptual-motor area of function to be a subheading under sensory integrative dysfunction.

Neurophysiological Rationale for Sensorimotor Integrative Therapy

Sensorimotor integrative treatment using a logical multisensory approach is based on knowledge of sensory and motor neurological development, sensorimotor interrelationships, and perceptual development that can be applied to various categories of CNS-impaired individuals. The common causes of CNS dysfunction are thought to arise from functional irregularities of unknown etiology, biochemical abnormalities, genetically atypical development, or frank brain trauma. The intent of treatment is to correct underlying dysfunction by providing selected sensory input of the type and amount necessary to advance CNS integration and organization.

DEVELOPMENT AS A BASIS FOR SENSORIMOTOR INTEGRATIVE THERAPY

Evaluation in sensorimotor integrative therapy is based partially on developmental considerations. Development encompasses the full range of human behavior.

The psychological and social areas have certain characteristic milestones of development, just as do the sensory, motor, and cognitive areas. Adequate sensorimotor and perceptual abilities are necessary for successful performance of many age-related developmental tasks in each of these areas of development. The concept that each stage of development provides a foundation for later stages is supported by observations of normal development.

Sensorimotor Development

Every person develops to a certain level or degree of skill in sensorimotor function. One child may progress smoothly through the stages of development while the developmental milestones of another may be delayed. Lack of progress may be due to such factors as abnormal neurological development or insufficient sensorimotor experiences, among other possible causes. For coordinate movement, one must have not only a functional nervous system but also adequate bone structure, muscle strength, and range of motion (O'Connell and Gardner, 1967). In the treatment of sensorimotor integrative dysfunction, knowledge of all facets of human movement and its development is necessary in order to understand and be able to attempt correction of abnormal movement conditions.

From the time of conception, factors begin to operate that will have a bearing on later coordinate movement. Prenatal development is being carefully studied by researchers to help in understanding the progression of normal motor development and the occurrence of abnormalities of movement (Campbell, 1974; Jacobs, 1967). Movement development in prenatal life, which is particularly influenced by the early-developing tactile and vestibular systems (see Chapter 3), assures that the normal infant will be born with a characteristic set of movements and responses. When studied closely, the movements of the young infant show a pattern (Stone and Church, 1979). Throughout the neonatal months, controlled voluntary movements will be superimposed upon the early reflexive movements. During infancy and early childhood reflexes will be inhibited and integrated into the motor system as

more advanced reflexes emerge. Neuro-muscular maturation occurs, and life experiences provide opportunities for motor planning and strengthening. Appropriate life experiences also assist sensory and perceptual development, and this leads to enhancement of motor development.

Waterland (1967) discusses three components of skilled movement: (1) sensory input from within and outside the body, (2) reflexes elicited in association with purposeful acts, and (3) voluntary movements that may be cortically directed. Poor or unskilled movement is said to be dominated by cortical control, while skilled movement is the result of integration and balance of willed and reflexive actions. Reflex movements can at times be appropriately used in treatment as a means of developing muscle tone and inhibiting antagonists, thus leading to more coordinate movement (O'Connell and Gardner, 1967; Huss, 1971).

A good environment stimulates, provides repetition to allow categorization and integration of perceptions, and gives opportunity for motor responses. Natural environmental experiences are sufficient for adequate development in most children, but some may need specially structured experiences. If one part of the network is missing, it must be artificially provided to elicit responses. Super (1976) found that motor milestones in normal infants (as creeping or walking) appeared earlier than expected when effective sensorimotor stimulation was provided during care practices, and Molnar (1974) demonstrated that motor milestones in infants appeared soon after the underlying reflexes affecting them developed. Treatment designed to bring about reflex maturation is often useful in sensorimotor integration therapy.

Perceptual Development

Researchers have detailed a partial hierarchy of perceptual abilities as they develop with age and experience, but age relationships for many abilities are not firmly established. Many gaps still exist in perceptual development knowledge.

The human infant is born with certain capacities that can enable him to begin making perceptual sense of his environment. Some of his capacities are merely reflexive survival skills—for example, sucking and grasp. Other capacities include inherent perceptual modes of action, such as a predisposition to track moving objects and attend to entire patterns or certain features of forms, and some apparent awareness of depth (Stone and Church, 1979). By using these capacities the infant increases the sensory input he receives and learns that certain consistent sensations follow various actions on his part. Experiences that are repeated give him an opportunity to test and retest his sensations and perceptions and to form concepts about his physical world. Novel situations allow him opportunities to expand his sensory awareness and capabilities. Sensory stimuli are essential to development, and lack of adequate stimulation can lead to impaired perceptual development (Silverman, 1974).

From these early beginnings, perceptual development progresses throughout childhood. A young child is perceptually dependent upon each stimulus, but cognitive development allows the child to advance to systematic methods of gathering information and developing generalizations and concepts. Concepts of same and different, of directions such as up and down, of categories of shapes, of objects appearing different at a distance, and so forth, require sensory impressions that are perceived in certain ways enough times to form accurate concepts about environmental stimuli.

Once sufficient concepts are formed, the child has a cognitive structure by which he can judge new perceptual experiences and either decide that they are consonant with old concepts or that they require explanation in order to fit with new concepts. The child also learns that illusions sometimes occur, such as of movement when there is none, of apparent color changes because of the level of the sun, and so forth. Misperceptions can result from inadequate or conflicting information, lack of sufficient intensity of a stimulus, overintensity (in which pain over-rides perception), blurring of visual stimuli, masking of auditory stimuli by other sounds, and similar conditions (Gibson, 1966). Children learn to attend to distinctive features of stimuli, they learn about invariant perceptual occurrences

that help them develop notions of perceptual constancy and permanence, and they develop higher-order structures and rules (Gibson, 1969). In addition, perceptual learning is enhanced through language, whereby perceptual features are labeled, explained, or described, and put into categories.

The same principles that seem to be operating in other kinds of learning are believed to operate in perceptual learning (Epstein, 1967). Validation through sensory experiences helps the child to learn truths about movement, touch, pressure, sight, sound, taste, smell, pain, and temperature. Sensations from one sensory modality are compared with sensations from other modalities, so that a total picture of the environment and its contents is formed by intersensory processes. *Intersensory integration* is a term sometimes used in reference to this process. Intersensory comparison ability improves with age in children (Bartley, 1969). (See Multisensory or Cross-Modal Stimuli, Chapter 3.)

Perceptual development trends occur because of the interaction of maturation and environmental experience. Gibson (1969) describes three trends in perceptual development: (1) discrimination becomes more specific, with fewer errors and decreasing reaction times; (2) attention strategies change, becoming more exploratory, systematic, selective, and exclusive; and (3) efficiency increases in gaining information from stimulation and in discovering relationships that stay constant despite certain changes, such as movements of an object or person, and so forth.

SENSORIMOTOR INTEGRATION ASSESSMENT

Purpose of Assessment

The purpose of assessment prior to sensorimotor integrative therapy using a multisensory approach is to pinpoint the performance deficits and, when possible, determine the presumed reasons for the problems noted. Other reasons for assessment in general are discussed in Chapter 2. Assessment procedures determine the nature of the symptoms, and interpretation of assessment results helps to relate the symptoms to underlying sensorimotor integrative deficiencies, when present.

Assessment Areas

Assessment prior to sensorimotor integration therapy should include an evaluation of:

1. Reflex and voluntary motor functioning, including developmental levels
2. Sensory receptor inadequacies
3. Central sensory integration deficiencies
4. Disorders of perception and perceptual developmental levels
5. Speech and language deficiencies
6. Academic strengths and weaknesses, if pertinent
7. Social and emotional functioning
8. Activity level.

Some of these areas of evaluation overlap. An ideal assessment requires interdisciplinary team participation. The individual working alone will be able to use assessment techniques for which he is qualified, seeking outside consultation when necessary.

Evaluation of perceptual abilities is difficult without a "normal" point of reference. Norms are available for certain standardized tests purporting to measure perceptual, perceptual-motor, and sensory integrative functions. However, many abilities cannot at this time be tested, and it is sometimes difficult with tests presently available to obtain a valid, clear picture of overall dysfunction.

Developmental tests allow the examiner to determine levels of development and to pinpoint areas of lag. A classic work was Gesell's developmental appraisal (Knobloch and Pasamanick, 1974), used primarily for evaluating motor, adaptive, language, and personal-social behavior in children from birth through the early childhood years. A number of developmental evaluations were developed with Gesell's work as a basis. Later researchers, such as White (1975) and Caplan and Caplan (1977), have published careful assessment charts for behavioral comparison during infancy and early childhood. One of the first comprehensive tests for newborn behavior was the test developed by Graham (1952). Rosenblith (1974) modified the Graham test and separated the items into subscores, which helped in finding more relations to later behavior.

Brazleton developed the Neonatal Behavioral Assessment Scale (Brazelton, 1973).

All of these scales help to determine which infants are likely to suffer from some type of developmental deficit as they grow. Delay in acquisition of many developmental milestones usually indicates underlying nervous system disorder, which may manifest itself in mental retardation, cerebral palsy, or less easily identifiable problems as some emotional disturbances or learning disabilities. However, rigid use of developmental charts can be a naive practice, since there are wide discrepancies in developmental behaviors in many normal children.

Determination of dysfunctional sensory systems is aided by tests of sensory, motor, sensory integrative, perceptual, and perceptual-motor development. Some psychometric, language, and academic evaluation instruments also provide information about sensory and intersensory functioning that is helpful in remediation. A list of some of these tests is provided in the Appendix. Catalogues from test publishing houses may be studied to determine appropriateness of various tests for particular problems.

Because of the evidence for a neurological basis in many cases of sensorimotor dysfunction, therapists utilizing a sensorimotor integrative approach include assessment of certain neurological signs in their evaluations. Some of these signs are the same as soft signs that will be discussed under the heading *Medical Evaluation*. Structured (partly standardized) and unstructured (informal) clinical observations give important behavioral clues to sensory integration and to reflex development. Some of these observations involve screening for immature reflex development and muscle tone and movement abnormalities, while others assess eye dominance and ocular movements. These observations are then taken into consideration during interpretation of sensory integrative and other tests.

Evaluation of Changes from Sensorimotor Integrative Therapy

Ongoing evaluation during the course of therapy provides evidence of positive change or lack of it. Observations of performance and responses to sensory stimuli are used to infer that changes in sensory integrative ability are occurring.

CNS normalization is indicated in part by (1) improvement of reflex development, (2) improvement of voluntary motor functioning, (3) improvement in perceptual and cognitive processes, and (4) signs of improved functioning of the various sensory systems. These might include greater tactile awareness or less tactile defensiveness, improvement of kinesthetic awareness and accuracy of movement, improvement of balance that shows more adequate vestibular system functioning, improvement of ocular control, improvement in differentiating and localizing sounds, and improvement in language abilities such as speech and reading.

Progress in treatment is shown not only by improvement in sensory and motor functioning but also by social-emotional changes that help the subject improve his self-concept and behave in more socially acceptable ways. Changes should be validated by re-evaluation using the same measurement instruments and methods used in initial assessments, with results recorded as objectively as possible on forms developed for the purpose.

Examples of Tests Used in Sensorimotor Integrative Assessment

Ayres developed the Southern California Sensory Integration Tests (1972) and the Southern California Postrotary Nystagmus Test (1975) to aid in assessment of children with sensory integrative dysfunction, and the interpretation of the results provides a basis for treatment planning. The tests have sometimes been used with adults, but results must be interpreted in a judgmental way, since the test was standardized only on children. Pretreatment and post-treatment test results provide comparison scores to show whether or not improvement has occurred.

Ornitz et al (1977) have detailed a behavioral evaluation for autistic children, which measures disturbances of perception, motility, and relating to persons or objects. The degree to which various fac-

tors in these categories are present is rated on a scale from 1 to 5.

Gerardot and Dossett (1977) have described a number of observations of physical appearance and psychomotor behavior that they found in autistic children. Although there is no standardized test to evaluate these characteristics, the information would be useful in assessing autistic children for sensorimotor integrative therapy.

Schroeder et al (1978) have developed The Schroeder, Block, Campbell Adult Psychiatric Sensory Integration Evaluation (SBC) as an aid to comprehensive assessment of sensory and motor responses of psychiatric patients. Although the test has no norms, procedures are precise enough to allow data collection and comparison of results among subjects who are evaluated by this assessment instrument.

Siev and Freishtat (1976) suggest assessment techniques for adults with cerebrovascular accidents (CVAs), using commercially available and clinic-designed tests. Some of these tests are nonstandardized, but they provide a means of detecting gross perceptual abnormalities commonly found in brain-injured persons.

Problems in Evaluation

Evaluation of persons with sensorimotor integrative dysfunction is difficult, presenting some unique problems. Responses may be unusual, and distractibility or hyperactivity may interfere with the testing process and preclude obtaining valid results. Observation of general behavior and performance on as many structured tasks as possible may be the only way to evaluate some of these persons. The comprehension required to perform many of the tasks on commercially available perceptual and sensory integration tests would be too advanced for general use with this population. In addition to problems in testing persons with limited mental ability, special adaptations must also be made for the deaf, persons with aphasia, those with certain motor handicaps, and so forth. The creative therapist can overcome some of these testing problems, but there will be persons who are impossible to test, just as there are those who are not feasible candidates for sensorimotor integrative therapy.

Academic Evaluation in Learning Disabilities

A number of tests have been used to determine areas of weakness in abilities necessary for academic performance. Many of these instruments assess the visual, auditory, and motor abilities that are needed for effective reading and writing. Vocal and written responses are studied to help define particular problems. Those tests purporting to measure reading abilities frequently evaluate function in combined sensory channels. They help the examiner assess the individual's ability to integrate incoming sensations and to make the appropriate sensory associations and matches. Characteristic patterns of responses have been related to specific sensorimotor integrative deficits. Some tests evaluate computational skills, but less is written regarding the contribution of specific sensory processing to abilities required in this area.

Labeling a child as learning disabled should be done after careful evaluation. Psychological effects of classifying a child can be unpredictable — sometimes favorable, sometimes unfavorable. Especially frightening to parents are terms such as neurological dysfunction or minimal brain dysfunction, given as reasons for a learning disability, even when accompanied by an explanation that the terms do not necessarily mean "damage, " only disordered or inefficient functioning.

How precise should a diagnosis be? Should children be given complete neurological and neurophysiological examinations to try to pinpoint areas of dysfunction? Would results of these examinations help in educational remediation, or are remediation theories and methods too ill-defined at present to benefit from in-depth neurological evaluations?

Denckla (1973) believes that neurological examination is useful in therapeutic programming for learning disabled children. A syndrome diagnosis, if possible, is a first step toward educational or pharmacological prescription. In addition, the neurologist can suggest relationships between childhood signs and known adult syndromes, especially when the same behavioral complaint is present. These comparisons are helpful in determining relevant brain mechanisms, Denckla believes. However, deQuiros (1978) believes that comparison with adult symptoms is not always valid, particularly in children below the age of 5. On the other hand, some educators seem to think that medical diagnosis can be bypassed (Adams, 1975; Divoky, 1973).

Black (1976) does not believe that there is any educational usefulness in using "brain-damage" labels. He found that, although children with suspected neurological dysfunction scored higher than those with documented neurological dysfunction on intellectual measures, there were no appreciable differences on perceptual, academic, and two of three behavioral variables in his study. Documented neurological dysfunction in his study included hemiplegia, cerebral palsy, and treated seizure disorders. Since both groups of children showed similar academic deficiencies, he believes that they should respond to similar remedial methods without the necessity of emphasizing differential diagnosis. In a study of 100 children with learning or behavioral problems or both referred because of suspected minimal brain dysfunction, Kenny and Clemmens (1971) found no significant commonality in results of medical or neurological examinations and electroencephalograms. Since final diagnosis was more dependent upon symptoms and psychological studies, they concluded that routine referral of learning disabled or behavior problem children for neurological examination or electroencephalograms is not necessary (Kenny and Clemmens, 1971). In any event, academic remediation programs are based more at present on educational test findings than on neurological findings. Educational labels must therefore be precise in order to be useful in remediation.

Thus, while identification of any individual with a learning disability is certainly important, so that remediation measures may be initiated, the advantage of differentiating those individuals with evident aberrant neurological signs from those without remains controversial.

Specific neurological and neuropsychological delineations of dysfunction would be helpful to occupational, physical, and speech therapists who work in schools. They may not be as helpful to many educators, unless they are interpreted in terms of teaching implications. The author believes that assessment of neurological functioning often leads to better understanding of learning, motor, and other behavioral problems, thus leading to better selection of remediation methods. For example, auditory-visual integration problems could make learning to read difficult, pathological reflexes might interfere with handwriting ability, and stereognostic deficits could hinder learning of geometric shapes by manipulation.

Medical Evaluation

Many children and adults referred to individual therapists or to clinics providing sensorimotor integrative therapy have been evaluated medically. Some may be under continuing close medical supervision for the duration of their therapy. Persons with diagnoses reflective of brain damage or minimal brain dysfunction have obviously received those labels from a physician. Physicians have become increasingly involved in evaluating children for suspected medical factors in learning disabilities, and evaluating both children and adults for such factors in emotional disturbances.

For a child, the medical history should include developmental, psychological, and social information. The parents' description of the child's behavior is important. A complete physical examination including a neurological assessment may be indicated, and tests for visual acuity, ocular movements, and color vision are frequently performed. Poor vision may interfere with school learning requirements.

Neurological examinations focus primarily on sensory and motor system functioning and on "hard" neurological signs. Hard signs are seen in cerebral palsy and cerebrovascular accidents, among numerous other conditions resulting from definite CNS lesions. Electroencephalographic (EEG) findings are at times abnormal or irregular in all of the conditions under study

in this chapter, but significance of the findings is often obscure. "Soft" neurological signs may indicate some neurological deviation from normal, but they do not localize lesions (Quitkin et al, 1976).

In addition to looking for hard and soft neurological signs and physical anomalies possibly associated with CNS dysfunction, other factors may be investigated. Allergies to some natural foods and intolerance to artificial additives have been implicated as possible causes of hyperactivity and distractibility in certain individuals. Biochemical studies in autistic and schizophrenic children and adults have sometimes revealed abnormalities (Schneider and Tarshis, 1975).

Physical anomalies are evaluated in some medical assessments and have been investigated in connection with a number of diagnostic conditions. Certain physical anomalies have been associated for many years with specific types of mental retardation. More recently, work has been done that suggests relationships between physical anomalies and mild conduct disturbances. In the realm of more severe behavioral problems, schizophrenic children are also reported to have a significantly higher incidence of physical anomalies than do normal children (Waldrop et al, 1968).

Multiple minor physical anomalies were found to be associated with hyperkinetic, aggressive, impatient, and intractable behavior in otherwise normal 2½-year-old children by Waldrop et al (1968). Anomalies in this study included two or more hair whorls, "electric hair" (hair that stands on end), epicanthus, hypertelorism, ear abnormalities, tongue abnormalities, high palate, and finger or toe abnormalities. These anomalies are commonly seen in children with Down's syndrome as well.

Physical anomalies have been found in association with certain abnormal motor manifestations in children, such as poor coordination, head banging, and hyperactivity, among other disturbances (Halverson and Victor, 1976). Minor physical anomalies mentioned in the cited article refer to head circumference beyond normal range, widely spaced eyes, epicanthal folds, curved fifth finger, and wide gaps between first and second toes.

It is believed by some researchers that physical anomalies may reflect embryological developmental errors (Halverson and Victor, 1976; Waldrop et al, 1968). Certain defects are hypothesized to be associated with genetic transmission or with teratogenic factors operating in the first few weeks of pregnancy. These same factors apparently also produce CNS abnormalities that may contribute to behavioral problems or developmental deviations.

Neuropsychological Evaluation

Detailed neuropsychological evaluations are frequently conducted on persons with known or suspected brain lesions. Neuropsychological measures are designed to assess brain-behavior relationships (Lezak, 1976). Behavioral indicators are sought through examination of intelligence, memory, and comprehension, as well as by the use of tests that may provide localization clues, information on language function, and other neurological evidence of dysfunction. Walsh (1978) describes some of the purposes of this form of assessment. Such measures help to establish neurological diagnosis by discerning cerebral impairments, with lateralization and localization of lesions possible in some instances. Subtle impairments that may be missed in neurological evaluation may be detected. Documentation of mental functions and deficits leads to increased understanding of patients' areas of difficulty and their rehabilitation needs. Through neuropsychological evaluation, effects of neurosurgery, drug therapy, and rehabilitation efforts can be evaluated by objective scientific means.

Swiercinsky (1979) lists eight factors in analysis of a neuropsychological battery of tests used for assessment of organic brain damage: general verbal information processing (considered representative primarily of dominant hemisphere functioning), spatial relations skill, visual motor coordination, bilateral tactile acuity, bilateral gross motor speed, motor strength, chronological age (reflecting maturation, experience, or other cerebral changes occurring as a function of age), and eye and hand dominance. This factor structure, because of exclusion of some available tests, did not include some areas found in previous analyses by other researchers — those of

receptive and expressive speech, auditory processing, memory functions, concentration, and symbolic or abstract information processing. Knowledge of these factors of neuropsychological functioning provides insight into behavior observed in brain-damaged individuals particularly. An interesting point is that Swiercinsky found behavioral similarities in this analysis of neuropsychological performance between brain-damaged patients and those having psychiatric disorders without labels of brain damage.

REVIEW OF THE LITERATURE

When reviewing the literature related to brain damage and minimal brain dysfunction, learning disabilities, emotional disturbances, and mental retardation one finds many similarities among the disorders. It would appear that the commonalities in these conditions are the result of neurological factors not yet fully understood, although a number of hypotheses have been advanced to explain the perceptual, cognitive, motor, and emotional problems individuals with these conditions experience.

Soft Signs as Indications of Dysfunction

It has become more common in recent years to see research reports including evaluation of soft signs in learning disabled and emotionally disturbed individuals, with inferences made that these signs may point to neurological dysfunction as the causative agent in these problems. Varied selections of soft signs are used by different researchers. It should be recognized that soft neurological signs are sometimes present in individuals demonstrating no apparent problems in life functioning.

Soft signs have been found to be more prevalent in persons with CNS dysfunction than in the general population. It is logical to expect more hard and soft signs in persons with known brain damage, but evidence indicates that there are also more neurological signs in persons with learning disabilities, mental retardation, and psychiatric disturbances (Hertzig and Birch, 1966, 1968). Minimal brain dysfunction (MBD) is therefore inferred in many research reports investigating these conditions. (The term minimal brain dysfunction has been generally reserved for those individuals who do not have severe enough damage to lower their intelligence to subnormal ranges (Clements, 1973).)

Critchley (1970) states that many soft signs are related to incomplete maturation of the nervous system, being more evident in younger children. He stresses that no set combination of deficits can be considered indicative of pathology. The consensus in the literature appears to be that no single soft sign can be associated, for example, with learning disabilities. Rather, groups of soft signs have been associated with academic learning problems, but the lists are inconsistent from study to study. However, some signs appear to be more predictive or indicative of dysfunction than others. With further research the lists should become more discrete and therefore more useful. Variations from normal by age are not yet fully defined, and precise criteria for evaluating the presence and intensity of the signs are not available for all signs.

In investigations with children having suspected MBD a variety of soft signs have been identified. DeHaven et al (1969) found that deficits of distal alternate motion rate were pertinent to the diagnosis of MBD. These motions were finger wiggle, finger-to-finger opposition, foot patting rate, and heel-toe walking with eyes closed. Twitchell et al (1966) showed that motor defects are common in children with minimal cerebral dysfunction. One abnormality noted by Twitchell et al was overpronation of the hands with arms outstretched, often in combination with wrist flexion and finger extension. This hand overpronation could be facilitated for testing purposes by light contact stimulation on the ulnar border, leading also to total arm raising in some cases. This pattern was identified as the avoiding response, and it was further evidenced by problems in making rapid alternating movements and performing serial opposition of the fingers and thumb. During alternating movements a pronation tendency was apparent, and in serial opposition flexion was

deficient and extension was exaggerated. Other difficulties included problems with visual fixation and search, facial and tongue movements, and, less commonly, heel-tapping and gait. Walking on the heels intensified postural abnormalities seen in the upper extremities. *Synkinesis* (involuntary movement of a body part occurring at the same time as a reflex or voluntary movement of another body part) was also commonly seen.

All of these motor symptoms are normal in the course of development, but should not be apparent beyond the ages when they normally disappear. Twitchell et al found none in normal children beyond 9 years of age.

An interesting association between soft signs and academic abilities has been noted. Galante et al (1972) found that all the poor readers in their study had at least six soft signs, whereas only a few children reading at or above grade level showed six or more. Eaves et al (1974), by testing sensation, cranial nerve function, nystagmus, associated movements, praxis, and other factors, correctly predicted kindergartners' later readiness for third grade.

Minimal Brain Dysfunction and Learning Disorders

Low birth weight has been studied as one possible cause of MBD. Some researchers have reported finding an association and others have not. Lee (1977) found that children who were of low weight at birth (less than 5 lbs or 2268 gm) scored lower on perceptual-motor performance tasks than did children of medium and high birth weights. The perceptual-motor categories measured included body image, balance, laterality, directionality, locomotor ability, and eye-hand coordination. Of these, the low birth weight children scored significantly lower on tasks involving body image, balance, and locomotor ability. The implication is that low birth weight may be associated with these problems because of possible neurological damage.

Minimal brain dysfunction syndrome and hyperactivity syndrome are sometimes used synonymously in the literature, although MBD is a term that encompasses numerous behavioral consequences, one of which may be hyperactivity. Hyperactivity is a frequent symptom of MBD, but normal activity level or excessively quiet behavior characterizes some individuals with known or suspected MBD (Hopkins and Smith, 1978; Small, 1973).

Minimal brain dysfunction is considered to be the underlying problem in many learning disabled and emotionally disturbed children and adults. Silver (1971) prefers the term neurological learning disability syndrome over MBD when referring to children having apparent neurologically based learning disabilities. He divides such children's problems into two basic areas: (1) relating to the environment and (2) receiving, processing, storing, and expressing information. Secondary emotional problems may also occur, he asserts. Silver further proposes that one form of the neurological learning disability syndrome may be the result of an inherited type of nervous system predisposing to a neurohumeral imbalance. The fact that certain brain hormones and peptides have been shown to improve attention and memory, among other abilities (Treichel, 1976), lends credence to such a theory.

Denckla (1973), in her neurology practice devoted to learning disabled children, has observed certain syndromes repeatedly: (1) behavior disorder with unfocused hyperactivity, distractibility, poor attention span and/or poor impulse control; (2) learning disorder in school subjects dominated by language content (including reading, spelling, verbal memorization, and following instructions); (3) learning disorder confined to language arts skills (reading and spelling); (4) learning disorder with complaints restricted to coordination skills (athletics, handwriting, self-care tasks); (5) learning disorder only in arithmetic (rare). Numbers 1 and 4 are frequently seen together as chief complaints; numbers 2, 3, and 5 are seen in combination with moderate frequency, as are numbers 1 and 2.

The combination of number 5 with difficulties in spelling, writing, and spatial relations ability is like a developmental Gerstmann syndrome. The Gerstmann syndrome in adults with acquired left parietal lobe damage includes deficits in writing (*agraphia*), calculating (*acalculia*), finger identification (*finger agnosia*), and right-left confusion. The "developmental" adjective is used to indicate that these four functions did not emerge when they were expected during maturation with age.

Sixty-four per cent of learning disabled children with difficulties confined to reading and spelling were right-handed, right-footed, and left-eyed for sighting. In this same example, Denckla determined that these right-handed children showed slowness of left hand finger movements in comparison to the right. Since right and left hand finger movements are normally virtually identical, this is a significant finding.

Sensorimotor integrative therapy has been widely used with learning-disordered children suspected of having minor neurological deficits. However, not all those with neurologically based learning disorders seem to benefit from therapy to enhance sensory integration. Evaluation is used to distinguish those who might benefit from those who would probably be better served by a special education program. Research by Ayres (1976), as reported later in the chapter, in the discussion of efficacy of sensorimotor integration treatment, elaborates some characteristics of candidates best suited for sensorimotor integrative therapy or special education programs.

Emotional Disturbances Associated with Learning Disabilities and Minimal Brain Dysfunction

Clements (1973) provides a list of the 10 most frequently cited characteristics of learning disabled children:
1. Hyperactivity
2. Perceptual-motor impairment
3. Emotional lability
4. General coordination deficits
5. Disorders of attention (short attention span, distractibility, perseveration)
6. Impulsivity
7. Disorders of memory and thinking
8. Specific learning disabilities (reading, arithmetic, writing, spelling)
9. Disorders of speech and hearing
10. Equivocal neurological signs and electroencephalographic irregularities (Clements, 1973)

It is immediately apparent from this list that emotional and other aspects of behavior are included along with learning difficulties.

Associations between emotional disturbances and learning disorders have been pointed out by a number of authors. Apparent perceptual-motor and sensory integrative dysfunction has been found in many children in both groups. Neurological signs indicative of possible dysfunction have been identified in children and adults with emotional disturbances.

Studies with children having emotional disturbance using the Ayres' Southern California Sensory Integration Tests (SCSIT) (1972) have resulted in interesting findings. Llorens, in a study of hospitalized emotionally disturbed children, found that all showed some degree of dysfunction. These children were selected for testing from the total inpatient population because of deficiencies in motor control and coordination as found during a routine occupational therapy initial evaluation. They also had learning problems, as determined by at least one year's retardation on standardized academic achievement tests. Llorens (1968) reports that perceptual-motor dysfunction was present at any given time in 50 to 75 per cent of the emotionally disturbed children admitted to their clinic over a six-year period. Llorens found both developmental apraxia and integration of body sides dysfunction in these hospitalized children, as well as problems with visual figure-ground, form and position in space, and tactile defensiveness (Llorens, 1968).

Weeks (1977) found sensory integrative dysfunction in a group of nine children with emotional problems severe enough to require hospitalization. Sensory integrative dysfunction was determined on the basis of individual testing on the Southern California Sensory Integrative Tests (1972).

Schizophrenia and Autism

Testing with schizophrenic and autistic children has demonstrated that they often appear to be deficient in perceptual-motor skills. Goldfarb (1964) has reported that schizophrenic children are not different in their visual and auditory *acuity* from normal children, but that they are impaired in organization of sensory stimuli into forms and patterns, ability to differentiate body cues (needed to develop body image), and are deficient in conceptual functions (higher processes). They are also inferior in psychomotor responses. Defective body image is a paramount characteristic of schizophrenic children (Fisher, 1970). Birch et al (1964) state that the argument for existence of a primary neurologic defect is most marked for schizophrenic patients who have histories of notable childhood behavior disturbances. Findings that differentiated this group of patients from other schizophrenic patients included memory disturbance, thinking disorders, low IQ, and preponderance of males, all of which hint at a nervous system defect.

Researchers have found an increased incidence of neurological signs in adult psychiatric patients, with the more severely ill demonstrating more signs, and schizophrenic patients evidencing relatively more than other types of psychiatric patients (Rochford et al, 1970; Quitkin et al, 1976; Mosher et al, 1971; Tucker et al, 1975).

The most commonly found soft signs in schizophrenic patients are deficits in stereognosis, graphesthesia, coordination, balance, gait, and movement, according to Tucker et al (1975). Hertzig and Birch (1966, 1968) have detailed the comparatively greater incidence and numbers of hard and soft signs in psychiatrically disturbed adolescents than in the normal population.

Soft neurological signs in a sizeable percentage of autistic children have included poor muscle tone or hypotonia, incoordination, hyper-reflexia, ankle clonus, hyperkinesis or hypokinesis, and strabismus. EEG abnormalities have been found in varying numbers of autistic patients. Rapid eye movement (REM) activity of REM sleep is reduced, and nystagmus is reduced (Ornitz and Ritvo, 1976).

Blau (1977) hypothesizes that children demonstrating *torque* (a tendency to draw circles in a clockwise direction with either hand, rather than counterclockwise) have a neural integrative defect in the corpus callosum that results in mixed cerebral dominance interfering with acquisition of social, language, and cognitive skills. In his 10-year follow-up study, he found that a significant proportion of children (11 out of 52 subjects) demonstrating torque at an average age of 9 years were later diagnosed as schizophrenic, while only one child of the 52 subjects in the no-torque group was later diagnosed as schizophrenic.

Many studies have supported the findings of minor neurological abnormalities and inability to screen out internal and external stimuli in schizophrenic patients (Pincus, 1974). Studies support the theory that the behavior of schizophrenics reflects disturbance of the sensory integrative functions of the brain (Pincus, 1974). A breakdown of homeostatic regulation or modulation of sensory input is considered to be important in autism (Ornitz et al, 1977; Johnston and Magrab, 1976). Autistic children and schizophrenic persons of all ages are unable to filter, order, and organize input. Inability to adequately process incoming sensory information may lead to withdrawal or other defense behaviors. Some behaviors of autistic children appear to be attempts to provide some types of sensory input (rocking, head banging, skin pinching, finger flicking) (Freedman, 1975). (See Maladaptive Behavior, Chapter 3 page 125.)

Autistic children, according to DeMyer (1975), generally test subnormal in intelligence but show more signs of neurological dysfunction than nonpsychotic mentally subnormal children. DeMyer suggests that visual-motor integration problems and dyspraxia-like symptoms may add to verbal comprehension difficulties in forcing emotional withdrawal. Ball-playing skills and imitation of body movements with the extremities were found to be worse in autistic children than in nonpsychotic subnormal children, and DeMyer wonders if visual-motor integration skills might be related to the integrational skills needed for verbal abstraction and reasoning. Fish and Hagin (1973) found retarded midline bimanual manipulation, which they classified as a visual-motor disorder, in infants who were born to schizophrenic mothers and 10 years later also had emotional problems or schizophrenia. The authors believe this may indicate that poor neurologic integration is a precursor of the disordered integration of vision and pro-

prioception noted in schizophrenic adults. Schizophrenic patients frequently show deficits in auditory-visual integration and show overinclusive thinking (Tucker et al, 1975). Abnormal vestibular function has been reported in schizophrenia and in autism (Pincus, 1974).

All of the research results just discussed give support to a rationale for using a multisensory approach in sensorimotor integrative therapy for certain emotionally disturbed individuals.

Vestibular Dysfunction

Several researchers have also implicated the vestibular system in learning disabilities. Ayres (1972a) has reported significant vestibular problems in a number of children with learning disorders. The vestibular system and related postural disturbances have a definite effect on learning disabilities, according to deQuiros (1976, 1978). His studies involved almost 2000 children who were tested within hours after birth and then followed for several years. He states that the learning disabilities associated with vestibular disturbances are often not noted until "soft signs" lead to a diagnosis of "minimal brain dysfunction" after a child begins school (deQuiros, 1976). Speech, and learning connected with human communication in children, were thought by deQuiros to be particularly affected by vestibular dysfunction. Reading requires intact vestibular centers and efficient vestibular-oculomotor pathways, according to deQuiros.

Rider (1973) found significantly lower scores in emotionally disturbed children than in a control group of normal children in all four positions of the labyrinthine righting tests of the Fiorentino reflex tests. Both the emotionally disturbed and the control children were enrolled in regular public school classes, but the emotionally disturbed children had been identified as such by a committee of counselors, psychologists, teachers, and the school principal. Optical righting was not significantly different in three out of four tests, leading one to believe that the emotionally disturbed children may use their eyes to compensate for poor labyrinthine responses. Rider suggests that inadequate reflex maturation or other sensory integrative defects may have caused the behaviors that led to the diagnosis of emotional disturbance (Rider, 1973). The findings of a number of researchers suggest a strong relationship between certain emotional disorders and learning disabilities.

Silberzahn (1975) reported the results of administration of the Southern California Sensory Integration Test to 87 children aged 5 through 9 years, who were referred to a child guidance clinic. Psychotic or severely emotionally disturbed children were not a part of this population. Silberzahn states that "children with CNS irregularities may present a clinical picture indistinguishable from the psychopathological and emotional symptoms of the psychogenic syndromes." She found considerable evidence of the postural and bilateral integration syndrome, as described by Ayres (1972), in these children. Postural and bilateral integration problems are considered to be closely associated with certain aspects of vestibular system dysfunction, and Silberzahn believes that a link between emotional development and the vestibular system is suggested. She stresses the need for sensory integration evaluation of children with behavior problems, particularly evaluation for disorders possibly stemming from vestibular dysfunction. She suggests that perhaps the reason she did not find many children with apraxia is that the symptoms of apraxia may be more easily identified and such children may therefore be treated as having minimal brain dysfunction rather than a behavioral disorder (Silberzahn, 1975). It is interesting that both Rider and DeMyer report praxis difficulties in the severely disturbed children they studied, whereas Silberzahn found few apraxic children in the child guidance population she studied.

It seems apparent from this review of the literature that behavior in certain psychoses and other emotional disturbances is affected by problems of sensory input, processing, and feedback. Information is not as complete with regard to more minor emotional disturbances. Emphasis is often placed on human interaction etiological factors, with sensory and motor factors — if mentioned — frequently being considered as characteristics without reference to significance in relation to the behavior displayed.

This survey of the literature reflects the focus of some clinicians and researchers on identification and treatment of emotionally disturbed individuals based on an understanding of possible underlying neurological causes of behavior.

Mental Retardation

Learning has been extensively studied in the retarded, to determine their manner of learning and the differences in their ways of learning from mentally normal persons. Attending processes, specifically learning to attend to the relevant dimensions of a problem, may be an important factor in learning by the retarded (Suppes, 1974). Suppes (1974) points out that verbal performance rather than simple difficulty with abstractions is the primary deficiency in retarded individuals. Mentally retarded children develop language in a sequence similar to that of normal children, but cognitive functions of language are not as well developed in them (Suppes, 1974).

Verbal coding has been shown to enhance the amount of perceptual information retained about objects by both normal and retarded children (Swanson, 1977). Thus it follows that deficiencies in verbal abilities would limit certain kinds of perceptual learning in retarded individuals particularly.

Motor performance of the mentally retarded tends to be worse than that of normal individuals (Dunn, 1978), and this motor deficiency extends as well to simple reaction times in response to both auditory and visual stimuli (Jones and Benton, 1968). Learning-disabled children having visual or auditory perceptual disturbances may perform as if they are retarded (Baumeister, 1967). Learning disabilities of some types may therefore be the result of neurological deficits similar to those occurring in mental retardation. Caution must be exercised in applying research from one area to the other, however, since aptitude treatment interaction studies show a number of learning differences between persons of high and low academic ability (Cronbach and Snow, 1977).

Research by Dunn (1954) indicates that retardates make less use of context clues than normal subjects of comparable mental age, and in speech they have more faulty vowels and sound omissions. Both groups seem to be similar in frequency of word reversals and faulty consonants, as well as having no significant differences in hand-edness, eye dominance, or mixed lateral dominance. Suppes (1974) reports that a number of studies found automatic se-quential responses to be deficient in re-tarded individuals, which he interprets as indicating that reading difficulties of the retarded are at a nonmeaningful automatic response level rather than at a meaningful level. Gordan and Panagos (1976) found that mentally retarded children with Down's syndrome acquired grammar at a reduced rate but in the same patterns as normal children and that the rate was associated with severity of retardation.

Association of Minimal Brain Dysfunction with Delinquent Behavior

Slight neurological abnormalities char-acteristic of MBD or of hyperkinetic be-havior syndrome have been noted in de-linquent children. Behavioral manifesta-tions are also similar, including hyper-activity, distractibility, short attention span, emotional lability, impulsivity, and learning disorders (Zinkus et al, 1979). Reading difficulties have been found to be common in delinquents. Zinkus et al (1979) found that a high percentage of their juvenile delinquent subjects exhibit-ed auditory processing deficits as well as visual-spatial and visuomotor deficits. Mixed eye-hand dominance was common among the subjects and was found to be associated with poorer academic skills in this study. These authors suggest that de-linquent behavior may sometimes begin because of poor perceptual and academic functioning leading to low self-esteem and eventual antisocial attitudes.

Certain social and emotional problems have been found to be associated with neurological signs or deficient perfor-mance on neuropsychological tests. Ber-man (1978) believes that he can identify children at risk for later delinquent behav-iors as early as third grade. Tests that he found useful from the Halstead-Reitan neuropsychological test battery (Reitan

and Bavison, 1974) included the Tactile Perception, Trailmaking test, and Speech Sounds Perception. Seventy per cent of the delinquent children he tested showed deficiencies on the Halstead-Reitan bat-tery. Berman noted that the neuropsycho-logical problems were manifested mainly in learning disabilities.

Association of Minimal Brain Dysfunction with Adult Behavioral Disorders

Wood et al (1976) surveyed literature that indicated an association of MBD with adolescent delinquents and underachiev-ers, and with adult impulsive character disorders, sociopathy, psychosis, hysteria, and alcoholism. Rather than agreeing that symptoms of MBD disappear before ado-lescence as others have suggested, these investigators suggest that the age decrease is slower than that, with possible disap-pearance of symptoms after the age of 40. Wender (1972, 1974) has hypothesized that MBD is caused by a genetically trans-mitted abnormality of monoamine metabo-lism. Adults studied by Wood et al (1976) responded favorably to the low dosages of methylphenidate, pemoline, and tricyclic antidepressants, which were administered differentially according to type of behav-ior.

Borland and Heckman (1976), in a 25-year follow-up study of hyperactive boys, also found that symptoms persisted into adulthood. Almost half of the subjects had problems of a psychiatric nature in adult-hood. In addition, the adult men in the study had not equaled the socioeconomic status of their brothers. Although symp-toms of hyperactivity had decreased in adulthood, the men continued to be rest-less, nervous, impulsive, often depressed, and prone to displays of temper.

ACADEMIC CONSIDERATIONS

Evaluation and Special Education in Learning Disabilities

The Education for All Handicapped Children Act (Public Law 94–142), which mandates special education and related services for handicapped children, became law in 1975. In it, handicapped children are defined as children who are:

mentally retarded, hard of hearing, deaf, orthopedically impaired, other health impaired, speech impaired, visually handicapped, seriously emotionally disturbed, or children with specific learning disabilities who by reason thereof require special education and related services (Department of Health, Education, and Welfare, 1977).

Each of these types of handicapping conditions is defined in the act. The definition for a learning disability is the only one included here, since the term has sometimes caused confusion.

"Specific learning disability" means a disorder in one or more of the basic psychological processes involved in understanding or in using language, spoken or written, which may manifest itself in an imperfect ability to listen, think, speak, read, write, spell, or to do mathematical calculations. The term includes such conditions as perceptual handicaps, brain injury, minimal brain dysfunction, dyslexia, and developmental aphasia. The term does not include children who have learning problems which are primarily the result of visual, hearing, or motor handicaps, of mental retardation, or of environmental, cultural, or economic disadvantage (Department of Health, Education, and Welfare, 1977).

The term related services referred to in the definition means:

transportation and such developmental, corrective, and other supportive services as are required to assist a handicapped child to benefit from special education, and includes speech pathology and audiology, psychological services, physical and occupational therapy, recreation, early identification and assessment of disabilities in children, counseling services, and medical services for diagnostic or evaluation purposes. The term also includes school health services, social work services in schools, and parent counseling and training (Department of Health, Education, and Welfare, 1977).

The individuals whose conditions are excluded in this definition of a specific learning disability may have similar learning difficulties, but their learning problems are believed to be secondary to their primary diagnosis. Educational evaluation and remediation methods, however, though not always mandated by law, apply to all children who have difficulty learning.

Learning disorder and *learning disability* are commonly used interchangeably throughout the literature, although at times the term disorder is used to indicate dysfunction in underlying psychoneurological processes that leads to a learning disability. A few authors use only learning disorder and refrain from using the term learning disability. The latter term is overwhelmingly favored in educational and government publications. In addition to broader terms used to indicate the problems underlying learning disabilities, such as neurological dysfunction, minimal brain dysfunction, or sensory integrative dysfunction, there are other terms that are more specific. Dyslexia, specific language disability, and such terms as agraphia, dyscalculia, apraxia are used to describe discrete aspects of a learning problem.

Conceptual, evaluation, and remediation dilemmas in learning disabilities can be discussed in several areas:

Etiology. The causes of learning disabilities of different types are difficult to pinpoint, and in many cases will never be known. Neurological damage or dysfunction may be a factor in etiology, but deficits in sensory receptors should also be considered, since poor hearing or vision may cause a child to show difficulties that appear similar to those caused by central dysfunction.

Diagnosis. If a label is to be given or a diagnosis made, interdisciplinary consistency and consistency in evaluating the same learning or behavior problems by those doing testing are necessary. Precise definitions of various problems must be developed, so that knowledge can advance more rapidly through comparison of information gained in different professions. Medical terms, for example, must be translated into educationally meaningful descriptions. Likewise, it is essential to understand educational problems from a neurological viewpoint, when pertinent, and to combine this information with educational assessment results.

Validity and Reliability. All measurement instruments used in assessing learning disabilities should be valid and reliable in order to assure accuracy of diagnosis and reasonable evidence of improvement or lack of it. Remediation methods should also be subjected to scientific scrutiny to prove their effectiveness.

Interpretation. After a thorough assessment has been made of the individual's learning assets and deficiencies, results must be interpreted in terms of current and expected behavioral manifestations that have a bearing on education and life functioning. Intervention strategies should be based on this analysis.

Teaching Implications. Since teachers are not medically trained, information about sensory integrative or sensorimotor problems provided to them must be put in terms they will understand and be able to use in an educational setting. Research relating sensorimotor integrative theory and therapy to educational problems is being increasingly produced. These findings should be reported in ways that will help educators understand the sensorimotor integrative problems of the children in their care. Treatment of learning problems for many years was based on trial and error with little neurophysiological rationale to guide remediation efforts. Despite that lack, many careful practitioners devised successful methods of helping children academically. This experimental knowledge, combined with basic CNS research and neuropsychological test findings, has helped to link performance manifestations with categories of CNS dysfunction.

In addition to therapy directed toward underlying disorders, there are a number of remedial efforts based on task analysis, learning styles, and environmental manipulation that merely require intelligent appraisal of the child and his learning needs. The therapist or teacher should examine the child's academic responses and productions, since many academic problems can be helped by carefully assessing task approach or performance, and providing new attack skills and training. The child may be able to overcome some learning disabilities with stronger basic instruction or helpful coping skills.

Remediation methods are becoming more sophisticated, as the results of research are applied in practical ways. Dilemmas still remain, however, in that aptitude-treatment interaction studies have demonstrated that aptitudes and learning styles vary greatly among individuals and among various ability groups (Cronbach and Snow, 1977). This complicates selection of remedial methods, since few methods can be shown to help all learners. It is helpful to assess learning style and to attempt to help the child overcome behavioral traits that interfere with his learning. Methods to help him overcome certain of of these hindering traits could include behavior modification or biofeedback training to assist the child in establishing inner control. Ozer (1978) advocates helping the child learn to modify his environment so that he is better able to cope with competing stimuli. The child should know the nature of his problem and be taught strategies to help him maintain attention and make school tasks and learning more manageable.

It need not be a secret from the child that alternative sensory approaches are being used to aid his learning. In fact, if he knows this, he may be able to help himself by using an orderly sensory approach, adding sensory modalities to help himself learn. For example, he might find that studying is made easier by a combination of reading, speaking aloud to himself, and writing.

Teachers might help a child control distractability by teaching him to reduce distracting stimuli in his environment when he is trying to concentrate. For example, when he needs to study, he can try to find a quiet, nonstimulating place. Children may also be taught to organize their work by planning a logical, sequential system of performance. In this way, they should learn to think ahead and plan how to proceed, rather than beginning in a disorganized fashion.

When possible, learning activities can be designed to require a purposeful response from the child. Enjoyable interventions with sensory stimuli increase motivation to respond adaptively.

Teachers should recognize the developmental nature of sensory and motor processes. Basic perceptual skills must be mastered before complex skills such as reading and writing can be effectively taught. Reading involves the ability to match or associate visual symbols with sounds. Problems can apparently occur in either of these primary sensory avenues (visual or auditory), or in the integration of the two forms of input. Some studies have favored teaching reading through the visual mode primarily, and others have favored the auditory mode (Saphier, 1973; Baker, 1975). Certain approaches to the teaching of reading provide a combination of sensory input including visual, auditory, kinesthetic, and tactile (Slingerland, 1971).

If educational methods used to alleviate learning disorders are not effective, referral to practitioners of sensorimotor integrative therapy (generally occupational and physical therapists) should be considered. Developmental stimulation of sensory and of motor processes through the methods these specialists employ might strengthen the sensory integrative and sensorimotor bases of much academic learning.

SENSORIMOTOR INTEGRATIVE TREATMENT

Sensory Normalization Techniques

The principles of the multisensory theory of neurorehabilitation (Chapter 3) apply to the patient population discussed in this chapter. It is an aim of therapy to improve the functioning of the various sensory systems and to enhance intersensory integration. Various techniques of sensory input have been developed for each sensory system, and detailed descriptions of their application in sensory or sensorimotor integrative therapy are given in other sources (Ayres, 1972; Montgomery and Richter, 1977; Knickerbocker, 1980; King, 1974). The creative therapist can readily develop similar activities once the basic concepts of treatment purposes are grasped.

Input to the earliest developing sensory systems, particularly the spinothalamic, spinoreticular, and vestibular systems, are considered to be the stimuli most likely to cause integration to occur among all sensory systems (Ayres, 1972). Proprioceptive (epicritic) stimuli through receptors in muscles, tendons, and joints also provide valuable sensory information. Kinesthetic awareness is gained partly through proprioceptive information and partly through cutaneous and visceral sensations (Bothelo, 1965). General proprioceptive input is often used as a means of encouraging acceptance of the concomitant touch input that might be intolerable to some subjects if provided separately.

All of the sensory information gained from these systems helps in developing perceptions and conceptions about the body's form and movement capabilities, and about body movements in relationship to space and the force of gravity. Use of olfactory and gustatory input in sensorimotor integrative therapy is not yet well defined, and as a result these sensory modalities are employed less often. The reader may refer to Chapter 3 for detailed information on the current uses of these modalities in therapy.

The importance of early-developing sensory systems does not negate the importance of the later-to-mature auditory and visual systems. Interpretation of input to these systems complements information gained from the other systems, as well as leading to percepts and concepts uniquely developed from auditory and visual information singly. It is easy to recognize the importance of auditory and visual input in assisting with movements, and to confirm the use of auditory and visual information for many cognitive activities. While auditory and visual inputs are not eliminated in early treatment, emphasis on them is generally reserved until the more basic normalizations occur. Sensory integration involving later-maturing systems is then presumed to occur more readily through therapy.

Motor Improvement Techniques

Motor improvement techniques rely heavily on attempted normalization of sensory systems, since motor planning and accurate responses require adequately functioning sensory systems. Higher level reflexes, which are frequently found to be inadequate or maturationally delayed, require the use of the types of sensory input that elicit them. Proprioceptive positioning, tactile stimuli, ocular changes, and vestibular stimulation are commonly used to elicit and strengthen reflexes deemed necessary in treatment of the person with CNS damage or dysfunction. Reflex-inhibiting postures and sensorimotor inhibition treatment techniques are used to inhibit reflexes that are present beyond the time when they should have diminished in strength and been integrated into voluntary motor functioning without interfering. Clinical experience demonstrates that lower level reflexes present beyond the appropriate age of disappearance can be inhibited and that higher level reflexes can be enhanced. Inhibition of reflexes can be done by using the Bobath reflex-inhibiting postures (Bobath, 1970), and by employing patterns opposite to the reflexes during active games and exercises (Ayres, 1972). Facilitation techniques may be used to improve the balance of power of muscles opposing the reflex-involved muscles and to decrease the power of reflex-involved muscles through reciprocal inhibition.

Body movement provides sensory input, as the movements create opportunities for the sensory receptors to be stimulated. For example, during movement the following may occur: head changes in space stimulate the vestibular apparatus in the inner ear; visual changes are received and interpreted; auditory, proprioceptive-kinesthetic, and tactile information allows the individual to estimate and adjust force, speed, and timing; air against the body, body hair displacement, and skin contact also provide information about the environment and the progression of the body in space.

Sensory input should be considered primary to developing proper motor skills, since motor responses are based on sensory information from the environment and from within one's body. Therapists, as well as persons responsible for training others in motor or sports skills, should thoroughly familiarize themselves with the reflexive basis of motor skills. Awareness of movements that will be difficult because of conflicting reflexes might bring to mind modifications of an activity to prevent the conflict. Such awareness might point to a need for control by cortical or subcortical means of the offending reflex-controlled body parts until the reflex is over-ridden during voluntary activity. Conscious control might be too difficult for certain individuals, however, particularly the mentally retarded (Montgomery and Richter, 1977).

Training in motor skills for persons suspected of having CNS dysfunction should not stress cortical or cognitive learning of the motions involved. A means of making learning of movements subcortical is to require purposeful actions in completion of tasks or activities, rather than giving verbal instructions to move body parts.

Adaptive behavior occurs more readily because of the need to fulfill a purpose. Sensations resulting from desired movements are transduced and stored in memory, to be used again when the same task is attempted. Repetitive practice of a sequential movement pattern eventually allows it to be done without conscious planning (i.e., subcortically), and at that point the movement is generally more coordinated than when performed with consciously planned actions. O'Connell and Gardner (1967) state that skill is achieved when a movement pattern becomes so automatic that a single stimulus can initiate the sequential responses necessary to complete the act. Ongoing motor performance requires sensory feedback from proprioceptive (including labyrinthine) and cutaneous receptors primarily, but with other receptors (such as visual and auditory) also playing a part.

Treatment Theories and Clinical Approaches

A number of individuals have developed treatment theories and clinical approaches in sensory or sensorimotor integrative therapy. One of the most important in creating interest in this area of practice was A. Jean Ayres, whose theory-based methods led to specialization by numbers of occupational therapists.

The sensory integrative neurobehavioral theory of Ayres (1972) holds that disordered sensory integration accounts for certain aspects of some learning disorders and that enhancement of sensory integration may make academic learning easier. This sensory integrative approach to treating learning disorders avoids teaching specific skills. Instead, the objective is to enhance the brain's ability to learn, after which academic and other tasks should become easier to master. The purpose, then, is to modify the neurological dysfunction that is hindering learning. Dysfunction is determined from the results of sensory integrative tests and other measures. This therapy is advocated as an adjunct to classroom instruction rather than a replacement or alternative.

While most of Ayres' evaluation and therapy methods were designed for use with children, treatment techniques based on Ayres' theoretical constructs, after being modified for age capabilities and acceptance, have been used to some extent with brain-injured, blind, mentally retarded, and psychiatrically disturbed adults (Siev and Freishtat, 1976; Baker-Nobles and Bink, 1979; Clark et al, 1978; King, 1974). Treatment techniques developed by others primarily for children are also being modified for use with adults.

King (1974) has used sensory integrative principles to develop treatment programs for adult schizophrenic patients. Process or reactive schizophrenics seem to be good candidates for therapy to enhance sensory integration, but paranoid schizophrenics, in her experience, do not seem to be good candidates.

King (1974) suggests use of recreational and noncompetitive game-type activities that are designed to enhance sensory integration. Task-oriented activities may be effective after the patient's level of functioning has been raised. Group activities as well as one-to-one therapy may be done. Therapeutic activities are chosen to counteract primitive reflex patterns and excessive flexion, adduction, and internal rotation patterns. Efforts are also made to increase joint range of motion. Activities involving bilateral heavy work patterns for the tonic muscle groups (as suggested by Rood) are believed by King to be beneficial. In addition, activities suggested by Ayres (1972) are sometimes utilized in programs for schizophrenic patients. Vestibular stimulation through motion involving head movement is an important component of King's recommended program, and proprioceptive and other forms of sensory input are also believed to be valuable.

Knickerbocker (1980) has developed a treatment approach that addresses school-related difficulties in a skill-development manner. She advocates analyzing processes involved in task performance and developing underlying subskills in a hierarchical manner that will lead to improved performance. Her "holistic," or comprehensive and unified, approach to evaluation and treatment of children with learning disorders involves both the development of underlying sensory and motor organization and the development

of foundation abilities more visibly related to academic performance (directionality, sequencing and problem solving organization, pre-reading skills, fine motor skills for handwriting, and so forth).

Treatment of adult cerebrovascular accident patients or those with perceptual dysfunction has been divided into three approaches by Siev and Freishtat (1976): (1) sensory integrative approach, (2) transfer of training approach, and (3) functional approach. The sensory integrative approach is similar to the approach recommended by Ayres (1972) for children. Since the perceptual problems in an adult with cerebrovascular accident or other brain damage are due to interference in already developed systems in a mature nervous system, not all of the treatment principles developed for children are considered valid. In addition, methods would require modification to allow for the physical and cognitive deficiencies of adult stroke patients. The transfer of training approach assumes that work on spatial or other perceptual tasks will lead to improvement in the abilities trained and that those abilities will then be available for use in functional performance of life skills. The functional approach involves teaching techniques of performing the actual life skill that perceptual problems are making difficult, with hints given on compensation for the problem or adaptation of the environment. Unfortunately, research is sparse regarding the relative efficacy of these approaches.

Schwartz et al (1979) suggest that the favored teaching approach for left hemisphere/aphasic patients is a visual, nonverbal method, using demonstration of tasks rather than verbal explanations that the patient will probably not remember. Persons with right hemisphere brain damage, on the other hand, would profit more from auditory verbal presentations. Simple verbal instructions that the patient repeats as he performs task steps are considered best for the latter type of patient.

Treatment Planning

In general, treatment planning should be specific to the individual, particularly with those who have severe dysfunction.

One-to-one therapy, however, is not always possible, and the therapist must then provide the best possible treatment under group circumstances, always monitoring and evaluating individual changes.

Although individuality in treatment *planning* is always important, certain treatment activities can sometimes be carried out with groups, if the groups are manageable and the individuals physically capable of group participation. For example, a room can be arranged so that each person can proceed from one supervised sensory stimulation activity to another, or group circle activities can be done with everyone receiving general proprioceptive, vestibular, tactile, visual, and auditory stimuli through various movements and accompanying sounds. These movements can include shaking, rolling, stretching, jumping, pulling, pushing, and head movements, and accompanying sounds can include foot tapping, self-patting, rhythmical music, singing, and so forth. Other activities, such as balloon volleyball and parachute games, have been used with groups to provide sensory input in an enjoyable atmosphere. Such programs, however, presuppose that those involved in them react favorably and with adaptive responses, indicating that their nervous systems are capable of organizing multiple simultaneous sensory stimuli.

Treatment, remedial, or coping strategies are developed according to need. Although the preferred strategy is to alleviate the underlying dysfunction, so that performance and emotional manifestations are normalized without supreme conscious effort, there are situations for which coping methods make academic, social, and motor performance activities easier until correction is effected. For patients in whom full correction proves to be impossible, coping ideas and aids may help the individual function more adequately.

EFFICACY OF SENSORIMOTOR INTEGRATION TREATMENT

Validation of the effectiveness of therapy is necessary for professional accountability. Support for the effectiveness of sensorimotor integrative therapy using a multisensory approach is provided by a collection of research results.

Carlsen (1975) reported on a program with young cerebral palsied children that utilized the approaches of Rood, Ayres, and the Bobaths to attempt to bring about integration on a gross sensorimotor level. It was found that spontaneous improvement occurred in fine motor activities, including activities of daily living skills, without specific training in such activities or skills. Children given traditional training in specific developmental tasks such as fine motor adaptive and self-care skills showed less gain.

Improvement in fine motor control and social and emotional behavior was noted along with improved reflex development and gross motor skills in a sample of 12 cerebral palsied children (aged 2 to 6) participating in 16 sessions of stimulation of horizontal and vertical semicircular canals over a period of four weeks (Chee et al, 1978). The authors suggested that the vestibulo-ocular reflex may have improved retinal image stability, thus helping to provide a stable background for movement. This study used only vestibular stimulation, rather than a complete sensory integrative program. In a similar study with Down's syndrome infants, approximately two weeks of daily rotatory stimulation in varying body positions resulted in improved motor skills (Kantner, 1976).

Clark and Shuer (1978) point out that there is a lack of research in the area of sensory integration therapy with retarded children and adults. They stress that appropriate measurement instruments need to be developed and tested, and that program effectiveness with different classifications of retardation should be investigated. However, some results of research and clinical application are available.

Norton (1975) demonstrated that sensory stimulation of the type employed in sensory integrative therapy caused improvement in profoundly retarded preschool children with multiple handicaps.

Clark et al (1978) compared the relative effectiveness of an operant approach (behavior modification), a modified sensory integrative approach, and a combination of both methods in bringing about improvements in 27 profoundly retarded institutionalized adults. Each of these programs resulted in similar gains in frequency of vocalization, frequency of eye contact, and quality of postural adaptation. The authors believed that their results supported the use of sensory integrative therapy with profoundly retarded adults, and they further mentioned that results of the sensory integrative program might have been even greater had their physical facilities not precluded the use of suspended equipment to provide more vigorous vestibular input. This study was a pioneering effort by speech and occupational therapists that validates the use of sensory integrative therapy with a population on whom primarily operant methods were previously used.

The effect of sensory integrative therapy or neuromotor development of trainable mentally retarded children was investigated by Montgomery and Richter (1977). Three groups of children participated in different motor programs for eight months, three times a week. The greatest gains on tests for reflex integration and gross and fine motor skills were shown by the children receiving sensory integrative therapy, and those children in the developmental physical education program showed greater improvement than those in the third group, who participated in an adaptive physical education program combined with an arts and crafts therapy program. Neuromotor development appeared to be improved more by activities facilitating postural responses than by specific motor skills practice.

Fiebert and Brown (1979), using only rotary vestibular stimulation, demonstrated that 10 CVA patients showed greater improvement in functional ambulation than 10 controls who did not receive this stimulation. Both experimental subjects and control subjects received a standard physical therapy program for this diagnosis once a day for two weeks, during which time the experimental subjects also received the rotary stimulation. The authors attributed this improvement to the relationship of vestibular function to the proprioceptive, visual, and motor systems, all of which are important in ambulation. While the authors suggested that vestibular stimulation is a beneficial therapeutic measure with this population, they did not discuss precautions, which must be considered.

Several authors have reported improvement in psychiatric patients after programs involving sensory stimulation. Davis and Ware (1967) saw improved facility in interpersonal relations and greater tolerance to frustration in a psychotic child given tactile and proprioceptive stimulation. Nitzun, Stapleton, and Bender (1974) noted improvements in behavior, body image, and intellectual attainments in psychiatric patients who participated in a movement and drama program.

Ayres and Tickle (1980) studied 10 autistic children, who were given one year of twice weekly sensory integrative therapy that provided somatosensory and vestibular stimulation and elicited adaptive responses. Changes attributed to therapy were noted in social-emotional functioning, language, and purposeful activity. Subjects showing the best response to treatment had initially shown that they were registering sensory input but failing to modulate it. In pretherapy testing these subjects had shown tactile defensiveness, gravitational insecurity, avoidance of movement, and an orienting response to a puff of air. More therapeutically responsive subjects had also shown some clinically observable nystagmus beats, rather than none as in some subjects. Therapeutic results were interpreted to mean that the therapy was more effective in helping the nervous system to modulate sensory input than in assisting the brain in registering or orienting to it.

Wolkowicz et al (1977) used a sensory integrative program based on the works of Ayres (1972) with four older autistic children (aged 11 to 18 years). After a treatment period lasting four months, in which the children were seen three times a week for 45 minutes per session, improvements were seen in motor and social behavior. The changes included increased eye contact and spontaneous vocalizations, increased social responses, reduced fear reactions, and participation in constructive activities in place of self-stimulatory behaviors.

King (1974) states that empirical studies show that chronic process schizophrenics function more adequately after gross motor treatment. Gains made in sensory integration tend to be relatively permanent and do not show the same regression effect as gains made through verbal therapies, she adds.

Jorstad, Wilbert, and Wirrer (1977) reported improvement in self-esteem, affect, socialization, and overall functioning in six chronic schizophrenics after three weeks to six months in a sensory integrative program. All were discharged, and at six months after discharge all had maintained their ability to function in a home or a board-and-care living situation. King (1974, 1978, 1979) believes that permanent changes in integrative capacities of chronic process schizophrenics is possible after programs incorporating sensory integrative treatment principles. Varied sensory input is provided through patient participation in activities allowing vestibular, tactile, proprioceptive-kinesthetic, visual, and auditory stimulation.

Levine, O'Connor, and Stacey (1977), in a study involving testing before and after a six-week program of sensory integrative types of activities daily for one hour with six chronic schizophrenic patients, found that scores increased on the measures used: Southern California Sensory Integration Tests, human figure drawing, Kephart's Double Circles, and a social-emotional rating scale. Weeks, Burack, and Barrett (1979) carried out a 12-week program of sensorimotor integrative movement therapy with two 45-minute sessions per week. Comparisons before and after therapy of raw scores on the Southern California Sensory Integration Tests showed that the experimental subjects showed significant improvement in a number of areas, whereas control subjects did not.

Few studies directly address academic improvement resulting from sensory integrative therapy. Because of conflicting research regarding academic improvement from commonly used "perceptual-motor" programs, educators may be reluctant to institute sensorimotor integrative programs until years of research illuminate the benefits and limitations of such therapy.

Behavioral and motor results of sensorimotor integrative therapy, while educationally relevant in many ways, are harder for administrators to justify financially. As more research is done and benefits are scientifically elaborated, decisions should be easier to make. At present, educators are being convinced of the value of this therapy by individual results rather than by extensive research.

Ayres (1976) attempted to determine which types of learning-disabled children respond well to sensory integrative therapy. Her research led her to conclude that sensory integrative therapy was most beneficial in promoting academic learning for children with hyporeactive nystagmus. Shortened duration nystagmus is believed by Ayres to reflect some vestibular system disorder that interferes with academic learning. Sensory integrative therapy appeared to enhance vestibular input processing and thereby changed academic achievement. Children with generalized neurological problems resulting in a low IQ, but with normal duration nystagmus, were helped the least by sensory integrative therapy. Children having left hemisphere dysfunction showed little academic improvements (although some made language gains), and might benefit more from special education programs than from a sensory processing program.

Educators have used a form of remediation resembling sensorimotor integrative therapy for many years, under the heading of multisensory approaches (Wiederholt, 1974). Multisensory presentations of educational material have been shown to be useful in helping children learn. Traditional classroom visual and auditory presentations have been supplemented with kinesthetic and tactual involvement on the part of the child. These methods have been used to prevent some initial learning problems, as well as to remedy difficulties, particularly in reading (Slingerland, 1971). Correction of reading difficulties helps a child succeed in other academic areas, since reading and auditory-language skills are necessary to some extent in all subject areas. It is likely that these methods are all that is needed for many children. Children who have more severe degrees of dysfunction in sensory integration affecting academic performance may not be sufficiently helped by the traditional or multisensory educational approaches. In the area of research regarding sensorimotor integration therapy, there are enough reports indicating positive results to encourage further use.

McKibben (1973) found that a 16-week sensorimotor integrative therapy program of three one-hour sessions per week with children having coordination or learning deficits or both resulted in improved motor planning ability and tactile perception. Retesting in two to three months showed that gains were maintained. In addition, parents and teachers reported positive changes in self-concept, self-confidence, academic performance, and peer relationships. All of the children in this study were of normal intelligence with no physical disabilities.

Ottenbacher et al (1979) found that learning disabled children with hyporesponsive postrotary nystagmus demonstrated reduced oculomotor control skills considered necessary for reading. After a long-term program of sensory integrative therapy (mean duration of 10.7 months, 2 hours per week) emphasizing vestibular-proprioceptive activities, duration of postrotary nystagmus increased and ocular fixation ability improved. The authors suggest that sensory integrative therapy may thus alleviate eye movement control deficits that may be associated with reading problems.

While moderation is indicated, some experimentation must take place in treatment if new, more effective methods are to be developed. Controlled research with adequate samples is, of course, a preferred means of achieving new insights into treatment effectiveness, but there are some problems unique to small numbers of children, and collection of sufficient numbers of patients for a sample might be difficult. Case study reporting of success in treating patients with unusual problems might help to disseminate information.

It can be seen that a multisensory approach to sensorimotor integrative problems is logically consistent with current neurophysiological information. Persons working with children and adults in the diagnostic categories of learning disabilities, mental retardation, brain damage, and emotional disturbance should study the latest experimental evidence of the results of sensory input on human performance.

Effective combinations and sequences of sensory input for encouraging rapid maximum correction have not been developed for all problems. Many years of research will be needed before the most efficacious treatment programs are developed. In the meantime, practitioners must use current knowledge sensibly for selected problems.

The desire to provide the most effective treatment at the lowest cost in time, money, and emotional stress should always be foremost in therapists' minds.

REFERENCES

Adams RR: Learning disabilities: a developmental approach. J Special Educ 9:158–165, 1975.

Ayres A: Sensory Integration and Learning Disorders. Los Angeles, Western Psychological Services, 1972.

Ayres AJ: Improving academic scores through sensory integration. J Learning Disabilities 5:336–343, 1972.

Ayres AJ: Southern California Sensory Integration Tests. Los Angeles, California, Western Psychological Services, 1972.

Ayres AJ: Southern California Postrotary Nystagmus Test. Los Angeles, California, Western Psychological Services, 1975.

Ayres AJ: The Effect of Sensory Integrative Therapy in Learning Disabled Children. Monograph, Pasadena, California, The Center for the Study of Sensory Integrative Dysfunction, 1976.

Bailey J, Meyerson L: Effect of vibratory stimulation on a retardate's self-injurious behavior. Psychological Aspects of Disability, Vol. 17, No. 3, 133–137, 1970.

Baker-Nobles L, Bink MP: Sensory integration in the rehabilitation of blind adults. Am J Occup Ther 33:559–564, 1979.

Bartley SH: Principles of Perception, 2nd ed. New York, Harper and Row, 1969.

Baumeister AA, Forehand R: Stereotyped acts. Int Rev Res Mental Retardation 6:55–95, 1973.

Baumeister AA: Mental Retardation. Appraisal, Education and Rehabilitation. Chicago, Aldine Publishing Co., 1967.

Benton AL (ed): Behavioral Change in Cerebrovascular Disease. New York, Harper and Row, 1970.

Berman A: Delinquency as a learning disability. Science News 114:180–181, Sept. 9, 1978.

Berry MF: Language Disorders of Children. The Bases and Diagnoses. Englewood Cliffs, NJ, Prentice-Hall, Inc., 1969.

Birch HG, Thomas A, Chess S: Behavioral development in brain-damaged children. Arch Gen Psychiatry 11:596–603, 1964.

Black F: Cognitive, academic, and behavioral findings in children with suspected neurological dysfunction. J Learning Disabilities 9:182–187, 1976.

Blau TH: Torque and schizophrenic vulnerability. Am Psychol 33:997–1005, 1977.

Bobath B: Adult Hemiplegia: Evaluation and Treatment. London, William Heinemann Medical Books Ltd., 1970.

Borland BL, Heckman HK: Hyperactive boys and their brothers. A 25-year follow-up study. Arch Gen Psychiatry 33:669–675, 1976.

Botelho SY: Proprioceptive, vestibular, and cerebellar mechanisms in the control of movement. The Child with Central Nervous System Deficit. Report of Two Symposiums. Washington, DC, U.S. Government Printing Office, 1965.

Brazleton TB: Neonatal Behavioral Assessment Scale. Philadelphia, J.B. Lippincott Co., 1973.

Bush WJ, Waugh KW: Diagnosing Learning Disabilities, 2nd ed. Columbus, Oh, C. E. Merrill Publishing Company, 1976.

Campbell S: The Developing Infant: Neuromuscular Maturation. The Comprehensive Management of Infants at Risk for CNS Deficits, Proceedings, 65–74. Chapel Hill, University of North Carolina, 1974.

Campbell SK, Wilson JM: Planning infant learning programs. Psy Ther 56:1347–1357, 1976.

Caplan F, Caplan T: The Second Twelve Months of Life. New York, Grosset and Dunlap, 1977.

Carlsen PN: Comparison of two approaches for treating the young cerebral-palsied child. Am J Occup Ther 29:267–272, 1975.

Chee FK, Kreutzberg JR, Clark DL: Semicircular canal stimulation in cerebral palsied children. Phys Ther 58:1071–1075, 1978.

Clark FA et al: A comparison of operant and sensory integrative methods on developmental parameters in profoundly retarded adults. Am J Occup Ther 32:86–92, 1978.

Clark F, Shuer J: A clarification of sensory integrative therapy and its application to programming with retarded people. Mental Retardation 16:227–232, 1978.

Clements SD: Minimal brain dysfunction in children. In S Sapir, A Nitzburg (eds): Children with Learning Problems. New York, Brunner/Mazel Publishers, 1973.

Clements SD, Lehtinen LE, Lukens JE: Children with Minimal Brain Injury. Chicago, National Society for Crippled Children and Adults, 1963.

Clements S, Peters J: Minimal brain dysfunctions in the school-age child. Arch Gen Psychiatry 6:185–197, 1962.

Cratty BJ: Perceptual and Motor Development in Infants and Children. New York, Macmillan, 1970.

Critchley M: The Dyslexic Child. Springfield, Charles C Thomas Publisher, 1970.

Cronbach LJ, Snow RE: Aptitudes and Instructional Methods. New York, Irvington Publishers, Inc., 1977.

Cruickshank WM, Bice HV, Wallen NE: Perception and Cerebral Palsy. Syracuse, NY, Syracuse University Press, 1957.

Davis A, Ware C: Sensory stimulation in the treatment of a psychotic child. Phys Ther 47:383–384, 1967.

DeHaven GE, Mordock JB, Loykovich BA: Evaluation of coordination deficits in children with minimal cerebral dysfunction. Phys Ther 49:153–157, 1969.

DeMyer M: The nature of the neuropsychological disability in autistic children. J Autism Child Schizophr 5:109–127, 1975.

Denckla MB: Research needs in learning disabilities: a neurologist's point of view. J Learning Disabilities 6:441–450, 1973.

deQuiros JB, Schrager L: Neuropsychological Fundamentals in Learning Disabilities. San Rafael, Ca, Academic Therapy Publications, 1978.

Divoky D: Toward a nation of sedated children. Learning, pp. 6–13, March 1973.

Dunn FM: A comparison of the reading process of mentally retarded and normal boys of the same mental age. Monographs of the Society of Psychological Development 19:7–99, 1954.

Dunn JM: Reliability of selected psychomotor measures with mentally retarded adult males. Perceptual and Motor Skills 46:295–301, 1978.

Eaves LC, Kendall DC, Crichton JU: The early identification of learning disabilities: a follow-up study. J Learning Disabilities 7:632–638, 1974.

Epstein W: Varieties of Perceptual Learning. New York, McGraw-Hill, 1967.

Fico JM, Brodsky HS: The effect of visual and tactual stimulation on learning of abstract forms. Psychonomic Science 27:264–268, 1972.

Fiebert IM, Brown E: Vestibular stimulation to improve ambulation after a cerebral vascular accident. Phys Ther 59:423–426, 1979.

Fields WS (ed): Neurological and Sensory Disorders in the Elderly. New York, Stratton Intercontinental Medical Book Corporation, 1975.

Fiorentino M: Normal and Abnormal Development. Springfield, Charles C Thomas Publisher, 1972.

Fiorentino M: Reflex Testing Methods for Evaluating CNS Development. Springfield, Charles C Thomas Publisher, 1973.

Fine MJ (ed): Principles and Techniques of Intervention with Hyperactive Children. Springfield, Charles C Thomas Publisher, 1977.

Fish B, Hagin R: Visual-motor disorders in infants at risk for schizophrenia. Arch Gen Psychiatry 28:900–904, 1973.

Fish B et al: The creator of schizophrenia in infancy: a ten-year follow-up report of neurological and psychological development. Am J Psychiatry 121:768–775, 1965.

Fisher S: Body Experience in Fantasy and Behavior. New York, Appleton-Century-Crofts, 1970.

Freedman A, Kaplan H, Sadock B (eds): Comprehensive Textbook of Psychiatry II. Baltimore, Williams and Wilkins Co., 1975.

Galante MB, Flye ME, Stephens LS: Cumulative minor deficits: a longitudinal study of the relation of physical factors to school achievement. J Learning Disabilities 5:75–80, 1972.

Gerardot JM, Dossett R: Autism: an approach to learning. Phys Ther 57:814–820, 1977.

Gibson EJ: Principles of Perceptual Learning and Development. New York, Appleton-Century-Crofts, 1969.

Gibson JJ: The Senses Considered as Perceptual Systems. Boston, Houghton-Mifflin Co., 1966.

Gillingham A, Stillman B: Remedial Training for Children with Specific Disability in Reading, Spelling, and Penmanship. Cambridge, Ma, Educators Publishing Service, 1965.

Gilroy J, Meyer J: Medical Neurology, 2nd ed. New York, Macmillan, 1975.

Goldfarb W: An investigation of childhood schizophrenia. Arch Gen Psychiatry 11:620–631, 1964.

Gordan WL, Panagos JM: Developmental transformational capacity of children with Down's syndrome. Perceptual and Motor Skills 43:967–973, 1976.

Graham F, Matarazzo R, Caldwell B: Behavioral

differences between normal and traumatized newborns: standardization, reliability, and validity. Psychol Monograph 70:17–33, 1952.

Grynbaum BB et al: Sensory feedback therapy for stroke patients. Geriatrics pp. 43–47, 1976.

Halverson C, Victor J: Minor physical anomalies and problem behavior in elementary school children. Child Dev 47:281–285, 1976.

Heasley BE: Auditory Perceptual Disorders and Remediation. Springfield, Charles C Thomas, 1974.

Hertzig ME, Birch HG: Neurologic organization in psychiatrically disturbed adolescent girls. Arch Gen Psychiatry 15:590–598, 1966.

Hertzig ME, Birch HG: Neurologic organization in psychiatrically disturbed adolescents. Arch Gen Psychiatry 19:528–537, 1968.

Hopkins HL, Smith HD: Willard and Spackman's Occupational Therapy. Philadelphia, J. B. Lippincott Co., 1978.

Hoskin TA, Squires JE: Developmental assessment: a test for gross motor and reflex development. Phys Ther 53:117–125, 1973.

Huss J: Sensorimotor Treatment Approaches in Occupational Therapy. Philadelphia, J. B. Lippincott Co., 1971.

Jacobs M: Development of normal motor behavior. Am J Phys Med 46:41–51, 1967.

Jimenez J et al: Prerequisites for perceptual evaluation of brain damage. Can J Occup Ther 43:165–167, 1976.

Johnston R, Magrab P: Developmental Disorders, Assessment, Treatment, Education. Baltimore, University Park Press, 1976.

Jones D, Benton AL: Reaction time and mental age in normal and retarded children. Am J Mental Deficiency 73:143–147, 1968.

Jordan D: Dyslexia in the Classroom. Columbus, Oh, C. E. Merrill Publishing Company, 1972.

Jorstad V, Wilbert D, Wirrer B: Sensory dysfunction in adult schizophrenia. Hospital and Community Psychiatry 28:280–283, April 1977.

Kantner R et al: Effects of vestibular stimulation on nystagmus response and motor performance in the developmentally delayed infant. Phys Ther 56:414–421, 1976.

Keats S: Cerebral Palsy. Springfield, Charles C Thomas Publisher, 1965.

Kenny TJ, Clemmens RL: Medical and psychological correlates in children with learning disabilities. J Pediatr 78:273–277, 1971.

Khanna JL Ed: Brain Damage and Mental Retardation. A Psychological Evaluation. Springfield, Charles C Thomas Publisher, 1968.

King LJ: A sensory integrative approach to schizophrenia. Am J Occup Ther 28:529–536, 1974.

King LJ: Occupational therapy research in psychiatry: a perspective. Am J Occup Ther 32:15–18, 1978a.

King LJ: Toward a science of adaptive responses. Am J Occup Ther 32:429–437, 1978b.

Kirk SA: Educating Exceptional Children, 2nd ed. Boston, Houghton-Mifflin, 1972.

Knickerbocker BM: A Holistic Approach to the Treatment of Learning Disorders. Thorofare, NJ, Charles B. Slack, Inc., 1980.

Knobloch H, Pasamanick B (eds): Gesell and Amatruda's Developmental Diagnosis, The Evaluation and Management of Normal and Abnormal Neuropsychologic Development in Infancy and Early Childhood, 3rd ed. New York, Harper and Row, Publishers, 1974.

Koppitz EA: The Bender-Gestalt Test for Young Children. New York, Grune and Stratton, Inc., 1963.

Lee AM: Relationship between birth weight and perceptual motor performance in children. Perceptual and Motor Skills 45:119–122, 1977.

Lerner JW: Children with Learning Disabilities. Theories, Diagnosis, and Teaching Strategies. Boston, Houghton-Mifflin, 1971.

Levine I, O'Connor H, Stacey B: Sensory integration with chronic schizophrenics: a pilot study. Can J Occup Ther 44:17–21, 1977.

Lezak M: Neuropsychological Assessment. New York, Oxford University Press, 1976.

Liemohn WP, Knapczyk DR: Factor analysis of gross and fine motor ability in developmentally disabled children. Research Quarterly 45:424–432, 1974.

Llorens L: Identification of the Ayres' syndromes in emotionally disturbed children: an exploratory study. Am J Occup Ther 22:286–288, 1968.

McKibben EH: The effect of traditional tactile stimulation in a perceptual-motor treatment program for school children. Am J Occup Ther 27:191–197, 1973.

Mack JL, Carlson NJ: Conceptual deficits and aging: the category test. Perceptual and Motor Skills 46:123–128, 1978.

Mayo Clinic: Clinical Examinations in Neurology. Philadelphia, W. B. Saunders Co., 1976.

Menkes MM, Rowe JS, Menkes JH: A 25 year follow-up study on the hyperkinetic child with minimal brain dysfunction. Pediatrics 39:393–399, 1967.

Milani-Comparetti A, Gidoni EA: Routine developmental examination in normal and retarded children. Dev Med Child Neurol 9:631–638, 1967.

Molnar G: Motor deficit of retarded infants and young children. Arch Phys Med Rehab 55:393–398, 1974.

Montgomery P, Richter E: Sensorimotor Integration for Developmentally Disabled Children: A Handbook. Los Angeles, California, Western Psychological Services, 1977.

Mosher LR, Pollin W, Stabenau, JR: Identical twins discordant for schizophrenia. Arch Gen Psychiatry 21:422–430, 1971.

Nitzun M, Stapleton J, Bender M: Movement and drama therapy with long-stay schizophrenics. Br J Med Psychol 47:101–119, 1974.

Noback C, Demarest R: The Human Nervous System, Basic Principles of Neurophysiology, 2nd ed. New York, McGraw-Hill 1975.

Norman DA: Memory and Attention. An Introduction to Human Information Processing, 2nd ed. New York, John Wiley and Sons, Inc., 1976.

Norton Y: Neurodevelopment and sensory integration for the profoundly retarded multiply handicapped child. Am J Occup Ther 29:93–100, 1975.

O'Connell A, Gardner E: Ingredients of Coordinate Movement. Am J Phys Med 46:334–361, 1967.

Ornitz E, Ritvo E: The syndrome of autism: a critical review. Am J Psychiatry 133:609–621, 1976.

Ornitz EM et al: The early development of autistic children. J Autism Child Schizophr 7:207–229, 1977.

Ottenbacher K et al: Nystagmus and ocular fixation difficulties in learning disabled children. Am J Occup Ther 33:717–721, 1979.

Ozer MN: The examination of "distractibility" in the child with learning problems. Clinical Proceedings. Children's Hospital National Medical Center 34:10–14, 1978.

Parmenter C: The asymmetrical tonic neck reflex in normal first and third grade children. Am J Occup Ther 29:463–468, 1975.

Pinkus JH, Tucker GJ: Behavioral Neurology. New York, Oxford University Press, 1974.

Platzer W: Effect of perceptual motor training on gross motor skill and self-concept of young children. Am J Occup Ther 30:423–428, 1976.

Quitkin F, Rifkin A, Klein DF: Neurological soft signs in schizophrenia and character disorders. Arch Gen Psychiatry 33:845–853, 1976.

Raskin RM, Baker GP: Tactual and visual integration in the learning processes: research and implications. J Learning Disabilities 8:108–112, 1975.

Reitan RM, Bavison LA (eds): Clinical Neuropsychology: Current Status and Applications. Washington DC, V. H. Winston & Sons, 1974.

Rider B: Perceptual-motor dysfunction in emotionally disturbed children. Am J Occup Ther 26:316–320, 1973.

Rochford JM et al: Neuropsychological impairments in functional psychiatric diseases. Arch Gen Psychiatry 22:114–119, 1970.

Rosenblith J: Behavioral Examination of the Neonate. The Comprehensive Management of Infants at Risk for CNS Deficit. Chapel Hill, University of North Carolina, 1974.

Saphier JD: The relation of perceptual-motor skills to learning and school success. J Learning Disabilities 6:583–592, 1973.

Schaltenbrand G: The development of human motility and motor disturbance. In OD Payton et al (eds): Scientific Bases for Neurophysiologic Approaches to Therapeutic Exercise. Philadelphia, F. A. Davis Co., 1977.

Schneider AM, Tarshis B: Physiological Psychology. New York, Random House, 1975.

Schroeder CV et al: SBC Adult Psychiatric Sensory Integration Evaluation. Second Experimental Edition. La Jolla, Ca, "SBC" Research Associates, 1978.

Schwartz RK: Olfaction and muscle activity: an EMG pilot study. Am J Occup Ther 33:185–192, 1979.

Schwartz R, Shipkin D, Cernak LS: Verbal and nonverbal memory, abilities of adult brain damaged patients. Am J Occup Ther 33:79–83, 1979.

Selkurt E: Basic Physiology for the Health Sciences. Boston, Little, Brown and Co, 1975.

Siev E, Freishtat B: Perceptual Dysfunction in the Adult Stroke Patient: A Manual for Evaluation and Treatment. Thorofare, NJ, Charles B. Slack, Inc., 1976.

Silberzahn M: Sensory integrative function in a child guidance clinic population. Am J Occup Ther 29:29–34, 1975.

Silver LB: A proposed view on the etiology of the neurological learning disability syndrome. J Learning Disabilities 4:123–133, 1971.

Silverman RE: Psychology, 2nd ed. Englewood Cliffs, NJ, Prentice-Hall, Inc. 1974.

Simonds J: Relationship between children's learning disorders and emotional disorders at a mental health clinic. J Clin Psychol 30:450–458, 1974.

Sister Kenny Institute: About Stroke. Minneapolis, Minnesota, Sister Kenny Institute, 1978.

Slingerland BH: A Multi-Sensory Approach to Language Arts for Specific Language Disability Children. A Guide for Primary Teachers. Cambridge, Ma, Educators Publishing Service, Inc., 1975.

Small L: Neurodiagnosis in Psychotherapy. New York, Brunner/Mazel Publishers, 1973.

Spache GD: Diagnostic Reading Scales. Monterey, Ca, California Test Bureau, 1963.

Stevens-Long J: Adult Life: Developmental Processes. Palo Alto, Ca, Mayfield Publishing Company, 1979.

Stoeling GBA, Van Der Werff Ten Bosch JJ (eds): Normal and Abnormal Development of Brain and Behavior. Baltimore, Williams and Wilkins, 1971.

Stone LJ, Church J: Childhood and Adolescence, 4th ed. New York, Random House, 1979.

Super C: Environmental effects on motor development: the case of "African infant precocity." Dev Med Child Neurol 18:561–567, 1976.

Suppes P: A survey of cognition in handicapped children. Rev Educ Research 44:145–176, 1974.

Swanson L: Effect of verbal and nonverbal short-term memory coding with normal and retarded children. Perceptual and Motor Skills 44:917–918, 1977.

Swiercinsky DP: Factorial pattern description and comparison of functional abilities in neuropsychological assessment. Perceptual and Motor Skills 48:231–241, 1979.

Treichel JA: Brain peptides and psychopharmacology. Science News 110:202–203, 1976.

Tucker GJ, Campion EW, Silberfarb PM: Sensorimotor functions and cognitive disturbance in psychiatric patients. Am J Psychiatry 132:17–21, 1975.

Twitchell TE et al: Transactions of the American Neurological Association 91:353–355, 1966.

Waldrop MF, Pedersen FA, Bell RQ: Minor physical anomalies and behavior in preschool children. Child Dev 39:391–400, 1968.

Walsh KW: Neuropsychology: A Clinical Approach. New York, Churchill Livingstone, 1978.

Waterland J: The supportive framework for willed movement. Am J Phys Med 46:266–278, 1967.

Weeks ZR: Effects of the vestibular system on human development. Part 1, Overview of functions and effects of stimulation. Am J Occup Ther 33:376–381, 1979.

Weeks ZR: Effects of the vestibular system on human development, Part 2. Effects of vestibular stimulation on mentally retarded, emotionally disturbed, and learning-disabled individuals. Am J Occup Ther 33:450–457, 1979.

Weeks ZR: An investigation of the relationship between sensory integrative dysfunction and emotional disturbance, Unpublished research, 1977.

Weeks ZR, Burack S, Barrett CE: An investigation of movement and behavior change in chronic schizophrenics. Unpublished research. 1979.

Wender PH: The minimal brain dysfunction syndrome in children: I. The syndrome and its relevance for psychiatry. II. A psychological and biochemical model for the syndrome. J Nerv Ment Dis 155:55–71, 1972.

Wender PH: Some speculations concerning a possible biochemical basis of minimal brain dysfunction. Life Sci 14:1605–1621, 1974.

White BL: The First Three Years of Life. New York, Avon Books, 1975.

Wiederholt JL: Historical perspectives on the education of the learning disabled: In L Mann, and D Sabatino (eds): The Second Review of Special Education, pp. 103–152. Philadelphia, JSE Press, 1974.

Wilentz JS: The Senses of Man. New York, Crowell Co., 1968.

Wolkowicz R, Fish J, Schaffer R: Sensory integration with autistic children. Can J Occup Ther 44:171–175, 1977.

Wood DR et al: Diagnosis and treatment of minimal brain dysfunction in adults. Arch Gen Psychiatry 33:1453–1460, 1976.

Zinkus PW, Gottlieb MI, Zinkus CB: The learning-disabled juvenile delinquent: a case for early intervention of perceptually handicapped children. Am J Occup Ther 33:180–184, 1979.

Additional References

Ayres AJ, Tickle LS: Hyper-responsivitiy to touch and vestibular stimuli as a predictor of positive response to sensory integration procedures by autistic children. Am J Occup Ther 34:375–381, 1980.

Benton A, Varniey N, de Hamsher C: Visual spatial judgment: a clinical test. Arch Neurol 35:364–367, 1978.

Caplan F: The First Telve Months of Life: Your Baby's Growth Month by Month. New York, Grosset and Dunlap, 1973.

Connors CK: A teacher rating scale for use in drug studies with children. Am J Psychiatry 126:884–888, 1969.

Davids A: Objective instrument for assessing hyperkinesis in children. J Learning Disabilities 4:499–501, 1971.

DeGangi GA, Berk RA, Larsen LA: The measurement of vestibular-based functions in preschool children. Am J Occup Ther 34:452–459, 1980.

Department of Health, Education, and Welfare Office of Education. Implementation of Part B of the Education of the Handicapped Act. Federal Register, Vol. 42, No. 163, Tuesday, August 23, 1977.

deQuiros JB: Diagnosis of vestibular disorders in the learning disabled. J Learning Disabilities 9:1 50–58, 1976.

Freeman B, Franke F, Ritvo E: The effects of response contingent vestibular stimulation on behavior of autistic and retarded children. J Autism Child Schizophr 6:353–358, 1976.

Madsen PS, Conte JR: Single subject research in occupational therapy: a case illustration. Am J Occup Ther 34:263–267, 1980.

Montgomery P, Gauger J: Sensory dysfunction in children who toe walk. Physical Therapy 58:1195–1204, 1978.

Montgomery P, Richter E: Effect of sensory integrative therapy on the neuromotor development of retarded children. Phys Ther 57:799–806, 1977.

Nelson D, Nitzberg L, Hollander T: visually monitored postrotary nystagmus in seven austitic children. Am J Occup Ther 34:382–386, 1980.

Ottenbacher K: Cerebral vascular accident: some characteristics of occupational therapy evaluation forms. Am J Occup Ther 34:268–271, 1980.

Ottenbacher K, Short MZ, Watson PJ: Nystagmus duration changes of learning disabled children during sensory integrative therapy. Perceptual and Motor Skills 48:1159–1164, 1979.

Siev E, Frieshtat B: Perceptual Dysfunction in the Adult Stroke Patient: A Manual for Evaluation and Treatment. Thorofare, NJ, Charles B. Slack Co., 1976.

Stilwell JM, Crowe TK, McCallum LW: Postrotary nystagmus as a function of communication disorders. Am J Occup Ther 32:222–228, 1978.

Troll LE: Early and Middle Adulthood. Monterey, Ca, Brooks/Cole Publishing Co., 1975.

Werry JS: Developmental hyperactivity. Pediatr Clin North Am 3:581–599, 1968.

APPENDIX 5–1 ASSESSMENT AREAS AND SOME REPRESENTATIVE TESTS

Reflex and Voluntary Motor Functioning, Including Developmental Levels

1. Bayley N: Bayley Scales of Infant Development. The Psychological Corporation.
2. Brazleton T: Neonatal Behavioral Assessment Scale. J.B. Lippincott Co.
3. Bruininks-Oseretsky Test of Motor Proficiency. American Guidance Service.
4. Denver Developmental Screening Test. Ladoca Project and Publishing Foundation, Inc.
5. Fiorentino M: Normal and Abnormal Development. The Influence of Primitive Reflexes on Motor Development. Springfield, Il, Charles C Thomas, 1973.
6. Fiorentino M: Reflex Testing Methods for Evaluating CNS Development. Second Edition. Springfield, Il, Charles C Thomas, 1973.
7. Gesell Developmental Schedules. The Psychological Corporation.
8. Hoskins T, Squires JE: Developmental assessment: a test for gross motor and reflex development. Phys Ther 53:117–125, 1973.
9. Milani-Comparetti A, Gidoni EA: Routine developmental examination in normal and retarded children. Dev Med Child Neurol 9:631–638, 1967.

Sensory Receptor Inadequacies

1. Auditory Acuity. Evaluation by a qualified audiologist may be indicated for persons demonstrating possible hearing problems and for those having language problems that may be due to poor discrimination of sounds from inability to hear well.
2. Visual Acuity. Examination by an ophthalmologist or optometrist is generally advisable.
3. Sensory Tests. Evaluations may be done to assess light touch, deep pressure, pain, temperature, two-point discrimination, vibration, position and movement awareness, smell, taste, and so forth. The examiner cannot be sure in all cases whether the deficiency is in the sensory receptors or in the CNS. Books describing neurological examinations explain how these clinical observations are made.

Sensory Integration Deficiencies, Disorders of Perception, and Perceptual Developmental Levels

1. Assessment of Sensorimotor Integration in Preschool Children. In DeGangi GA, Berk RA, Larsen LA: The measurement of vestibular-based functions in preschool children. Am J Occup Ther 34:452–459, 1980.
2. Bender-Gestalt Test. American Orthopsychiatric Association, Inc.

3. Benton A, Varniey N, de Hamsher C: Visual spatial judgment: a clinical test. Arch Neurol 35:364–367, 1978.
4. Developmental Test of Visual-Motor Integration. Follett Educational Corporation.
5. Frostig Developmental Test of Visual Perception. Consulting Psychologists Press.
6. Minnesota Paper Form Board Test. The Psychological Corporation.
7. Motor-Free Visual Perception Test. Academic Therapy Publications.
8. Purdue Perceptual Motor Survey. C. E. Merrill Publishing Company.
9. SBC Adult Psychiatric Sensory Integration Evaluation. "SBC" Research Associates.
10. Siev E, Freishtat B: Perceptual Dysfunction in the Adult Stroke Patient: A Manual for Evaluation and Treatment. Thorofare, NJ, Charles B. Slack Co., 1976.
11. Southern California Sensory Integration Tests. Western Psychological Services.

Speech and Language Deficiencies

1. Goldman-Fristoe-Woodcock Test of Auditory Discrimination. American Guidance Service.
2. Jansky J: The Jansky Screening Index. 120 East 89th Street, New York, NY 10028.
3. Jordan Oral Screening Test, Jordan Written Screening Test, Jordan Auditory Screening Test. In Jordan DR: Dyslexia in the Classroom. Columbus, Oh, C. E. Merrill Publishing Co., 1972.
4. Illinois Test of Psycholinguistic Abilities. Urbana, Il 61801. University of Illinois Press.
5. Slingerland Screening Tests for Identifying Children with Specific Language Disability. Educators Publishing Service, Inc.
6. Wepman Auditory Discrimination Test. Western Psychological Services.

Academic Strengths and Weaknesses°

1. Goodenough-Harris Drawing Test. Harcourt Brace Jovanovich.
2. Gray Oral Reading Test. Bobbs-Merrill.
3. Peabody Picture Vocabulary Test. American Guidance Service.
4. The Pupil Rating Scale for Learning Disabilities. Grune and Stratton.
5. Quick Test. (Intelligence) Psychological Test Specialists.
6. Slosson Intelligence Test (SIT) and Slosson Oral Reading Test. Slosson Educational Publications.
7. Wide Range Achievement Test. Guidance Associates of Delaware.

Social and Emotional Functioning

1. Behavioral examination for autistic children. In EM Ornitz et al: The early development of autistic children. J Autism Child Schizophr 7:207–229, 1977.
2. Mental Status Examinations. These assessment examinations consist of interview questions and observations that help to assess such factors as appearance or mannerisms, speech, orientation, intellectual or thought disturbances, affect, attitude, social functioning, and observable motor involvement or activity level. Numerous adaptations are commonly used in psychiatry and neurology, and forms are available for both children and adults.
3. Preschool Attainment Record. American Guidance Service.
4. Vineland Social Maturity Scale. American Guidance Service.

Activity Level

1. Connors CK: A teacher rating scale for use in drug studies with children. Am J Psychiatry 126:884–888, 1969.
2. Rating Scale for Hyperkinesis. In A Davids: Objective instrument for assessing hyperkinesis in children. J Learning Disabilities 4:499–501, 1971.
3. Werry-Weiss-Peters Activity Scale. In JS Werry: Developmental hyperactivity. Pediatr Clin North Am 3:581–599, 1968.

APPENDIX 5–2 PUBLISHERS' ADDRESSES FOR TESTS IN APPENDIX 1

1. American Guidance Service, Publishers' Building, Circle Pines, Minnesota 55014.
2. American Orthopsychiatric Association, Inc., 1790 Broadway, New York, NY 10019.
3. The Bobbs-Merrill Company, Inc., Publishers, 4300 West 62nd St., Indianapolis, In 46206.
4. Consulting Psychologists Press, Inc., 577 College Ave., Palo Alto, Ca 94306.
5. Educators Publishing Service, Inc., 75 Moulton St., Cambridge, Ma 02138.
6. Follett Publishing Company, 1010 West Washington Blvd., Chicago, Ill 60607.
7. Grune and Stratton, Inc., 111 Fifth Ave., New York, NY 10003.
8. Guidance Associates of Delaware, 1526 Gilpin Ave., Wilmington, De 19806.
9. Harcourt Brace Jovanovich, Inc., 757 3rd Ave., New York, NY 10017.
10. La Doca Project and Publishing Foundation, Inc., East 51 Ave. and Lincoln St., Denver, Co 80216.
11. J. B. Lippincott Company, East Washington Sq., Philadelphia, Pa 19105.
12. Charles E. Merrill Publishing Company, 1300 Alum Creek Dr., Columbus, Oh 43216.
13. The Psychological Corporation, 304 East 45th St., New York, NY.
14. Psychological Test Specialists, Box 9229, Missoula, Montana 59801.
15. "SBC" Research Associates, Psychiatric Occupational Therapy, 8314 Paseo Del Ocaso, La Jolla, Ca 92037.
16. Charles B. Slack, Inc., 6900 Grove Rd., Thorofare, NJ 08086.
17. Slosson Educational Publications, 140 Pine St., East Aurora, NY 14052.
18. Western Psychological Services, 12031 Wilshire Blvd., Los Angeles, Ca 90025.

°Including intelligence tests not requiring special qualifications to administer.

CHAPTER 6

THERAPEUTIC RELAXATION

Shereen D. Farber, MS, OTR, FAOTA

A major emphasis of the text to this point has been to synthesize a conceptual model for treatment of CNS deficits and related problems. This frame of reference for neurorehabilitation addresses patients who have suffered a nervous system insult and attempts to reduce the sequelae *(secondary prevention)* while improving adaptive responses. It seems intuitively obvious that *primary prevention* (the identification of risk factors and subsequent modification of environment or behavior or both designed to block the occurrence of a disease) should receive priority whenever possible. The intent of this chapter is to explain the use of therapeutic relaxation modalities to relieve stress and promote such primary and secondary prevention. General information regarding the nature of stress and psychosomatic illness will be included along with specific assessment and treatment techniques.

BACKGROUND

According to Selye (1974, 1976), *stress* can be defined as the body's nonspecific response to any demand. In stress studies, Selye noted a *general adaptation syndrome* with three components: an alarm reaction following exposure to harmful stimuli, a stage of resistance that produced increased defenses to the stressor, and a stage of exhaustion leading to disease or in extreme cases, death. Stress has been characterized as the most prevalent health problem in America (Rosch, 1979). A number of experts believe that there is an intimate relationship between chronic stress and the manifestation of disease (Thomas, 1977; Rosch, 1979; Rogers, Dubey, Reich, 1979; Selye, 1974).

One must be able to differentiate between the stressor (the agent causing harmful bodily reactions) and the responses of the individual. The same agent may produce deleterious effects in one individual while motivating a second to reorganize his behavior to increase personal productivity. Variations in reactions are due in part to cultural, environmental, genetic, and physiological factors (Rosch, 1979). Positive events such as promotions, graduation from an educational program, and pleasurable experiences may induce a stress reaction. Selye (1974) calls these positive stress reactions "eustress;" he labels responses from aversive stimuli as "distress." Eustress and distress must be balanced. D. A. Tubesing, President of Whole Person Associates in Duluth, Minnesota, is quoted by Bolch (1980) as comparing stress to the tension placed on a violin string. Optimum tension produces a nice sound from the string, whereas excess tension can cause the string to snap.

One must also consider stress in relationship to its effect on the body's homeostasis (Cousins, 1979). Vital body functions should be in balance with each other. Stress can interfere with energy restoration and immune responses (Cousins, 1979; Rogers, Dubey, Reich, 1979). A main goal of the multisensory treatment approach as described in Chapter 3 is to enhance autonomic nervous system (ANS) homeostasis. Many of the therapeutic relaxation procedures included in this chapter have been observed to facilitate such homeostatic and restorative processes (Benson, 1973, 1976).

Psychosomatic Disease

The author views illness and wellness as a continuous process in which various etiological factors may cause an individual to move from a wellness state to emotional, physical, or psychosomatic dysfunction (Fig. 6–1). This view was initially influenced by the work of Lewis (1953), who thought of health as a single concept and believed that it was impossible to use different criteria for physical and mental health. For the purpose of this chapter, psychosomatic illness is defined as any bodily disease process arising from psychogenic factors.

Illness and Personality

A variety of disease patterns have been described for patients with characteristic personality traits or diagnostic conditions. Eastwood (1975) reports, for instance, that patients suffering from psychiatric illness demonstrate more physical complaints than do other people.

In 1974 Friedman and Rosenman described two basic behavioral types: A and B. The *type A* person is portrayed as a stress externalizer likely to suffer from hypertension, obesity, strokes, and ulcers. This type of individual is frequently hard-driving and success oriented, having free-floating hostility and time urgency (pushed to do more in less and less time). Type A persons claim they "don't have time to relax." They function on the sympathetic side of the ANS continuum.

The *type B* individual is resistant to stress and has a balanced response to life's demands. People with type B behavior live longer than those with type A. They learn to relax after stressful periods. Ro-

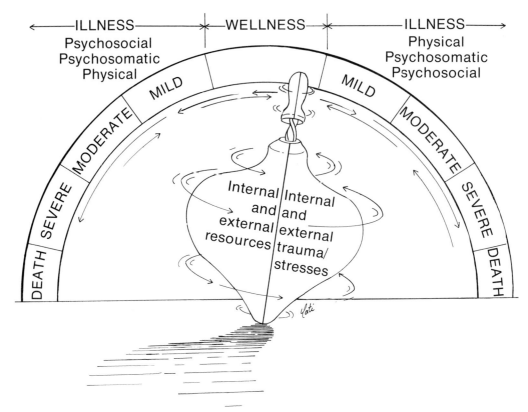

ILLNESS ← | → WELLNESS ← | → ILLNESS
Psychosocial Psychosomatic Physical
Physical Psychosomatic Psychosocial

MILD MODERATE SEVERE DEATH

Internal and external resources

Internal and external trauma/ stresses

Figure 6–1.

senman and Chesney (1980) also describe a *type X* personality characterized by behavior having equal components of types A and B.

Arnold Fox, an expert in stress management, in an interview with Pike (1980) presents still another personality type — *type C*. Those with type C personalities are internalizers likely to cause changes in their immune responses that result in development of conditions such as cancer, colds, depression, and impotence. Fox believes that these individuals turn their negative feelings inward; the result is adrenal gland stimulation and production of cortisone, which is an immunosuppressant. Lewis (1975) describes a "cancer personality" with behavioral traits similar to Fox's type C personality.

ASSESSMENT TOOLS

Physical Examination. As with all other effective types of treatment, assessment of stressed patients is necessary before specific treatment can be planned.

One of the best ways to begin the therapeutic relaxation assessment is by referring the patient to a physician for a complete physical examination. This protects the therapist from such situations as trying to help a tense patient reduce the number of headaches he suffers when those headaches are the result of a condtion such as a tumor, which requires immediate medical treatment. It may also prove reassuring to the patient. The physician and the therapist must communicate about the results of the examination, with the physician pointing out any necessary precautions.

Identification of patients at risk for severe stress reactions is a high priority in primary prevention programs. Physicians normally screen vital signs during the physical examination. When the physician finds patients demonstrating imbalance in autonomic function (hypertension), referral for therapeutic relaxation should be considered with medical treatment as a means to help prevent cerebrovascular accident or heart attack. Relaxation therapy complements pharmacological intervention. The author recognizes that medication may quickly reduce the patient's hypertension, but if the patient's lifestyle does not promote health, the medication alone may not be enough to protect the patient from illness. In addition, physicians may be tempted to prescribe medication to treat a patient's specific symptoms instead of helping the patient understand that his lifestyle or method of coping with stress may be unhealthy. Many patients who take a wide variety of medication experience adverse drug interactions. While a pill may quickly temporarily remove a symptom, it decreases the immediacy of assuming responsibility for changing pathological personal habits.

Screening. There are *stress inventories* and *rating scales* that can be employed to assist in screening those at risk (Holmes and Rahe, 1967; Rosenman and Chesney, 1980). The author has developed a checklist to facilitate screening patients (Appendix 6–1). Patients showing an imbalance between work and play-leisure activities frequently become ill. The emotional and physical history is included to give the therapist some insight into the patient's coping methods.

If a patient has a history of many of the illnesses on the checklist, or if members of his immediate family have had many diseases, one might assume that the patient and family use illness as a way to cope with stress. For this type of patient, illness provides a rest from responsibility. Unfortunately, while psychosomatic illness may allow a patient a rest from a demanding schedule, it does cause damage to the body and is therefore maladaptive.

Initial Interview. The initial interview, as discussed in Chapter 2, is used to help establish rapport, to further screen the patient and to obtain an occupational history, and to initiate the educational program. The therapist then explains the purposes of therapeutic relaxation. During this time it is especially important that the therapist set a positive example of good health habits if the patient is to accept the idea of therapeutic relaxation. If the therapist appears tense and displays unhealthy habits, the patient is not likely to be convinced that therapeutic relaxation is worthwhile.

Stress Diary and Dietary Assessment. The stress diary is one method of helping a patient become aware of his body responses, life schedule, habits, diet, and so on. The patient is given a small spiral note pad and asked to set it up as illustrated in Figure 6–2. The left side of the page is used to list key descriptions of sensation or emotion experienced during the morning, afternoon, and evening. Examples of typical recorded statements for this section include:

8:00 Awoke — headache, anxious
10:00 Sore throat

The right side of the notebook page is used for the anecdotal record and diet for the day. For example:

8:00 Awoke — remembered neuroanatomy test scheduled for 10:00
10:00 Took test
11:00 Went to anatomy lab
11:30 Took break — had chocolate bar for lunch
1:00 Bad headache

The patient is asked to keep the stress diary for a two-week period; this forces him to take the first step toward assuming responsibility for his actions. Many individuals, after keeping a stress diary, report a new awareness of unhealthy patterns.

After a two-week period, the therapist analyzes the diary with the patient. The number of specific symptoms is quantified and the results plotted on graph paper. Comparison of symptoms, patterns, and daily events helps the therapist and the patient come to conclusions regarding changes that might improve the patient's health. Either a dietician or a nutritional biochemist may be consulted to analyze the diet.

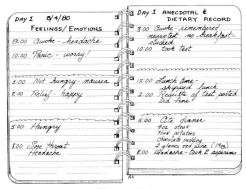

Figure 6–2.

Other diagnostic baseline activities may be conducted to complete the patient's assessment profile, including diagnostic use of electromyography (EMG), evaluation of physical conditioning, and frustration tolerance assessment. The patient and the therapist then plan a realistic therapy program on the basis of the patient's needs, interests, abilities, and limitations.

THERAPEUTIC RELAXATION PROCEDURES

The Patient's Responsibility. The single most important aspect of treatment for distressed patients is to help them to understand the nature of stress, distress, eustress, psychosomatic illness, and hypochondria (imaginary ill health) and then to encourage them to assume responsibility for *gradually* changing unhealthy aspects of their lives. Instead of coming to grips with fundamental causes of stress, many stressed patients become accustomed to visiting family physicians for each new physical manifestation of the stress. Likewise, "pill popping" may be an ingrained habit.

As part of the educational program, patients are assigned reading materials on stress and its management (see the recommended reading section of the bibliography). They are then required to read this material and participate in patient education classes as the first phase of therapeutic intervention.

Group Education Classes. Patient groups are limited to six members per session to facilitate maximum group interaction. During one initial group meeting the author overheard an impatient gentleman state, "I hope this doesn't take too long. I only have six hours available to learn to relax." Another group member laughed and said, "You sure are a classic type A!" Thus the door was opened for a dynamic discussion. Experts in nutrition, physical conditioning, creativity, and related areas may be invited to contribute to group sessions as is appropriate.

Individual Therapeutic Program. In conjunction with group therapy, individual programs are designed in which one-on-one therapy is ongoing. The therapist continually assesses the patient's progress. It may take several months to find the correct combination of relaxation activities, physical conditioning, diet, and work load to effect maximum stress resistance. There seems to be no one formula that works universally; however, successful programs seem to require elements of relaxation and physical conditioning. Patients are urged to make gradual changes because any change, even a change for the better, can be stressful.

Therapeutic Relaxation Activities. Since things that reduce stress for some people may increase it for others, the therapist must have a large "bag of tricks" from which to select the most appropriate activity for a given patient. Certain activities are not relevant for given patient populations. For example, when conducting a therapeutic relaxation program for psychiatric patients, the author recommends:

1. Avoiding use of fantasy exercises with those lacking reality orientation.
2. Avoiding use of deep breathing exercises with patients suffering from chronic schizophrenia; these patients seem to start breathing on a cortical level instead of subcortically. They may stop breathing or begin hyperventilating.

Certain types of physical exercise may be contraindicated for patients with specific physical disabilities. An example of this includes any activity stressful to joints for a patient with rheumatoid arthritis.

The following list of activities is by no means complete. Many excellent references are now available to provide further programming ideas. In general, a repetitive, rhythmical activity (as discussed in Chapter 3) is calming. Many techniques discussed in Chapter 3, such as maintained pressure, slow rolling, and slow stroking, are also effective for those in need of therapeutic relaxation.

Before learning any of the specific relaxation activities the patient must understand that a person makes his own schedule; his schedule should not make him. He alone is responsible for making necessary changes in his lifestyle. Also, he cannot make relaxation occur but instead must learn to let it occur. Patients are cautioned not to make relaxation another job. It is best to plan relaxation activities into the schedule several times per day so that the harmful effects of stress are not allowed to build up.

AEROBICS. Cooper (1968) is credited with initiating a total body conditioning program that is designed to improve heart and lung function while toning up the entire body. Once the "athlete" is conditioned, activities are done at a given rate for a given distance. This forces an increase in the heart rate. Specific tables and instructions are included in Cooper's text. Jogging, swimming, bike riding, walking, and jumping rope can all provide aerobic exercise and are repetitive activities. The therapist must be careful to advise that the patient initiate an aerobic program slowly after medical clearance. Many patients try to overdo exercise in their desire to get into condition immediately. As stated earlier, the ideal stress reduction program contains elements of physical conditioning and appropriate relaxation activities.

AUTOGENIC TRAINING. This relaxation technique was originated by J. H. Schultz (Schultz and Luthe, 1959) as a result of Dr. Schultz's experiments using hypnosis with psychosomatically ill patients. Schultz taught patients to progress from being hypnotized to effective self-hypnosis. The patient must have a positive attitude about his ability to learn the technique if he is to be successful and must have an important reason (compelling motivation) to learn autogenic training. The patient must learn to surrender himself to the process instead of making an excessive effort. Patients are encouraged to find a comfortable position, focus on self-relaxation, and transport themselves into the organ they wish to influence. Since digestion appears to interfere with the process, one should wait at least two hours after eating before initiating autogenic training.

BIOFEEDBACK. Biofeedback is a process of monitoring various unconscious physiological functions — for example, blood pressure, heart rate, skin temperature, muscle tone, and brain waves — for the purpose of normalizing autonomic function and for muscle re-education. Biofeedback is frequently used in combination with other activities such as progressive relaxation or fantasy exercises. Many health professionals, including psychologists, dentists, and occupational and physical therapists, use biofeedback as either a diagnostic or treatment modality. Biofeedback technicians also work under the direction of qualified health professionals.

Each health practitioner may use the equipment in a unique manner according to his professional background, interest, and experience. Biofeedback offers the distressed patient immediate information regarding body and mind states. This can enhance the effectiveness of therapeutic techniques. Therapists using biofeedback are encouraged to join national and state biofeedback societies that provide continuing education and help ensure quality care through specific certification.

CONVERTING ENERGY. The purpose of this technique is to help a patient learn to move from a negative state of mind to a more positive one. The patient is interviewed and asked about happy experiences he has had. Then, while the patient is deep breathing (see section of this chapter on deep breathing), he is asked to focus on the energy around him. The patient is given the following directions: "Let your attention drift to the energies around you, such as those required to grow plants and trees. Feel that energy. Think of a time when you were very happy, young, and strong." The therapist can use whatever fantasy is most meaningful to the patient. This helps the patient convert to a more personal form of energy. After the patient is breathing deeply and flowing with his positive image, he is asked to think of an experience during which energy was destructive to him. Following this fantasy, the patient learns to shift from negative energy experiences to positive ones. Mastery of this technique will allow an individual to change his mental state from a negative to a positive one.

YOGA. This science, practiced for thousands of years, helps to tone up the body, gain control over individual muscles, and improve the function of various body systems. There are several types of yoga, including a meditation process and a type that is primarily exercises. Yoga should be done under the supervision of a trained individual; some of the exercises can be stressful and may be contraindicated for some individuals.

DEEP BREATHING. This technique is a part of yoga practice that allows an individual to relax, to totally fill his lungs, and to normalize autonomic function (Benson, Beary, Carol, 1976). Deep breathing can be done in combination with many other relaxation techniques such as progressive relaxation, converting energy, fantasy exercises, and massage. Figure 6–3 shows the steps involved in the process. The patient is given the following instructions:

1. Assume a comfortable position. Clothing should be nonrestrictive.

2. Place your palms on your abdomen.

3. Make sure that your nasal passages are clear; one should ideally breathe air in through the nose for purification.

4. During inhaling: air should first fill the lower lungs, forcing your abdomen out; your hands should move slightly apart. Then continuing to inhale, expand your chest up and out; raise your shoulders and hold. This inhaling process can be done to the count of 4 in an even, rhythmical pattern.

5. Exhaling is also done to 4 counts and is just the reverse of inhaling.

It may take a patient several weeks of practice before he can do deep breathing in combination with other relaxation tech-niques. At first, many patients may have to find a quiet environment so that they can relax without distraction. The experienced deep breather can use this technique under any circumstances. For example, the author was attempting to unwind following a long, busy day by deep breathing. Her twin daughters decided that it would be great fun to take a ride on Mom's tummy! Deep breathing continued without interruption.

DIET. Many foods have been identified by a number of experts as capable of causing adverse physical and emotional reactions. Monosodium glutamate (MSG), red wine, cheddar cheese, and chocolate have all been reported to cause headaches. The therapist should work with a nutritional biochemist or dietician who has studied diets in relation to stress to advise the patient about foods to avoid. In addition to the type of food a patient eats, the way he eats is also important. The diges-

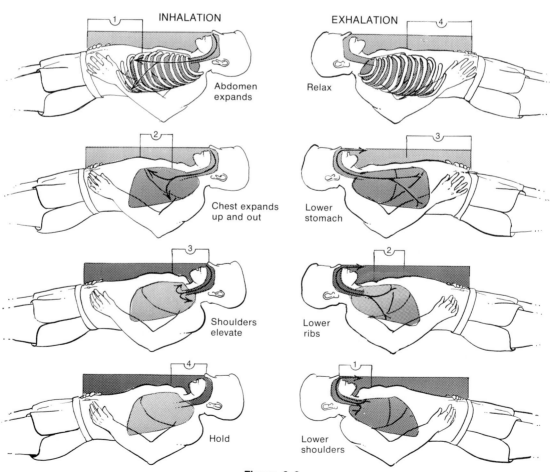

Figure 6–3.

tive process is dominated by the parasympathetic division of the ANS, as mentioned earlier in this text. If the patient attempts to eat on the run or has a stressful eating environment, he may compromise parasympathetic function.

DIFFERENTIAL RELAXATION. During activity, the individual is encouraged to take an inventory of tensions within his body. He is taught to differentiate between those tensions needed to carry out activity (primary tensions or tone) from those that are not necessary (secondary tensions or tone). He is taught to relax unnecessary tensions while continuing the activity. Biofeedback may be used during the activity to monitor muscle tone. An example of this process is when typing a paper, the typist is taught to stop and shrug his shoulders approximately every 20 minutes. He should tighten muscles in the shoulder region in all planes of motion including elevation, retraction, protraction, flexion, and extension. After tightening or contracting each muscle, the individual then slowly releases tone in each muscle group. It is often helpful to have the typist lean over from the waist, allowing his arms to hang down (see Fig. 3–10). This may facilitate the tonic labyrinthine inverted response to first promote relaxation and then excite trunk extensors.

CREATIVE EXPRESSION. Many people have a strong need to create something that is uniquely their own. Those individuals who are driven by this need seem to select occupations that require creativity. Those who ignore this need and structure their lives with experiences lacking in creative outlets may become distressed. The therapist should explore the patient's need to be creative along with the opportunities for creativity within the patient's lifestyle.

FANTASY EXERCISES. A variety of fantasy exercises can be utilized during deep breathing to accomplish different purposes. A fantasy exercise can be conducted with a group followed by a group discussion. Fantasy can also be used by an individual as a form of creative outlet or self hypnotism. It should not be used with patients lacking reality orientation.

MASSAGE. When excessive muscle tone builds in various body regions, the stressed patient experiences discomfort that can complicate behavior. Massage is one method of reducing the tone in a given area. Physical therapists are professionally trained in this technique, but family members can also learn to massage the stressed individual. The patient himself can massage accessible body areas. Besides reduction of spasm in a muscular group, massage involves the psychological benefits of touching and being touched.

MEDITATION. Benson (1976) has studied the effects of meditation on body processes. Meditation has been found to be successful in lowering respiratory rate, heart rate, blood pressure, oxygen consumption, and muscle tension while increasing brain alpha waves. Meditation involves repetition of a sound, word, or phrase that is said silently or chanted. The word may have meaning or be meaningless. In order to meditate successfully, the individual must assume a comfortable position in a quiet environment. He must also develop a passive volitional attitude. The meditation process is frequently done in conjunction with deep breathing — on exhaling, the individual says (silently) the word he chooses. He allows himself to relax, redirecting his attention if he should actively begin to think about something else. This process should be continued for about 20 minutes. Meditation should not be done within two hours of eating because digestion seems to interfere with the technique. Too much meditation may cause hallucinations in some individuals.

MOVEMENT. Movement in general is important in helping our body clear its waste and to stimulate endocrine gland activity, release tension, tone up muscles, and so on. Dance is one good way to incorporate movement into a therapeutic relaxation program; in aerobic dancing the elements of aerobic conditioning are combined with typical dance steps. Anaerobic exercise (short spurts of exercise such as running sprints) may be helpful in improving body flexibility and coordination. When a patient is using movement as a relaxation technique, he is encouraged to *let* movement occur instead of trying to make it occur. For example, when an individual is sweeping the floor using a push broom, he should allow the broom to float away from his body instead of fighting the movement needed for pushing.

Shaking is a warm-up procedure that releases tension and relaxes muscles. The individual should let his hands and arms hang at his sides loosely. He should vigorously shake his total upper extremities. The same technique can be done with the lower extremities. Shaking generally produces a warm, tingling feeling.

PROGRESSIVE RELAXATION. This technique was developed by Jacobson (1939, 1957, 1964) and has been used by many therapists in conjunction with deep breathing. The patient is asked to contract the muscles in his feet and then slowly release the contraction. This is repeated a second time. Each set of muscles progressing from the feet rostrally, is contracted and then slowly relaxed. The concept behind this procedure is that when a patient voluntarily contracts a muscle over excess muscle tone, he can release some of the hypertonicity as he relaxes the muscle.

RECOGNITION OF TENSION. A basic procedure in relaxation therapy is learning to recognize when tension is developing within the body. The patient is taught to avoid allowing unnecessary tension to build in any muscular group. As tension is increasing in a muscle, the patient uses the process just described of further tightening the muscle and then relaxing it. In addition, the patient can give himself suggestions that the muscle is getting loose, soft, limp, warm, or any other appropriate suggestion. It is important for a patient to know the parts of his body that usually develop too much tone during the course of the day, such as the upper back and neck. Taking an inventory of tone several times daily is a recommendation.

REFERENCES

Benson H, Beary JF, Carol MP: The relaxation response. *In* J White and J Fadiman (eds): Relax. New York, Dell, 1976, pp. 67–76.

Benson H, Rosner BA, Marzetta BR: Decreased systolic blood pressure in hypertensive subjects who practiced meditation. J Clin Invest 52:8a, 1973.

Bolch J: How to manage stress. Reader's Digest July 1980, p. 81.

Cooper K: Aerobics. New York, Bantam Books, 1968

Cousins N: Stress. JAMA 242:459, 1979

Eastwood MR: The Relation Between Physical and Mental Illness: The Physical Status of Psychiatric Patients at a Multiphasic Screening Survey. Toronto, University of Toronto Press, 1975.

Friedman M, Rosenman RH: Type A Behavior and Your Heart. Greenwich, Cn, Fawcett Publications, 1974.

Holmes TH, Rahe RH: The social readjustment rating scale. J Psychosom Med 11:213–218, 1967.

Jacobson E: Progressive Relaxation. Chicago, University of Chicago Press, 1939.

Jacobson E: You Must Relax. New York, McGraw-Hill, 1957.

Jacobson E: Anxiety and Tension Control. Philadelphia, J. B. Lippincott Co., 1964.

Lewis A: Health as a social concept. Br J Soc 4:109, 1954.

Lewis HR, Lewis ME: Psychosomatics: How Your Emotions Can Damage Your Health. Los Angeles, Pinnacle Books, Inc., 1975.

Lipowski ZJ (ed): Psychological aspects of physical illness. Advances in Psychosomatic Medicine 8. London, 1972.

Mason JW: Specificity in the organization of neuroendocrine profiles. Frontiers of Neurology and Neuroscience Research. Toronto, Neuroscience Institute, 1974.

Pike A: Stress from drugs to nutrition . . . how one M.D. handles it. Let's Live, April, 1980.

Rogers MP, Dubey D, Reich P: The influence of the psyche and the brain on immunity and disease susceptibility: A critical review. Psychosomatic Medicine 41:147–164, 1979.

Rosch PJ: Stress and illness. JAMA 242:427–428, 1979.

Rosenman RH, Chesney MA: The relationship of type A behavior pattern to coronary heart disease. Activ Nerv Sup (Praha) 22:1–45, 1980.

Schultz JH, Luthe W: Autogenic Training: A Psychophysiological Approach to Psychotherapy. New York, Grune and Stratton, 1959.

Selye H: Stress Without Distress. Philadelphia, J. B. Lippincott Co., 1974.

Selye H: The Stress of Life. New York, McGraw-Hill, 1976.

Thomas CB: Habits of Nervous Tension: Clues to the Human Condition. Baltimore, 725 Wolfe St., 1977.

Recommended Reading

Benson H, Kleeper M: The Relaxation Response. New York, William Morrow and Co., 1975.

Blain T: Goodbye Allergies. Secaucus, NJ, Citadel Press, 1965.

Eichenlaub JE: The Minnesota Doctor's Home Treasury of Unusual Stress Easers and Strong Shields Against Emotional and Physical Upset. New York, Award Books, Prentice Hall, Inc., 1964.

Foman L: Lilias Yoga and You. WCET TV, 2222 Chicasaw St., Cincinnati, Ohio 45219.

Freedman L, Galton L: Freedom from Backaches. New York, Simon and Schuster, 1976.

Gould H: Headaches: Causes, Treatment and Prevention. New York, Barnes and Noble, 1973.

Hittleman R: Yoga — 28 Day Exercise Plan. New York, Bantam Book, 1969.

Masters R: How to Control Your Emotions. Lincoln, NE, Foundation Books, 1974.

Miller DE: Body Mind — The Whole Person Health Book. Englewood Cliffs, NJ, Prentice Hall, 1974.

Stevens B: Don't Push the River — It Flows By Itself. Moab, UT, Real People Press, 1970.

Viscott D: Bad moods: how to handle them. Today's Health, March 1974.

White J, Fadiman J (eds): Relax. New York, Dell, 1976.

Yafa SH: Stress. Playboy, February 1975.

APPENDIX 6-1 STRESS SCREENING INVENTORY

Vocational/Avocational Balance

	Yes	No	Comments
1. Regularly works more than 45–50 hrs/wk			
2. Frequently brings work home			
3. Feels pressured at work			
4. Reports that he/she has no time for hobbies			
5. Reports that he/she has no outside interests			
6. Reports that he/she does not know how to relax			
7. Feels guilt when not working			
8. Turns hobby into another job			
9. Enjoys hobbies, home life, and relaxation time			

Emotional-Physical History

Include summary of current medical condition as reported by physician.

	Yes	No	Comments
1. Previous history:			
a. allergies			
b. arthritis			
c. asthma			
d. blood pressure: high			
low			
normal			
e. cancer			
f. colitis			
g. constipation			
h. diarrhea			
i. dizzy spells			
j. functional bowel disease			
k. heart disease			
l. headaches			
a. cluster			
b. menstrual			
c. migraine			
d. tension			
m. mental illness			
n. nausea			
o. nervousness			
p. psoriasis			
q. ulcer			
r. urinary frequency			
s. weight fluctuation			
t. other			

Personal Habits

1. Smoking
   amt./wk.
   past history
2. Drinking
   amt./wk.
   past history

Appendix continued on following page

APPENDIX 6–1 STRESS SCREENING INVENTORY *(Continued)*

Personal Habits *(Continued)*

3. Medication taken daily
4. Physical exercise: amt./day/time
   a. jogging
   b. walking
   c. swimming
   d. jumping rope
   e. specific exercises
   f. bike riding
   g. other
   h. no exercise

	Quantity/Wk	Comments
5. Usual diet – common foods		
a. beer		
b. buttermilk		
c. candy		
d. canned foods		
e. cheese (processed)		
f. chocolate		
g. coffee		
h. cola beverages		
i. eggs		
j. fruits – fresh		
k. fried foods		
l. ice cream		
m. margarine/butter		
n. meats/poultry/fish (fresh)		
o. meats – processed		
p. milk		
q. pastries		
r. salt		
s. sugar		
t. tea		
u. vegetables – fresh/frozen		
v. vegetables – canned		
w. whole grains (bread)		
x. wine		
red		
white		
y. yogurt		
z. other:		

	Yes	No	Comments
6. Eating habits			
a. eat 3 meals a day			
b. eat small amounts 5 or more times a day			
c. snack			
d. eat leisurely meals			
e. eat rapidly			
f. chew food thoroughly			
g. crave sweets			
h. sneak food			
i. overeat – stuff self			
j. drink fluids during the day			
k. enjoy eating			
l. eat because it is necessary			
m. always on a diet			
n. can eat anything			
o. other:			

CHAPTER 7

ADAPTIVE EQUIPMENT

Shereen D. Farber, MS, OTR, FAOTA
With a section on splint construction by
Judith Hunt Kiel, MS, OTR

The purpose of this chapter is to include a representative sample of adaptive equipment that has been successfully utilized in the multisensory approach. For most of the equipment included in the chapter, the following information will be provided: neurophysiological rationale, indications, contraindications and precautions, and methods of construction or commercial source.

Ideally, all adaptive equipment used in neurorehabilitation should meet the following six criteria. The equipment should:
1. Stimulate appropriate neurophysiological mechanisms
2. Enhance adaptive behavioral response formation
3. Not produce aversive responses anywhere in the body
4. Be dynamic instead of static whenever possible to allow the patient to move appropriately within the equipment
5. Allow normal sensory processes to occur
6. Prevent deformity.

It is not always possible to meet every one of these criteria, but an attempt to do so is recommended.

SPECIFIC ADAPTIVE EQUIPMENT

Orthokinetic Cuff

History and Neurophysiological Rationale. Julius Fuchs, an orthopedic surgeon, originally designed the orthokinetic cuff and described its rationale and construction in several professional journals (Fuchs, 1927; 1951). His early work was further studied and detailed by a number of others (Blashy, Harrison, and E. Fuchs, 1955; Blashy and R. Fuchs, 1959; Rider, 1970; Neeman, 1971; Farber, 1974).

Dr. Fuchs intended to create a dynamic device designed to increase range of motion at the joint distal to the orthokinetic cuff without danger of the total immobilization and pain frequently caused by static devices. The orthokinetic cuff was constructed with an active field made from a stretchy material that was placed over the muscle belly to be stimulated (the agonist). The remainder of the cuff was composed of an inactive (or relatively inactive)

field, which was placed over the antagonist. The contraction and relaxation of the agonist during movement caused the active field to expand and provided minute pinching action to the dermatome over the agonist muscle. The underlying agonist was thus facilitated by this exteroproprioceptive stimulation.

Renate L. Neeman (1971) described an adaptation of Dr. Fuch's original cuff, which was then further adapted by Farber (1974). A continuous foldover method of construction was utilized by both Neeman and Farber with an active field and a relatively inactive field. A 2:4 ratio foldover of active to relatively inactive field or a 3:6 ratio foldover was used. This means that in the 2:4 ratio, for example, the active field is two layers thick, while the relatively inactive field has four layers. (For further discussion, see the heading *Methods of construction*.)

When the active field is placed over an agonist, the therapist must consider the primary and secondary motions of that agonist. It is possible that more than one cuff may be needed to counter an undesirable secondary muscular action. For example, if a patient has foot drop during gait, an orthokinetic cuff placed below the knee with the active field over the anterior tibialis will facilitate dorsiflexion at the ankle. Since the anterior tibialis not only causes dorsiflexion but also inversion, a smaller cuff should be placed proximal to the ankle with the active field facilitating the peroneal musculature; this promotes eversion. The two cuffs together will facilitate a balance of dorsiflexion in a more neutral foot position appropriate to normal gait.

Indications. Orthokinetic cuffs are activated by motion. It is therefore most effectively used to enhance range of motion in patients having some voluntary motion. An orthokinetic segment may also be used as a strap for a splint (see dynamic orthokinetic wrist splint section of this chapter) and for the triceps of patients who are positioned in dynamic hemiplegia slings.

Contraindications and Precautions. It is inappropriate and ineffectual to use an orthokinetic cuff on a patient who has fixed contractures and total paralysis. There are several major precautions for use of orthokinetic cuffs. The therapist must be sure the patient or his caregivers or both apply the cuff correctly. If the active field is incorrectly placed, undesired muscular action will result. Secondly, the patient wearing an orthokinetic cuff should be followed closely to assure continued cuff fit. The author has noted an increase in girth (circumference) in the extremity on which a cuff has been placed; this may cause the cuff to become too tight and subsequently cut off circulation. Finally, extreme care should be taken to assure adequate baseline range of motion assessments so that one can determine if the cuff is having the desired effect. Biofeedback with electromyography can also be used to evaluate the muscular tone of the agonist and antagonist.

Method of Construction*

Ace bandage is used for the cuff. The width varies depending on the muscle

*Designed by S. Farber and R. Chapman.

belly size and the age of the patient. Two to six inches is the width range normally used for adults and one half to four inches is the range for children. Velcro is used for the fastening and the cuff is assembled and sewn on a sewing machine. The patient's extremity and the elastic must be carefully measured (Fig. 7–1).

1. Measure the circumference of the extremity and then measure the width of the belly of the agonist at the level of the motor point (area of maximum electrical activity for the muscle).

2. Subtract the agonist belly width from the circumference. This yields the measurement for the inactive field. Add two inches to the inactive field figure to provide for a foldover closure.

3. Multiply the inactive field figure (with the two inches added) times four (for the 2:4 ratio cuff) or times six (for the 3:6 ratio cuff).

4. Then multiply the active field times

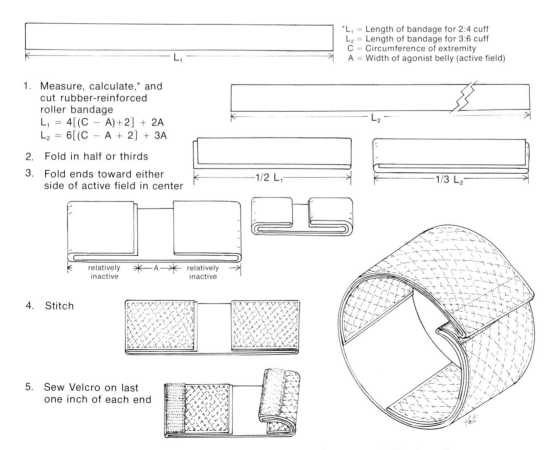

1. Measure, calculate,* and cut rubber-reinforced roller bandage
   $L_1 = 4[(C - A)+2] + 2A$
   $L_2 = 6[(C - A + 2] + 3A$

2. Fold in half or thirds

3. Fold ends toward either side of active field in center

4. Stitch

5. Sew Velcro on last one inch of each end

*L_1 = Length of bandage for 2:4 cuff
L_2 = Length of bandage for 3:6 cuff
C = Circumference of extremity
A = Width of agonist belly (active field)

L_1

L_2

1/2 L_1

1/3 L_2

relatively inactive — A — relatively inactive

Figure 7–1. Construction of continuous foldover orthokinetic cuffs.

two (for the 2:4 ratio cuff) or times three (for the 3:6 ratio cuff).

5. Add the two sums together. This will yield the total length of the elastic required for folding.

To fold: For the 2:4 ratio cuff, fold the total length in half. For the 3:6 ratio cuff, fold the total length in thirds. Then bring the ends in toward the center and place the ends and the fold on either side of the active field (see Fig. 7–1). Stitch the relatively inactive field as shown in Figure 7–1. Sew Velcro on the last one inch of each end for closure.

Orthokinetic Wrist Splint for Flexor Spasticity

History and Neurophysiological Rationale. The idea for the splint was originally conceived by A. Joy Huss, MS, OTR, RPT, FAOTA, and designed and constructed by T. Kay Carl, OTR, in the late 1960s. It was adapted in 1974 and again in 1980 by Judith Hunt Kiel, MS, OTR, who has written the orthokinetic splint construction section of this chapter.

The splint (Fig. 7–2) is designed to decrease flexion hypertonicity by several mechanisms. The hard cone and the lip on the forearm bar place pressure into the insertions of the wrist and hand flexors. This is inhibitory to them and reciprocally facilitory to the hand and wrist extensors. As extension is facilitated, the splint's dynamic wrist joint allows the movement in extension to occur. The orthokinetic segments used as straps in three places on the splint further enhance the extensor reaction. The hard material of the forearm bar provides maintained pressure into the volar arm surface, either inhibiting the flexors or causing them to adapt owing to the unchanging nature of the maintained pressure stimulus.

Indications. This splint is most effective for patients who have at least minimal voluntary extension in the upper extremity with flexor hypertonicity.

Contraindications and Precautions. The splint may not be effective for patients with total paralysis, fisted hands, severe thumb-in-palm deformities, or severe ulnar or radial deviation. Attempts to open the patient's hand via appropriate therapeutic sequences (see Chap. 3) should be made before splinting such deformities. Lining the forearm bar of the splint with foam is contraindicated because the foam may facilitate the flexors since it is soft and changes shape according to the degree of pressure exerted against it. Foam also holds in moisture and warmth, increasing the likelihood of skin breakdown.

The splint is difficult to fit properly; thus, the therapist must be sure the patient's wrist joint is lined up with the wrist joint of the splint. Placing a groove in the hand cone for the thumb is recommended to relieve pressure in the web space.

As with any splint, wearing time must be gradually increased. The splint is not designed to replace therapy. During treatment time, the splint should not be worn; the therapist must be able to facilitate wrist and hand extension patterns utilizing appropriate methods described in Chapter 3.

Construction Methods

by Judith Hunt Kiel, MS, OTR

MATERIALS FOR SPLINT PATTERN. To make a pattern and measure for this splint, the following materials are required: paper towel, pencil, tape measure, bandage tape, scissors, and ruler.

FOREARM BAR PATTERN

1. Place the pronated arm flat on a paper towel that has been opened and smoothed to one layer. The patient's fingers should be flat and be approximately ¼ in apart at the distal end of the hand. The entire arm, from fingertips to elbow, should be resting on the paper towel (Fig. 7–3). The pattern of the arm being splinted will be traced on the paper towel. The paper towel can be placed diagnally under the arm or taped to a second paper towel if it is not large enough to accommodate the tracing.

2. After making certain that there is no ulnar or radial wrist or finger deviation, trace around the hand and arm to the elbow. Be sure when tracing around the arm that the pencil is held perpendicular to the table so that the arm size will not be distorted (Fig. 7–4). It is not necessary to

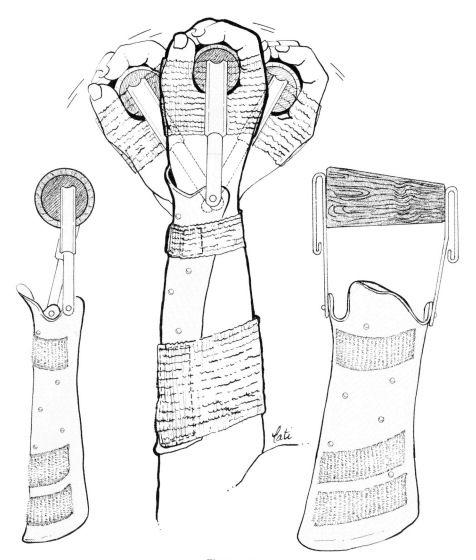

Figure 7–2.

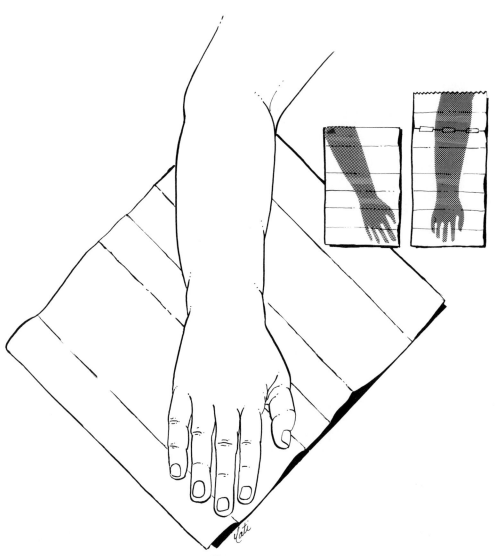

Figure 7–3.

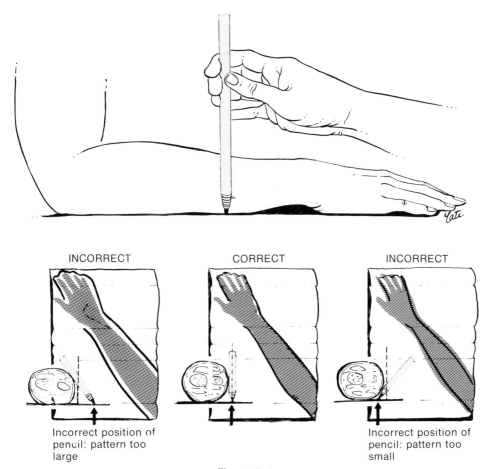

INCORRECT   CORRECT   INCORRECT

Incorrect position of
pencil: pattern too
large

Incorrect position of
pencil: pattern too
small

Figure 7–4.

trace around each finger for this splint (Fig. 7–4). Do not trace the thumb. Stop at the bottom of the web space, proximal to the metacarpal (MC) of the index finger, then begin again at the base of the first MC. There will be an open space in the finished tracing where the thumb would have been (Fig. 7–5).

3. Without moving the hand, mark the axis of the wrist joint on the radial and ulnar sides and mark the desired proximal length of the forearm bar (Fig. 7–5).

Note: In order to provide the longest lever arm possible and still not obstruct elbow motion, splints usually extend onto the forearm two thirds of the distance from the axis of the wrist joint to the elbow. The forearm bar of the orthokinetic wrist splint needs to be slightly longer than two thirds of the distance from the wrist joint axis to the elbow in order to ensure that the most proximal orthokinetic strap covers the bellies of the long wrist extensors. This distance can be established by measuring with a ruler from the elbow to the axis of the wrist joint, then mathematically determining slightly more than two thirds of the distance. You will notice that if the olecranon process is used to determine the elbow rather than the flexion crease, the

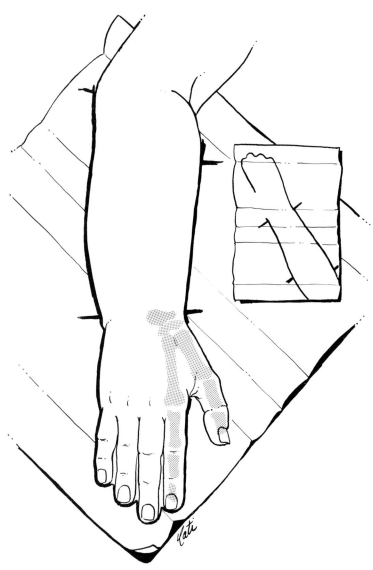

Figure 7–5.

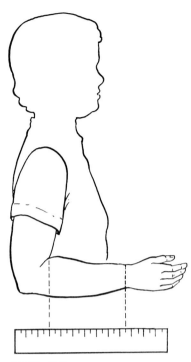

Figure 7-6.

distance is longer. There will be a better result if the elbow flexion crease is used as the measuring point (Fig. 7–6). With some practice, it is possible to estimate the length rather than using a ruler and determining it mathematically. The length of a completed forearm bar pattern should be checked by holding the pattern in place while the elbow is flexed to see that sufficient range of motion will be available with the splint in place. If elbow flexion is hampered by the length needed on the forearm bar, the pattern can be shortened on the radial side to prevent loss of range of motion.

4. Continuing to leave the arm stationary, tape the paper towel around the arm.

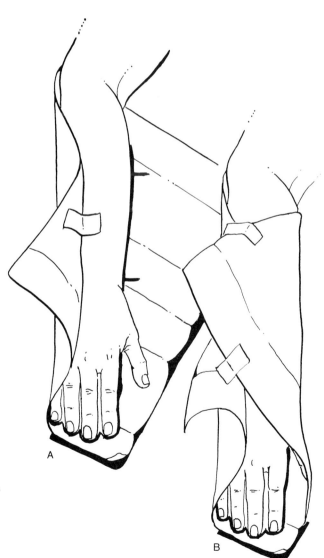

Figure 7-7.

It is helpful to tape the paper to the arm as well as to the paper itself (Figs. 7–7A, B).

5. Carefully hold onto the hand and paper towel, keeping the palm from sliding or rotating on the towel as you pick it up to look at the palmar surface. Trace the flexion crease and the thenar crease onto the paper towel.

a. Flexion Crease. Keeping the patient's thumb in an adducted, slightly extended position, have him (or help him) flex his metacarpal-phalangeal (MP) joints into 90 degrees flexion. Attempt to keep the paper towel from wadding or folding in the palm. Draw a line on the flexion crease with the hand in this position. *Note:* The flexion crease is neither the distal palmar crease nor the proximal palmar crease but is a line that must not cross either the bony joint or the crease caused by that joint. The flexion crease will be some combination of these two lines (Fig. 7–8A).

b. Thenar Crease. Have the patient hold all his MP joints in full (180 degrees) extension. Place his thumb in abduction. Trace the thenar crease. The line that is needed for making splints should stop at the point where it intersects the flexion crease (see previous paragraph). It should not extend through the web space (Fig. 7–8B).

6. Remove the paper towel from the patient's arm and transfer the markings that are currently on both sides of the paper towel to one side. It is usually easier to transfer the flexion crease and thenar crease lines rather than the entire tracing of the arm with all of the other notations (Fig. 7–9).

7. To provide sufficient curving contour in the forearm bar of the splint, add width to the sides of the forearm. Usually one half of the distance up the sides of the forearm is a satisfactory width for a volar

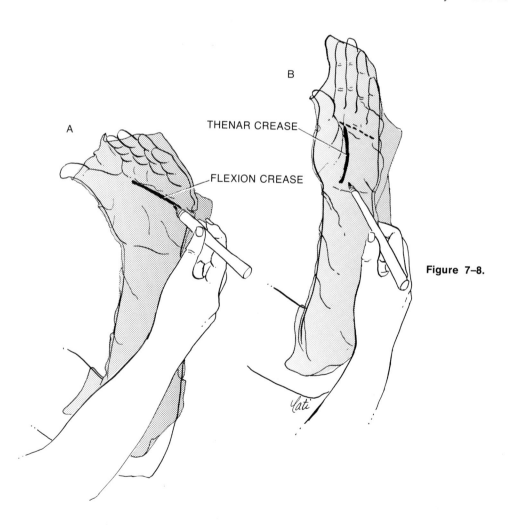

THENAR CREASE

FLEXION CREASE

Figure 7–8.

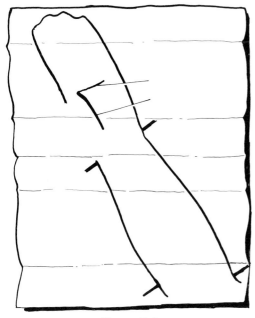

Figure 7–9.

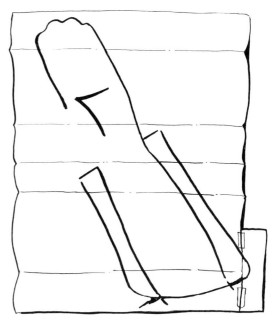

Figure 7–10.

splint. To determine how much width to add, lay the forearm on a flat surface. Measure the thickness of the forearm from the flat surface to the top of the arm at a point one half the distance between the elbow flexion crease and the axis of the wrist joint. Divide this measured distance by two and add the resulting measurement to each side of the traced forearm from the mark indicating the axis of the wrist joint to the mark indicating the correct length of the forearm bar. Again, with experience, this distance can be estimated rather than figured mathematically. *Note:* Frequently one corner of the pattern does not fit onto the paper towel. When this happens, the situation can be corrected either when tracing the pattern onto the plastic or by taping a small piece of paper towel where it is needed.

8. Round the corners formed where the width lines and the length lines intersect (Fig. 7–10).

9. Extend both lateral width lines distal to the axis of the wrist joint. The length of these lines should be to the middle of the length of the first and fifth metacarpal bones, respectively.

10. Draw rounded tabs on the distal end of the splint pattern that are entirely outside the drawn borders of the hand. The length should be from the middle of the first and fifth metacarpal bone to ¼ in to ½ in (depending on patient size) proximal to the axis of the wrist joint. The width of these tabs must not be less than ½ in, but for large children and adults can be as wide as ¾ in to 1 in (Fig. 7–11).

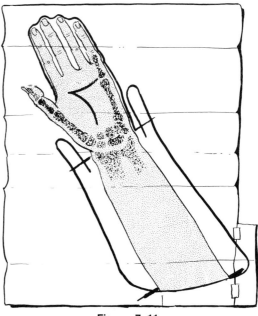

Figure 7–11.

11. Curve the proximal ends of the lines for the tabs at the wrist toward the medial portion of the hand and distally to meet in the center and make a "lip" that will cover the flexor tendon insertions. In order to be sure of covering all of the flexor tendon insertions, this lip must cover the proximal end of the third, fourth, and part of the fifth metacarpal bones and the capitate, hamate, lunate, triquetrum, and the ulnar half of the navicular carpal bones. The lip must not extend into the palm (transverse arch area) nor put any pressure on the thenar eminence (Fig. 7–12).

12. Check the forearm bar pattern for fit: proximal length should be long enough that the proximal elastic cuff can facilitate the muscle bellies of the wrist extensor muscles. Elbow flexion should not be hampered. The forearm bar width must entirely cover the wrist flexor muscle bellies but not cover the wrist extensor muscle bellies. The lip at the distal end must cover the insertions of the wrist flexor muscles. The tabs on the lateral borders of the distal end must curve around to the sides of the hand and be large enough to allow a hole to be drilled at the axis of the wrist joint with enough plastic surrounding the hole to hold a rivet securely as well as be heated and positioned in a way that none of the rivet or tab will touch the hand (Fig. 7–13).

MEASUREMENTS NECESSARY IN ADDITION TO THE PATTERN

1. The diameter of a circle formed by placing the thumb and index finger in a

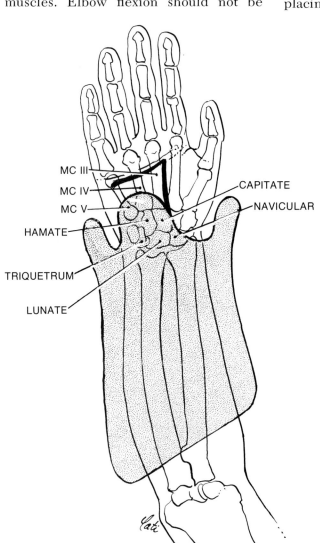

MC III
MC IV
MC V
HAMATE
TRIQUETRUM
LUNATE
CAPITATE
NAVICULAR

Figure 7–12. Forearm bar fit.

position approximating tip prehension; the fingers should not touch (Figure 7–14).

2. The diameter of an imaginary circle on the ulnar side of the hand with an arc of the circle being formed by the curve of the little finger in a functional position (Fig. 7–15).

3. The distance from the axis of the wrist joint on the radial side of the hand to the center of the circle described in #1 above (Fig. 7–14).

4. The distance from the axis of the wrist joint on the ulnar side of the hand to the center of the circle described in #2 above. This measurement will be shorter than the measurement described in #3 above (Fig. 7–15).

ASSEMBLING THE SPLINT

1. Equipment necessary to make the splint includes: power saw, belt sander, power drill, sewing machine, heat gun, wood file (fine tooth, half-rounded), drill bits (3/32, 7/64, 1/8, 9/64, 5/32 in.), countersink, appropriate drawing device for plastic used.

2. Materials necessary to make the splint include: rigid plastic (Kydex, Royalite, Bioplastic BX), cylindrical piece of wood (diameter of circle described in Figure 7–16), two screws (6 ga., 1 in length), two rivets (pop rivets or aluminum less than 1/2 in shank length, 1/8 in shank diameter), pieces of elastic to be used in each of three places (one wide enough to cover the proximal phalanx, the MP joints, and at least one half of the metacarpal bone; one wide enough to cover the muscle bellies of the wrist extensors; and a narrow strip usually about 1 in wide to be used at the

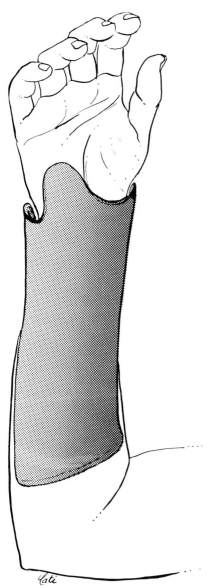

Figure 7–13. Forearm bar.

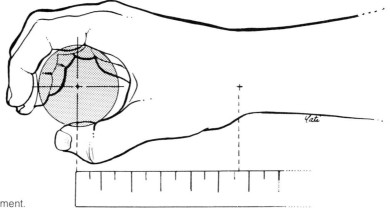

Figure 7–14. Radial measurement.

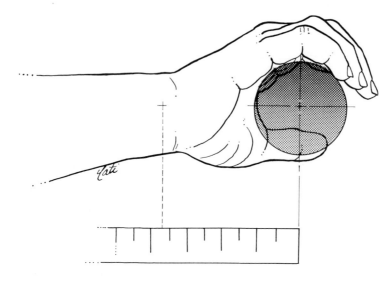

Figure 7–15. Ulnar measurement.

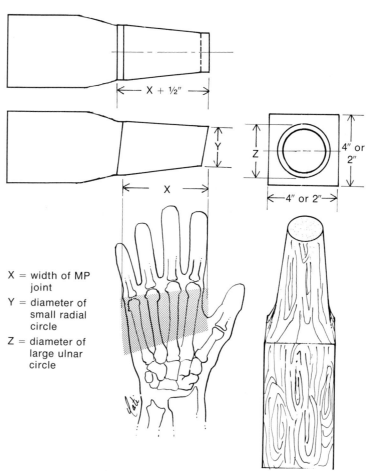

X = width of MP joint

Y = diameter of small radial circle

Z = diameter of large ulnar circle

Figure 7–16. Splint hand cone.

wrist), loop Velcro (standard backed), hook Velcro (pressure-sensitive back is recommended), fine sandpaper, medium-to-coarse steel wool, varnish, or a can of spray enamel or varnish.

MAKING THE SPLINT

1. Using the cylindrical piece of wood, make a cone to fit the hand. If a dowel rod is not available in the necessary size, a rectangular or square piece of wood may be sawed and sanded into the proper shape.

Sand with a belt sander one end of the cylindrical piece of wood so that its diameter is the size of the smaller circle on the radial side of the hand as described in 1. on p. 238, 239. The diameter of the cone should gradually taper from the size of the small radial circle to the size of the large ulnar circle at a length that equals the width of the MP joints (Fig. 7–16).

When the sanded end is the correct size the dowel can be cut to a length ¼ to ½ in longer than the width of the MP joints. The large end of the cut dowel must have a diameter the size of the diameter of the large circle on the ulnar side of the hand.

Place the cone in the patient's hand with the small end of the cone on the radial side of the hand. Trace the size and placement of the thumb onto the cone.

File a groove in the cone to provide a place for the thumb to rest in order to prevent pressure in the webspace.

Sand the entire cone so that it is very smooth and all splinters are eliminated.

Finish the cone with two to three coats of varnish or spray enamel.

2. Trace the paper pattern for the forearm bar onto the rigid plastic and cut it out using a power saw.

3. Cut two straight rods from the same plastic used for the forearm bar. These rods should be the width of the tabs on the lateral sides of the forearm bar. The length of one of these rods should be equal to the measurement as explained on p. 239, Figure 7–14, plus the width of the elastic that will cover the proximal phalanx, the MP joints, and one half of the metacarpal bones; plus 1½ in to allow for curves, screws, and rivets. The length of the second rod should be equal to the measurement as explained on p. 240, Figure 7–15, plus the same amount added for the first rod.

4. Finish the edges of all three plastic pieces with a file, sandpaper, and steel wool until the edges are smooth.

5. Drill ventilation holes in the forearm piece using the ⅛ in bit. These holes should be at least 1½ in apart and no closer to the edge than 1 in. No ventilation holes should be placed in the tabs or in the lip at the wrist area.

6. While the forearm bar is still flat, drill a hole using the ⅛ in bit centered in each tab. These holes must be in exact line with the axis of the wrist and should be ¼ to ⅜ in from the distal end of the tab. Countersink both of these holes on the surface that will be near the patient's skin.

7. Drill a hole in one end of each of the two rods. These holes should be 9/64 inch in size and should be centered on the rod ¼ to ⅜ in from the end of the rod. You will notice that the hole in the tab is smaller than in the rod. This is so that the connecting rivet will not pull through the tab hole, but the larger rod hole will allow joint movement at the wrist.

8. Rivet the rod to the tab with the rod on the outside of the tab. That is, the tab will be the thing closest to the patient. The head of the rivet should be on the outside of the splint and the shank should be pounded flat into the countersunk area in the forearm bar leaving no sharp edges to hurt the patient.

9. Using the heat gun, heat the forearm bar including the lateral tabs. It is not necessary to heat the rods that have been riveted to them.

The radial and ulnar sides of the forearm bar should be molded so that they are flush with the patient's skin. The proximal end should be lipped slightly away from the patient's arm to prevent pressure.

The distal end of the forearm bar should be lipped so that when the wrist is flexed there is pressure placed on the insertions of the flexor muscles; however, there should be no points or sharp edges that would cause soreness from the pressure on the insertions.

The tabs at the wrist (which have the rods attached to them) should be pulled away from the skin, beginning slightly proximal to the wrist. The plane of the tabs must be perpendicular to an imaginary axis going through the carpal bones in order to allow free movement of the wrist joint.

10. When the plastic portion of the splint fits the patient correctly, the straps may be put on the splint to simplify fitting the rest of the splint.

11. Assemble the straps and position them on the forearm bar (Fig. 7–17). The elastic straps should go around the circumference of the arm with slight stretch. They should meet in the center of the volar surface with no overlap. Velcro loop should be sewn on the two ends of the elastic; be sure that none will be covering the extensor muscle bellies. Velcro hook should be placed across the entire width of the forearm bar.

An elastic strap wide enough to cover the wrist extensor muscle bellies entirely should be placed at the proximal end of the splint. The distal end of the wide strap can be made more narrow in order to make the strap fit more smoothly and allow for the conical shape of the forearm.

A narrow elastic strap should be placed at the distal end of the forearm bar to go around the wrist and provide greater stability for the splint. If desired, a piece of narrow elastic can be sewn into a circle that would be the correct size at the wrist. Then a small piece of Velcro can be sewn on the inside of the seam to prevent slippage.

12. Place the forearm bar with attached rods on the patient, in the proper position, with the straps fastened. Place the wooden cone in the patient's hand; remember that the small end of the cone belongs on the radial side of the hand. *Note: While fitting the splint, it is not necessary to passively extend the wrist.*

13. Move the rods into a position where they cross the center of the cone ends. You will notice that the radial rod does not lie flat against the cone. The ulnar side should fit properly or be very near the correct position.

14. In order for the radial rod to meet the cone and avoid causing any pressure on the patient's hand, an S-shaped curve must be put in the rod (Fig. 7–18). The S-shaped curve is formed by heating the portion of the radial rod just distal to the radial tab to which it is riveted. Make a slight bend in the rod at this point that will make the rod parallel to the first metacarpal bone.

The second bend of the S-shaped curve should be placed at the level of the distal end of the first metacarpal bone. Heat the portion of the rod that passes this area and bend the rod back toward the cone until it lies flat against the radial end of the cone.

15. When both rods are positioned correctly to cross the middle of the cone ends, mark the rods where they lie over the

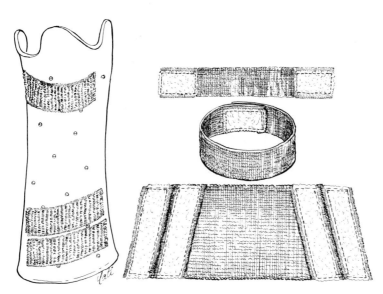

Figure 7–17. Splint straps.

center of the cone end. Also put a mark on the center of each end of the cone.

16. With the splint removed from the patient, drill one hole in the center of each end of the cone. If a 6-gauge screw is to be used, a 3/32 in bit should be used.

17. Drill a centered hole in the two rods at the level of the marks made in #16. In order to assure that the rods form a freely moving joint with the cone, a 5/32 in bit should be used. These two holes should be countersunk in the plastic on the side away from the cones in order to avoid having the patient scratched by the screw.

18. Screw the rods onto the cone. Be sure that they are left loose enough to allow for free movement at this joint.

19. If there is stiffness in any of the four joints, heat them in order to simultaneously move them through their range of motion while the splint is off the patient's

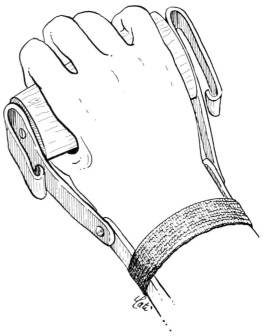

Figure 7–19. Rod loops.

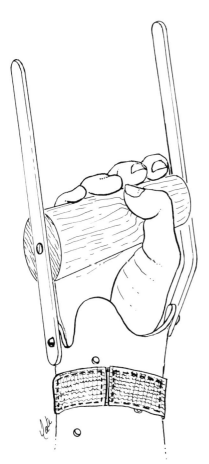

Figure 7–18. Splint rods.

hand. Continue moving the cone up and down until the plastic is cool.

20. Bend the part of the rods distal to the screws back toward the proximal end to make a loop that will hold the finger elastic in place (Fig. 7–19). A second loop should be bent into the ends of the rods ¼ to ½ in length. When bending these loops, place a tongue blade inside the bend to avoid making the curve too sharp and causing breakage.

21. The elastic designed to go around the fingers and cone should be wide enough to cover the proximal phalanx, the MP joint, and at least half of the metacarpal bone. The length of this elastic should be enough to go completely around the cone (without the fingers) with just a slight stretch. One inch should be added to allow the elastic to overlap and be sewn to form a circle. The overlapping ends should be sewn on a sewing machine.

22. Place the elastic around the hand after the splint has been put in place. Tuck it under the loops to prevent slippage (Fig. 7–20). *Note:* It is a good idea to make two sets of elastic straps and finger elastic, so that the splint can be worn while the extra straps are washed.

244

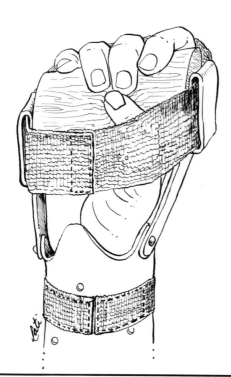

Figure 7–20. Wrist and finger elastic.

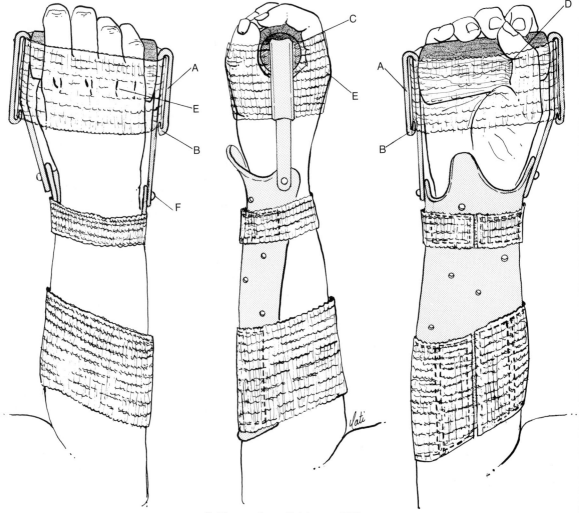

Putting on the splint (see p. 245).

SAMPLE OF INFORMATION GIVEN TO THE PATIENT'S FAMILY: CARE OF AN ORTHOKINETIC WRIST EXTENSION SPLINT

(Patient's Name) has been provided with a splint to help relax the tight muscles in his forearm and hand. If this splint is worn according to the instructions, it can help him use his hand and make it easier to keep his fingers loose so that they may be kept clean more readily.

Every day, the splint should be cleaned with *cold* water and soap. If any dirt has collected in the holes, it should be cleaned out well. The elastic on the arms may be washed as needed, but be careful not to stretch it too much, and let it dry in a relaxed position. The elastic around the fingers may be removed for washing by gently lifting the loop of plastic that holds the elastic in place (A in the drawing) and sliding the elastic toward his wrist. Wash this elastic in the same manner that the elastic on the forearm was washed. After it is washed and dried, it may be replaced by reversing the above procedure. Be sure that the edge of the elastic is inside the hook (B in the drawing) to prevent it from slipping out of place.

HOW TO PUT THE SPLINT ON

1. Be sure the splint is clean and dry. You have been provided with two sets of straps so that while one set is being washed, the splint can still be worn with the second set of straps on it.
2. Place the wooden cone in the palm of his hand, being certain the cone is touching the back of the web space (C in the drawing). (If the wrist is allowed to bend down it will be easier to open the fingers to put the cone in his hand). There is a groove made in the wood where his thumb should rest (D in the drawing).
3. Place the elastic smoothly over his fingers and thumb. It should cover the knuckles closest to his wrist (E in the drawing) (metacarpal-phalangeal). Be careful that the edge of a seam is not pressing onto a finger or thumb and causing soreness.
4. Move the plastic forearm piece up to meet his arm. The joints of the splint should be directly across from where his wrist bends (F in the drawing).
5. Place the elastic around his forearm. The wider strap goes close to the elbow. The elastic needs to have slight stretch, but not enough to cause pain. There will be a mark left on the arm where the elastic was (similar to the mark left by a watch). Unless you are specifically told otherwise, the strap should meet itself on the underside of his arm.
6. It may be more comfortable for the patient if he wears the top of a thin cotton sock or stockinette on his arm, or a very thin piece of gauze may be used to line the splint.
7. If there is a problem with perspiration, baby powder or a dry spray deodorant may be used.

(Instructions for contacting the therapist should be provided in case there is a problem with the splint.)

The forearm bar may be made of a soft plastic that has a lower forming temperature such as Polyform, Polyflex, Kay Splint, or Orthoplast if the directions are altered in the following manner.

FOREARM BAR PATTERN ADJUSTMENTS

1. Leave out steps 9 and 10 on page 237 and draw the "lip" that is described in step 11 (page 238).
2. Connect the lip to the sides of the forearm bar by tapering the edge of the lip out to the lateral sides of the splint pattern. This will have to be measured carefully to be sure that the sides will not put pressure on the radial or ulnar styloid processes (Fig. 7–21).
3. In checking the forearm bar pattern for fit, do not worry about curving of the tabs on the lateral border of the distal end and size large enough to accommodate a hole (p. 238).
4. When making the splint, trace the paper pattern for the forearm bar onto the soft plastic.
5. The tabs made of a rigid plastic must be added to the forearm bar that is made from a soft plastic. The length of these tabs should be from the middle of the first and fifth metacarpal bone to ¼ to ½ in (depending on the patient's size) proximal to the axis of the wrist joint, with additional length on the proximal end that is a curved piece of rigid plastic (Fig. 7–22). The width of these tabs must not be less than ½ in, but for large children and adults can be as wide as ¾ to 1 in. These tabs should be cut at the same time and from the same plastic as the rods described in 3, p. 241. Be sure to mark which tab is ulnar and which is radial.
6. Finish edges of the rods and the tabs with a file, sandpaper, and steel wool until the edges are smooth.
7. Heat the forearm bar and form it on the patient's arm using the fitting guide-

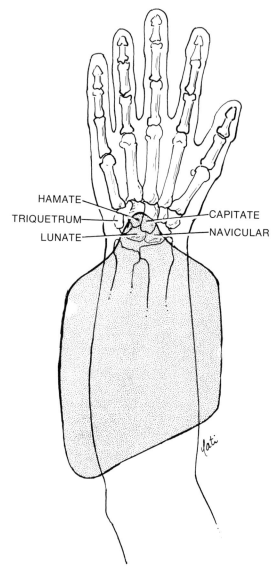

HAMATE
TRIQUETRUM
LUNATE
CAPITATE
NAVICULAR

Figure 7–21. Soft plastic forearm bar.

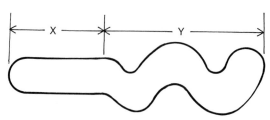

X = distance from center of MC bones to ¼"–½"
proximal to axis of wrist joint

Y = ½ length of forearm bar

Figure 7–22. Curved rigid plastic.

lines described in 9, page 241. At this time it is not necessary to pull the tabs at the wrist away from the skin.

8. Drill a hole with the ⅛ in bit centered ¼ to ⅜ in from the end of each tab. Countersink both of these holes on the surface that will be near the patient's skin.

9. Drill holes in the rods and rivet them to the tabs as described in 7 and 8 on page 241.

10. Heat the tabs one at a time and position them correctly on the forearm bar. It is not necessary at this time to heat the rods that have been riveted to the tabs. Be sure that the rods are placed on the outside, away from the patient's skin. Mold the curved part of the tab so that it lies flat against the forearm bar; the straight part should extend beyond the distal end of the splint so that it fits in the same manner that the tabs fit when made as part of the original forearm bar. When the tabs are both positioned correctly, a piece of the forearm bar plastic should be placed over the curved tab that rests on the forearm bar. In this way the tabs are securely sandwiched between two pieces of plastic and cannot move. When sticking the soft plastic together, be sure that both pieces of plastic are clean and dry. The forearm bar should be heated only slightly on the outside surface, while the top piece of plastic is heated thoroughly. *Note:* In the process of sandwiching these pieces of plastic, the tabs may be held stationary by using tape or manually holding them. Also, the heat of the tab when it is formed may temporarily stick it to the soft plastic long enough to get the second piece of plastic in place.

11. If ventilation holes are desired, they should be drilled or punched into the forearm bar at this time. Ventilation holes should be at least 1½ in apart and no closer to the edge than 1 in. No holes should be placed in the tabs that extend distal to the forearm bar or on the lip at the wrist area.

12. Continue making the splint as described previously, beginning with 10 on page 242.

Figure 7–23 shows the completed version of this splint, constructed from soft plastic.

Portions of the preceding section by Judith Hunt Kiel were adapted from her text (see references).

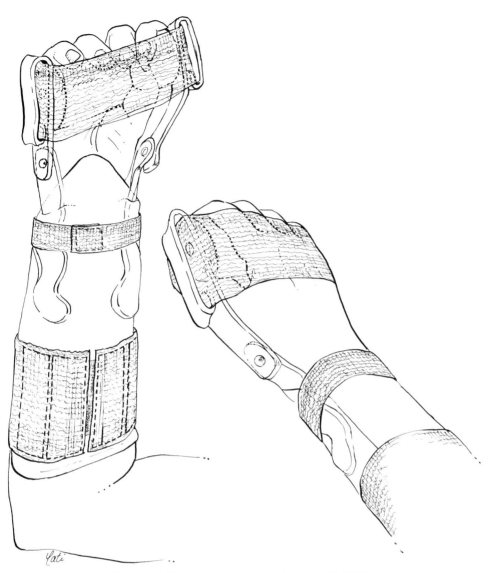

Figure 7–23. Dynamic splint made from soft plastic.

Other Commonly Used Splints

The *resting pan splint* and the *simple cock-up splint* are two splint designs frequently ordered by physicians for upper motor neuron–damaged patients. Many therapists empirically report that these splints and other similar static devices do not effectively reduce flexor hypertonicity. Neurophysiologically, theorists cannot exactly agree on which mechanisms are operating at the level of the secondary endings in the muscle spindle, Renshaw cells, or lower motor neurons when maintained stretch is applied by these devices.

There have been very few studies done to date measuring splint design effectiveness for patients with upper motor neuron damage. It would seem that controlled studies in this area would benefit many patients. Questions to be addressed include: What is the effectiveness of a static splint as compared with a dynamic splint for a patient with upper motor neuron pathology? Which is more beneficial, a dorsal or a volar splint? What effect does the type of splint material used (hard or soft) have on the pattern facilitated by the splint?

A study by Zislis (1964) compared the effects of two hand-wrist splints (one dorsal, one ventral) in the management of a patient having spastic hemiplegia. The volar splint promoted full extension and abduction of the fingers and was the more beneficial design for the patient studied. Zislis concluded that flexor inhibition may result from volar cutaneous or pressor receptors and from extension and abduction of the fingers. The dorsal splint did not produce the desired pattern.

Wheelchair Adaptations

Patients are forced to spend time in wheelchairs for various reasons. With the adaptive equipment presented in this chapter, a wheelchair *can assist the active therapy program* by neutralizing primitive reflexes and facilitating specific musculature.

Positioning Principles. For patients dominated by primitive reflexes, decerebrate posture, abnormal tone, or movement patterns, it is essential that an adapted wheelchair aid in accomplishing the following: normalize body alignment, reduce abnormal feedback secondary to faulty positioning mechanisms, neutralize primitive reflexes, facilitate appropriate motor behavior, and provide comfort and security.

One must understand that the chair *alone* will not help the patient reach these therapeutic goals, but it should complement the therapeutic program. Patients in need of an active neurorehabilitation program should not spend many hours in a wheelchair. Wheelchairs should be used primarily for transportation and positioning during feeding.

Examining components of positioning normal persons will assist the reader in understanding necessary adaptations for patients with a variety of problems. For maximum comfort and support in sitting, the normal person should position himself so that the hips are at 90 degrees flexion and placed all the way back in the chair, thighs are slightly abducted to widen the base of support for the trunk, and thighs are supported by the chair surface, leaving at least one inch of space behind the knees to avoid pressure into the popliteal area. His trunk is centered in midline, and the head and neck are centered over the trunk. Elbows are supported in 90 degrees flexion and knees are positioned at 90 degrees of flexion. The person's feet are firmly supported on a flat surface allowing a 90 degree flexion at the ankles.

Normal persons tend to shift their weight and modify their position frequently, depending on the comfort of the chair, length of sitting time, body alignment, and so forth. One common positional variation assumed by those sitting in a chair that is too deep for them is to slide their hips forward to the edge of the seat while leaning back. This places extreme strain on the lumbar spine. It would be more advisable to select a chair with less seat depth or to modify the chair by inserting a pad behind the back than to strain the lumbar spine in this manner.

Many variations are utilized in positioning patients with sensorimotor deficits. These will be presented in the following discussion. In general, the slingback canvas seat, commercially available in most wheelchairs, is not recommended for long-term use because it is hot and tends to promote internal rotation and adduction of the thighs.

Wooden Back and Seat Inserts.* Order the wheelchair without the canvas upholstery if possible. A wooden back and seat are then constructed to fit the specific wheelchair. Figure 7–24 shows a basic wooden back insert. According to Waterman (1978), the wooden seat back for a patient with head balance extends from the buttocks up to the level of C7 vertebra.

Various adaptations to the standard back are used, depending on the patient's needs and problems. If the patient requires a headrest, the back can be extended past the C7 level and can be reclined as needed as long as the seat is inclined to a matching angle (Waterman, 1978) (Fig. 7–25). The center of the back can be cut away to allow for protruding vertebral spines and then webbing straps, foam, and upholstery can

---

*Much of the information in this section originated from the work of Anita Slominski, OTR, FAOTA and Patricia Griswold, MS, OTR, of the Cerebral Palsy Clinic, Indiana University Medical Center, 1100 West Michigan Street, Indianapolis, IN 46223.

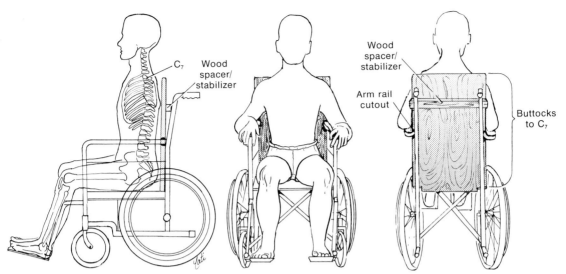

Figure 7–24. Standard wheelchair back.

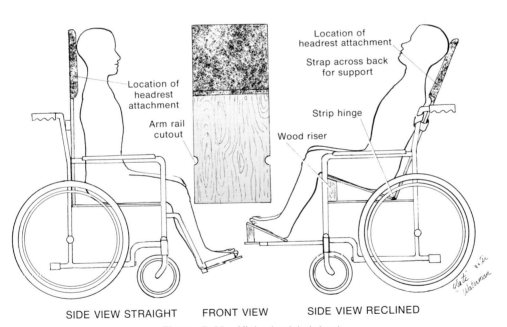

SIDE VIEW STRAIGHT   FRONT VIEW   SIDE VIEW RECLINED

Figure 7–25. High wheelchair back.

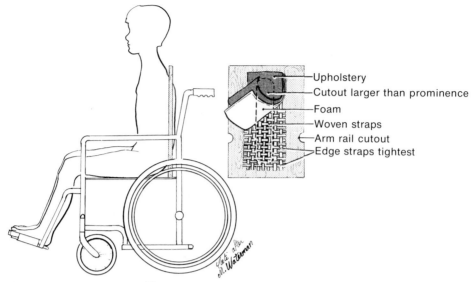

Figure 7–26. Seat back with cutout.

be placed over the cut-out area (Fig. 7–26). Scoliosis pads can also be used to assist in correcting trunk alignment (Fig. 7–27). The placement of scoliotic pads is critical to safe positioning of a patient. The pad must not exert pressure into the brachial plexus; therefore, it must be at least 1½ inches below the axilla. As depicted in Figure 7–27, pressure counter to the scoliotic curves is exerted by the pads. Hip pads may be used to narrow the back of the

seat and further stabilize the hips (Fig. 7–28). A seat belt that crosses the hips is used as another means of stabilizing the hips in the wheelchair.

Dynamic dental dam or Theraband straps are recommended to assist the patient in maintaining his trunk balance (Farber, 1974; Montgomery and Gauger, 1978). Figure 7–29 shows one method of attaching the straps to the wooden seat back. The neurophysiological rationale behind using

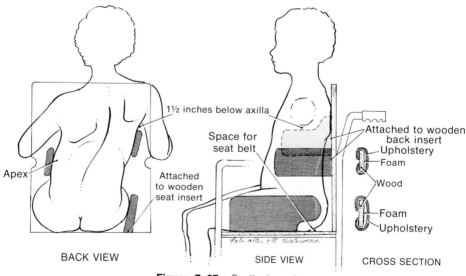

Figure 7–27. Scoliosis pads.

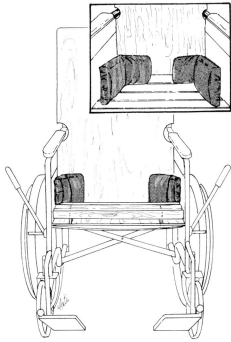

Figure 7–28. Hip pads.

a dynamic trunk support system is that the straps push the patient's trunk in a downward and inward direction, facilitating an upward and outward pattern as the patient resists against the straps. Montgomery and Gauger (1978) use a vest with the same strapping method as demonstrated in Figure 7–29. The straps must be positioned so that they cross under the sternal notch. The weight of the dental dam or Theraband used varies with the strength of the patient's back extensors. The patient must be supervised when wearing a dynamic trunk support system to assure adaptive responses and to avoid fatigue.

A basic flat wooden seat insert may be fitted into the bottom of the wheelchair (Fig. 7–30) or a wedge seat or rolled seat may be used (Fig. 7–31). The rolled slatted seat provides the patient with a contoured, comfortable seat that promotes femoral abduction and hip flexion. According to Waterman (1978), "The distance between the highest and lowest points (of the seat) is called the rise, which should not exceed 1

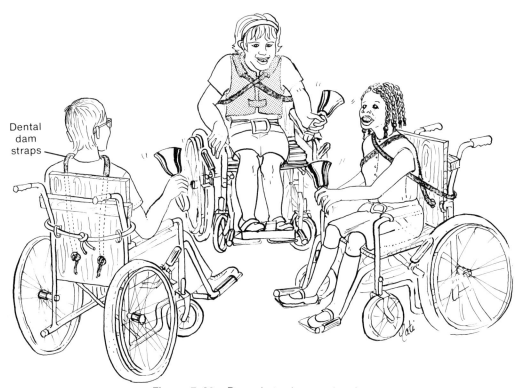

Dental dam straps

Figure 7–29. Dynamic trunk support system.

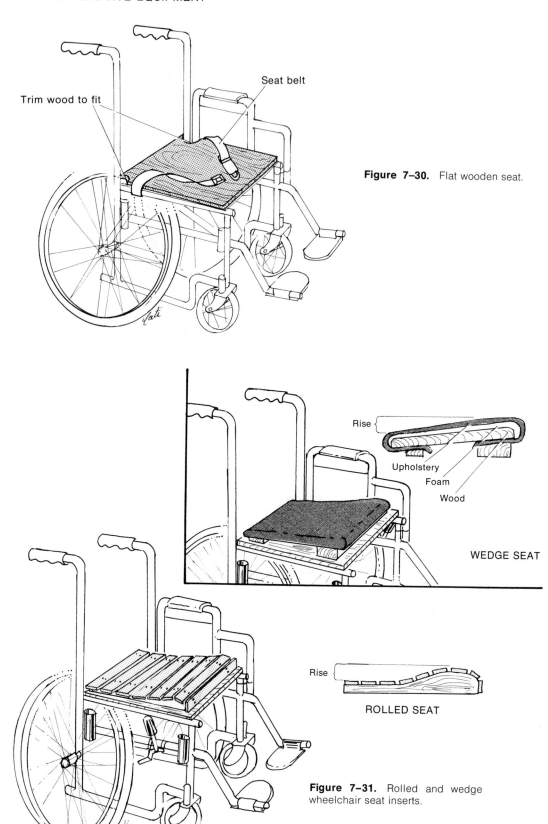

Trim wood to fit

Seat belt

Figure 7–30. Flat wooden seat.

Rise

Upholstery

Foam

Wood

WEDGE SEAT

Rise

ROLLED SEAT

Figure 7–31. Rolled and wedge wheelchair seat inserts.

inch per foot of length." The wedge seat also promotes a small degree of hip flexion.

Headrests. For patients requiring additional head support, the static or dynamic headrest may be attached to the wooden back.

General rules for use and construction of static head supports: Head supports should not be used continuously to position a patient's head. He should be given the opportunity to work toward active head balance on a daily basis. Static head support systems should be used for patients who completely lack or who have minimal head control. A static head support should be constructed so that it positions the patient's head between the occipital processes and the shoulders without exerting any pressure into the back surface (the occipital area of the head). Pressure in this region could set off the tonic labyrinthine in supine reflex and cause subsequent extensor tone throughout the body (Fiorentino, 1973). Unfortunately, the extensor tone that is facilitated by this occipital pressure is nonfunctional for a

good sitting posture because it promotes an extensor thrusting pattern.

Figure 7–32 shows an adaptation of the Slominski-Griswold design for a *static headrest*. It is designed so that the occipital region of the skull is free of pressure and the headrest is inclined down over the shoulders to prevent inappropriate trunk rotation. A solid piece of high-density open cell urethane foam is used to pad the wooden headrest frame and is covered by a cloth upholstery (Waterman, 1978).

The dynamic head support system designed by the author is shown in Figure 7–33. The neurophysiological rationale for this is: when the patient is positioned with his chin in slight ventroflexion, if his head falls forward or to either side he quickly stretches his neck extensors or his sternocleidomastoid muscles. This facilitates those muscles, returning the patient's head to midline.

The dynamic head support system is used for patients who are beginning to develop head balance and control.

When positioning the patient's head, it is critical that the neck flexors not be on

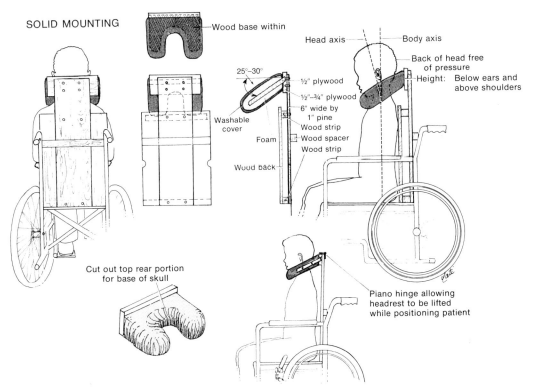

Figure 7–32. Slominski-Griswold static head rest and adaptations.

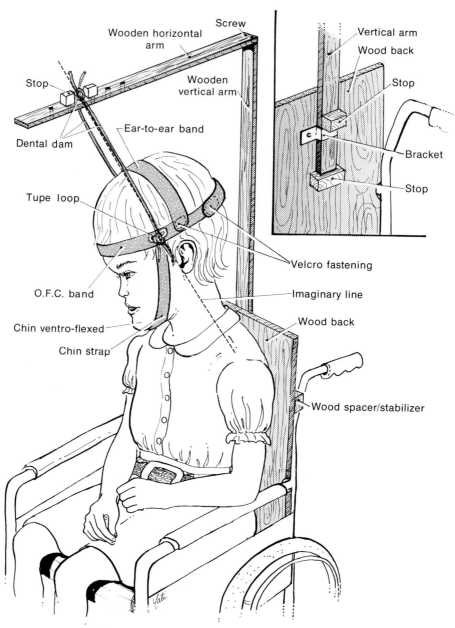

Figure 7–33. Farber dynamic head support system.

stretch or they may actually be facilitated during use of this support system. To avoid this problem, be sure to ventroflex the patient's head. An imaginary line is drawn from the patient's shoulder tip, through the tube loop, to the overhead support. Drawing this imaginary line will help the therapist determine the appropriate point of attachment for the tourniquet rubber hose or dental dam or Theraband straps.

Method of construction: The head sling consists of three major parts.

1. The head unit includes 1 to 2 in wide webbing band which goes around the occipital-frontal circumference (OFC) and has a Velcro closure allowing for OFC adjustment. The OFC band also has loops on it above and anterior to each ear in order to attach the head unit to the overhead support via the rubber hose. A sec-

ond webbing band is attached to the OFC band posterior to each tube loop and goes across the top of the head. It may also have a Velcro attachment to allow for adjustment. A third strap, attached with Velcro, is placed under the chin.

2. Tourniquet hosing, dental dam, or Theraband is used to attach the tube loops bilaterally to the overhead support.

3. Overhead support unit is a perpendicular device with one vertical arm inserted into a bracket on the back of the chair and a horizontal arm (forming a 90-degree angle to the vertical arm) going over the patient's head. It may be constructed from metal or wood. Stops may be placed on the overhead arm to keep the tourniquet hose in the desired attachment location.

The static headrest and dynamic head support system can be interchanged as the patient is progressing in acquisition of head balance. Initial use of the dynamic head support system should be closely monitored by the therapist to be sure that the patient does not fatigue while wearing the device.

Footrest. It is often necessary to dorsiflex the footrest to the same angle as the hips in order to break up abnormal extensor tone (Fig. 7–34). An elastic strap may be used over the top of the foot to further enhance dorsiflexion.

If the patient has a strong positive supporting reaction, pressure into the ball of the foot could reinforce plantar flexion (Fiorentino, 1973). Thus it may be necessary to construct the dorsiflexed footrest so that the ball of the foot is free from pressure and extending over the footrest.

Lap Tray. The lap tray provides a patient with additional trunk support. The elbows should rest on the tray at approximately 90 degrees flexion. It may be necessary to pad the area of the tray where the elbows rest in order to avoid pressure to the elbows (Fig. 7–35). A rim around the tray prevents objects from slipping off the work surface.

Femoral Abduction Devices. Achieving femoral abduction in sitting is desirable because it widens the base of support for the trunk. Many CNS-damaged patients have spastic adductors that cause

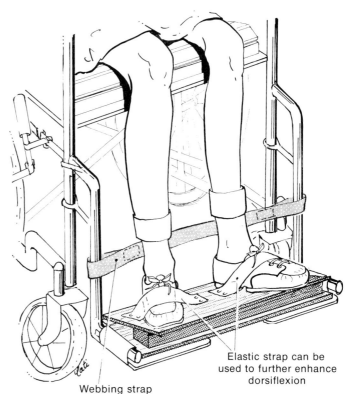

Figure 7–34. Dorsiflexion footrest.

Webbing strap

Elastic strap can be used to further enhance dorsiflexion

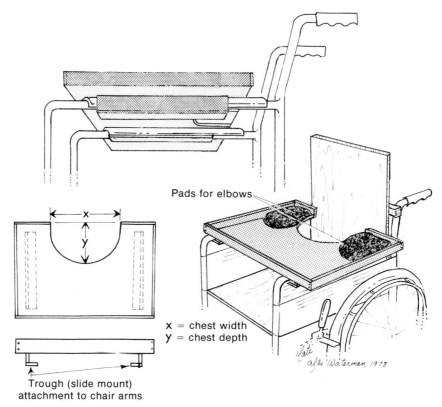

Pads for elbows

x = chest width
y = chest depth

after Waterman, 1978

Trough (slide mount)
attachment to chair arms

Figure 7–35. Lap tray.

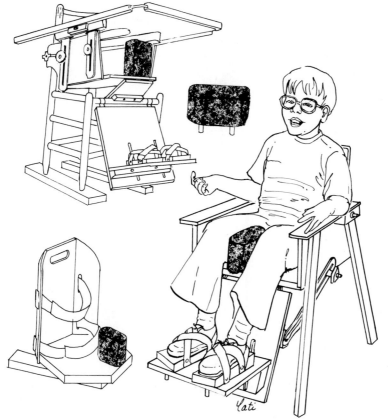

Figure 7–36. Abduction posts in commercially available seating devices.

difficulty in sitting and hip subluxation. Some commercially available sitting devices provide posts between the thighs designed to inhibit adduction (Fig. 7–36). The author has not found these posts to be totally effective with spastic patients as compared to use of the rolled seat. In many cases, the patient tightly adducts against the post, which then resists the adduction pattern. Adduction is subsequently reinforced. If the rolled seat alone does not reduce adduction, the therapist may try placing a Theraband strap around the patient's thighs (Fig. 7–37). The strap pulls the patient into abduction, causing a facilitation of the abductors. An alternative method to facilitate abduction is to use two Theraband straps. One is placed around the left thigh and attached to the right wheelchair arm while the second is placed

around the right thigh and attached to the left wheelchair arm (Fig. 7–37).

The patient who has a hip subluxation or dislocation should not be abducted dynamically because it could be painful. Only patients who respond to manual resistance into adduction with an abduction pattern should be fitted with these dynamic straps. The therapist should use these dynamic straps only when the patient is supervised. They should be worn for short periods of time, making sure that they do not cut off circulation.

Additional Designs and Reference Sources for Wheelchair Positioning. Many additional designs for positioning are available, including use of bolster chairs, relaxation chairs, box inserts, corner chairs, and so on. The reader is referred to the following additional re-

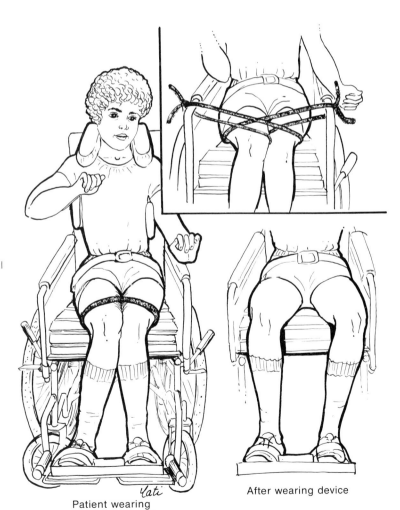

Figure 7–37. Dynamic femoral abduction devices.

Patient wearing
one abduction device

After wearing device

sources: Dicarlo and Forbis, 1977; Dunkel and Trefler, 1977; Fulford and Brown, 1976; Montgomery and Gauger, 1978; Robinault, 1973.

Currently, many rehabilitation equipment companies also manufacture adjustable seating devices or wooden seats that are well designed. The reader should consult the following manufacturers for additional information:

Cleo Living Aids
3957 Mayfield Rd.
Cleveland, OH 44121

Everest and Jennings
1803 Pontius Ave.
Los Angeles, CA 90025

The Equipment Shop
P.O. Box 33
Bedford, MA 01730

J. A. Preston Corp.
71 Fifth Ave.
New York, NY 10003

Rifton Equipment for the Handicapped
Division of Community Playthings
Hutterian Society of Brothers
Rifton, NY 12471

Fred Sammons, Inc.
Box 32
Brookfield, IL 60513

This list is by no means comprehensive but is meant to introduce the novice to commercial positioning equipment. In order for a therapist to evaluate the appropriateness of equipment depicted in a catalogue, he or she must thoroughly understand positioning principles. Often a commercial enterprise is willing to work with a therapist to adapt a design to meet a specific patient's needs. This may prove to be less expansive than custom design and manufacture by the therapist. Obviously, there are some patients whose problems are so complex that only custom design and manufacture are indicated.

Other Positioning Devices

The Side Lyer. The J. A. Preston catalogue stocks a side lyer. This device is useful in breaking up decerebrate posturing. Figure 3–47 shows an alternative method of positioning a patient in sidelying using sand bags, hard cones for the hands, special tennis shoes and a knee pad. By flexing a patient on his side, the effects of the tonic labyrinthine in supine reflex and decerebrate posturing are reduced. The patient is also conditioned for sitting by this type of positioning. As with any bed positioning, the patient should be repositioned every few hours.

Footboards. Footboards are commonly used devices to prevent foot drop secondary to disuse or to the sheets pulling down on the dorsum of the foot. Some hospital beds even have built-on footboards. The neurophysiological rationale is that the footboard maintains the ankle at 90 degrees but exerts pressure into the ball of the foot. *Caution:* In patients having upper motor neuron damage, this stimulus may facilitate the positive supporting reaction and produce plantar flexion (Fiorentino, 1973). Therefore a footboard may actually stimulate the pattern one is trying to prevent.

Special Shoes. As discussed earlier, high-topped tennis shoes are used to position the patient's ankles at 90 degrees. Figure 3–47 and Figure 7–38 show these shoes. If the patient is placed in these shoes immediately after head injury, equinus deformity can frequently be prevented.

For facilitating weight bearing during a play or activity sequence, the "shoe 2″ × 4″ device" is used (Fig. 7–39). The neurophysiological concept behind use of this device is the same as for the tennis shoes. The patient is able to bear weight at the heels and develop sit-squat to stand patterns or weight shifting without facilitating the positive supporting reaction. This device may be used during the squat-inversion sequence shown in Figure 3–14.

In construction, the size and depth of the board used vary with the patient's height and foot size. The taller the patient, the longer and deeper the board should be to provide clearance for the feet and stability. Long, sturdy screws with flat heads are used to secure leather or other durable shoes to the board. The screws are inserted down through the heels into the board. A countersink is used to ensure that the heads of the screws will not bother the patient. A felt pad may be glued in over the screws if necessary. The front section of the shoe is cut away so that the toes and balls of the feet are free.

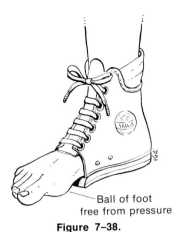

Ball of foot
free from pressure

Figure 7–38.

Slings and Related Devices. Shoulder subluxation is one of the most serious management problems in treating a patient with upper motor neuron damage. The shoulder probably subluxates for several reasons, including the weight of a heavy edematous extremity and muscular imbalance that accompanies upper motor neuron damage. Although some studies have been conducted measuring the effectiveness of various static slings in reducing or preventing subluxation, as yet, the author knows of no study which has compared the effectiveness of static and dynamic slings.

Robins (1969) discusses four major reasons one should avoid using hemiplegia slings. (1) The sling may interfere with body image. (2) It holds the arm in a flexed position, reinforcing the flexion position and seemingly inhibiting the triceps. (3) A sling may interfere with postural support during various activities. (4) A sling may impede the development of a good gait pattern. Obviously, the ideal situation would be to begin treatment immediately after a patient is stabilized following a cerebrovascular accident or related head trauma. Early involvement in an active neurorehabilitation program promoting

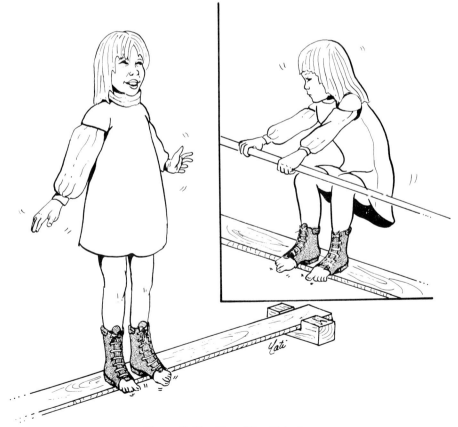

Figure 7–39. Shoe 2″ × 4″ device.

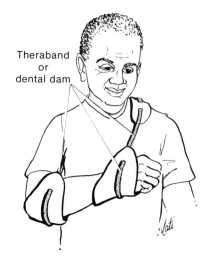

Figure 7–40. Standard cuff sling transformed into dynamic sling.

balanced tone at the shoulder may eliminate the need for a sling. Realistically, this is frequently impossible. Many patients are not even referred for therapy until muscle imbalance has already developed.

Ritt and Belkin (1980) studied four commonly used static slings, including the cuff type sling, clavicular strap, figure 8, and shoulder saddle designs. All slings were measured for proper fit before and after activity. Ritt and Belkin found that the traditional static cuff sling best maintained shoulder alignment but facilitated abnormal flexor pattern. It is hoped that Ritt and Belkin's excellent study presented at the national convention of the American Occupational Therapy Association in Denver, Colorado, April, 1980, will soon be published.

The *cuff sling* can be transformed into a dynamic sling for patients with an edematous upper extremity (Fig. 7–40). Theraband (heavy duty) is substituted for the webbing strap traditionally used. The elbow should be positioned at more than 90 degrees of flexion so that the biceps are not on stretch. Once the patient is positioned in this device, x-rays of the shoulder are recommended to determine if the device is correcting the subluxation.

The orthokinetic splint discussed earlier in the chapter can also be combined with Theraband and a saddle-sling design to make a *sling-splint*. The saddle is positioned over the affected shoulder. One dynamic strap comes from the back of the saddle, crosses the triceps and acts as an orthokinetic segment, and is tied to a "D" ring added to the outside surface of the proximal end of the forearm bar behind the orthokinetic segment strap (Fig. 7–41).

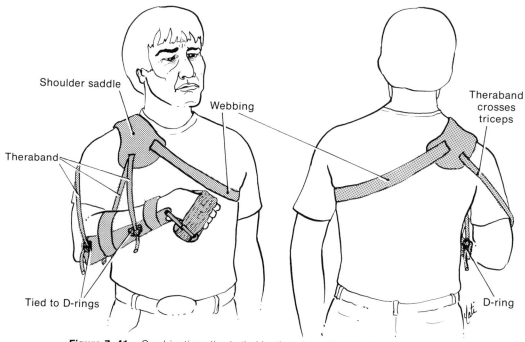

Figure 7–41. Combination sling/orthokinetic wrist splint (designed by Farber).

Two Theraband straps come from the front of the saddle, one to the proximal end of the forearm bar on the inner side (the side nearest the patient's trunk) to a "D" ring, and one strap to a "D" ring on the outer surface positioned directly proximal to the orthokinetic wrist strap. A webbing strap goes from the front of the saddle, across the chest, and under the opposite axilla to attach to the back of the saddle (Fig. 7–41). The elbow must be flexed at more than 90 degrees to ensure that the biceps muscle is not on stretch.

Another dynamic sling was originally designed by Mary Jo Winsinky, RPT, and adapted by the author (Fig. 7–42). This sling is designed to give a quick stretch to the triceps; as the triceps contracts, it does so against resistance provided by one of the dynamic straps. The hard hand cone inhibits flexors by exerting pressure into the insertions of the wrist and finger flexors.

The sling is used for patients who are free of shoulder pain but have a muscular imbalance with hypertonicity in the internal rotators, flexors, adductors, and prona-tors. It is most effective when used during gait or a similar activity, but it can also be used by a patient during a moderately active exercise such as propelling a wheel-chair.

This sling does not work well at reducing subluxation in patients having a heavy edematous extremity. It is also uncomfortable for a patient having shoulder-hand syndrome because the shoulder saddle is placed over the affected shoulder. If the patient's hand rolls over the cone into excessive flexion, or if excessive radial or ulnar deviation occurs at the wrist, the sling should not be used.

Theraband or dental dam is used for the hosing. A saddle is cut out of leather and two slits are cut into it to allow the hosing to pass through. Once the hosing is inserted, a square of Ping-Pong paddle rubber is glued to the inside saddle surface over the hose. The Ping-Pong paddle rubber keeps the saddle from slipping on the patient's shoulder. A hand cone is constructed from Polyform, Polyflex, Kay Splint, or Ortho-plast; a groove must be placed in the cone on the radial side for the thumb. The hose

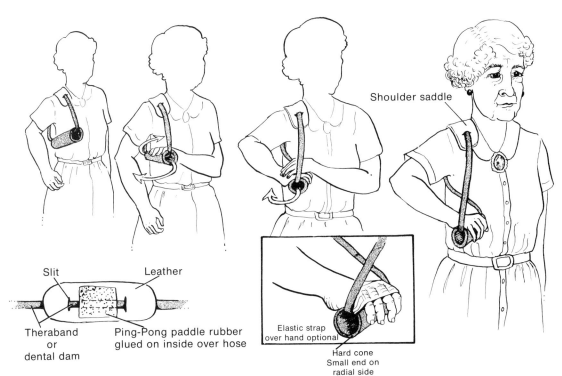

Figure 7–42. Winsinky dynamic hemi-sling (adapted by Farber).

is then tied inside the cone; the elbow is positioned at more than 90 degrees of flexion. An orthokinetic strap can be added to the cone to help keep the hand on the cone.

Instructions for Use. It is critical that this sling be correctly positioned on the patient. The sling is placed upon the shoulder with the cone hanging inferior to the axilla and with the small end of the cone pointing back away from the patient (Fig. 7–42). The cone is then rotated so that the small end turns to the patient's midline and ends up pointing forward. The small end of the cone should end up on the radial side of the hand.

Note: This sling is very confusing to patients and caregivers alike. If it can be correctly fitted and if the patient (or caregiver) can put it on correctly, it has proved to be an effective device. The therapist must remember that many patients become perceptually disoriented following a cerebrovascular accident and ease of sling application may be a major consideration.

Vestibular Input Equipment

THE FARBER-RADABAUGH HORSE. This piece of equipment was originally designed by the author and constructed and adapted by Jeffrey Radabaugh, OTR. The roller chair forces the patient to sit in abduction, which improves trunk support. Dynamic straps can be added to the back to further enhance trunk support (see Fig. 7–29). The roller chair "horse" can be mounted on a rocker platform so that righting and equilibrium responses can be stimulated.

The patient must have some trunk balance in order to use this equipment. The horse should not be used if it causes adversive responses or if the patient has severe hypotonicity in midline extensor musculature.

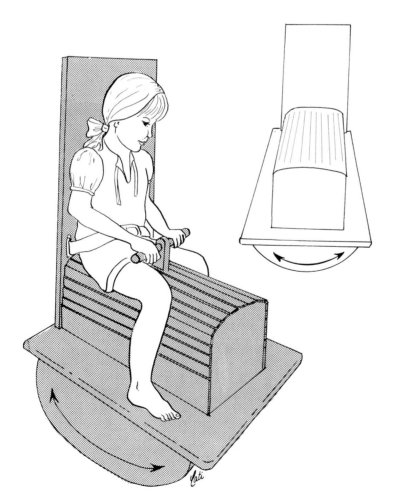

Figure 7–43. Farber-Radabaugh horse.

The horse is constructed from wood and is varnished. The slats on the roller chair should be closely spaced. Dimensions of the horse vary depending on the patient's size.

Note: The horse can be mounted on the rocker platform so that the rocking motion is in an anteroposterior direction or in a side-to-side direction. The platform should be large enough to safely support the roller chair unit (Fig. 7–43). The patient should be able to sit on the horse with his feet flat on the rocking platform.

THERAPY BALLS. Therapy balls can be ordered from a number of manufacturers (listed at the end of this section). They come in a variety of sizes and materials (Fig. 7–44). Therapists use therapy balls for inverting patients, facilitating righting and equilibrium responses and for many gross motor activities. When ordering a therapy ball, the therapist should consider the average height and weight of patients treated at a given facility. The ball should be large enough to support an inverted patient without allowing his hands to touch the mat surface. Inflating devices with which to quickly add or remove air are also available from the manufacturers.

BOLSTERS. Like therapy balls, bolsters come in an extensive range of sizes. Some bolsters are mounted on floor stands; some are free standing or are suspended from chains to make bolster swings (Fig. 7–45).

CEILING SUPPORT SYSTEMS. Many pieces of equipment that provide movement are suspended from the ceiling. Extreme caution should be exercised when equipment is suspended to avoid injury to the patient. Southpaw Enterprises Inc. carries a complete line of vestibular input equipment, including a manual on ceiling support application. The address of this company is listed at the end of this section.

THE MARX SIT'N SPIN. This is another useful device for vestibular input for children. It encourages active participation on the part of the patient. The Sit'n Spin is available in most toy stores.

SCOOTER BOARDS AND CREEPERS. These devices are used by many therapists to facilitate movement in prone position. Creepers and scooter boards (Fig. 7–46) can be easily constructed and are also commercially available. (See the list of manufacturers at the end of this section.)

TRICYCLES. Tricycles are used extensively in the multisensory approach to neurorehabilitation for children and for adults. The patient can actively participate

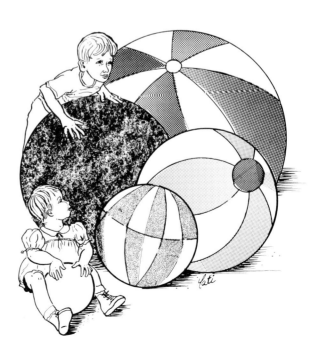

Figure 7–44. Therapy balls.

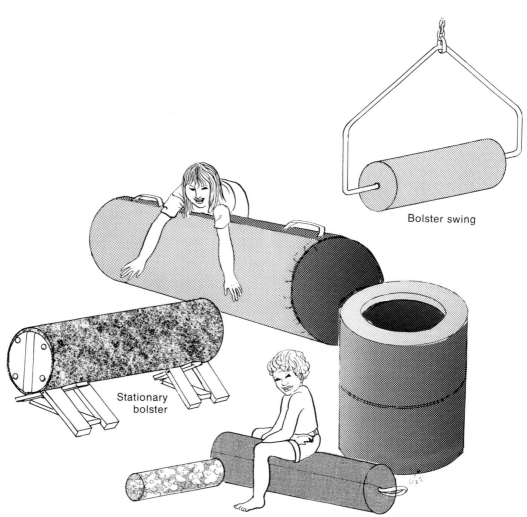

Bolster swing

Stationary
bolster

Figure 7–45. Bolsters.

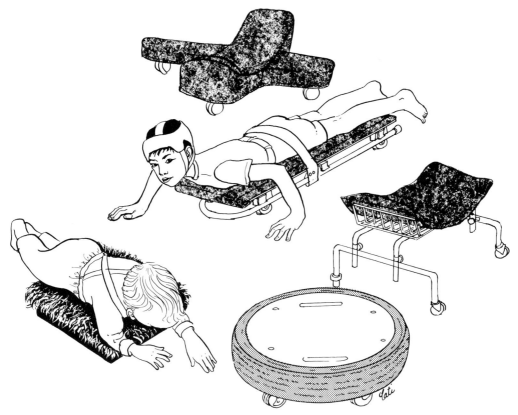

Figure 7–46. Scooter boards and creepers.

in creating the movement stimulus, and using a tricycle promotes a good reciprocal pattern. Adapted tricycles (Fig. 7–47) are available from The Equipment Shop, Cleo Living Aides and Community Playthings. (Addresses are at the end of this section.)

INFANT WALKER. The infant walker (Fig. 7–48) is one piece of equipment that is widely misused by parents of normal and developmentally delayed children. Infants are frequently placed in walkers before they establish co-contraction patterns at proximal joints. The infants learn to reciprocate and bear weight before they are ready to be upright. In addition, many infants who spend large amounts of time in walkers miss the sensory experience of belly crawling and creeping on the floor. The author recommends avoiding general use of infant walkers.

ADDITIONAL VESTIBULAR EQUIPMENT. It is not possible to list every piece of equipment used for vestibular input. Many types have been designed by cre-

ative therapists and manufacturers. The therapist is reminded of the precautions to vestibular input listed in Chapter 3. The following manufacturers have a complete line of equipment useful for vestibular therapy:

Cleo Living Aids
3957 Mayfield Rd.
Cleveland, OH 44121

The Equipment Shop
P.O. Box 33
Bedford, MA 01730

J. A. Preston Corp.
71 5th Ave.
New York, NY 10003

Rifton Equipment for the Handicapped
Division of Community Playthings
Hutterian Society of Brothers
Rifton, NY 12471

S. D. E. Co.–AMPRO Corp.
P.O. Box 6300
1340 N. Jefferson St.
Anaheim, CA 92807

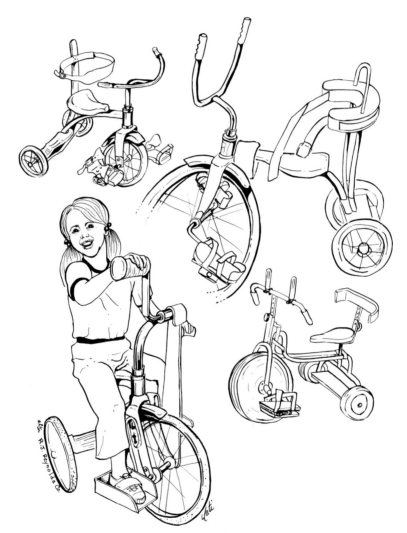

Figure 7–47. Adapted tricycles.

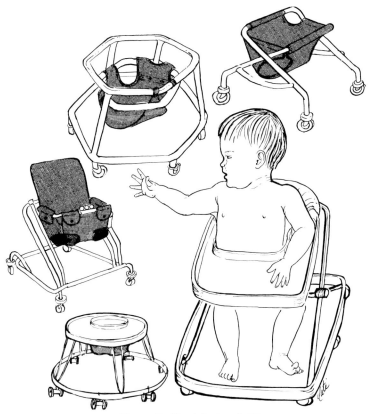

Figure 7–48. Infant walkers.

Fred Sammons, Inc.
Box 32
Brookfield, IL 60513

Southpaw Enterprises Inc.
2909 Edgemoor Lane
Moraine, OH 45435

ORAL FACILITATION DEVICES. The squeeze bottle with a modified mouth shell has been effective in promoting sucking. It is constructed from a Clairol applicator bottle (or similar plastic squeeze bottle), fish tank hose, and Aquaplast. The neurophysiological rationale for the device is that the Aquaplast mouth shell (Fig. 7–49) provides maintained pressure over the orbicularis oris muscle thus promotoing sucking. Since the squeeze bottle creates a vacuum once the patient seals his lips around the straw, liquid is drawn up into the patient's mouth.

In construction, place a piece of paper over the patient's mouth in order to trace a pattern for the mouth shell. Push a small amount of the paper between the patient's lips to make a slight shelf in the mouth shell. Trace around the mouth, leaving a notch for the nose. The shell is shaped like the mouth shield around a NUK brand pacifier. Transfer the pattern to the Aquaplast splinting material. Heat the small square of Aquaplast and cut out the shell with scissors. Shape the Aquaplast over the patient's lips, pushing a small amount of the splinting material between the patient's lips. Hold the material in place until it hardens. Remove it from the patient's mouth and place it in ice water for a few minutes. Then use a heat gun directed to the middle of the mouth crease and heat a small section. Push a wooden dowel rod that is the same diameter as the "straw" through the heated spot. When the hole cools, insert a length of fish tank hose (to be used for the straw) and reheat the same spot in the mouth crease. This will cause the mouth shell to bond to the plastic of the fish tank tube. Insert the other end of the straw into the squeeze bottle after cutting it on an angle. Instruct the patient to wash the mouth shell in cool water.

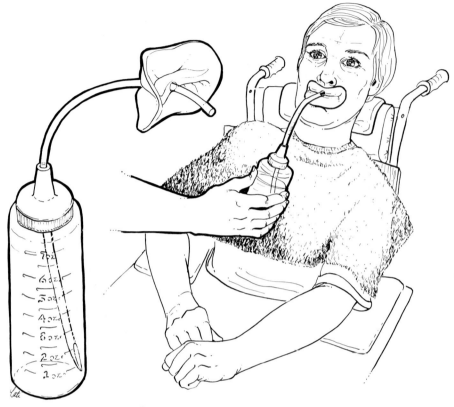

Figure 7–49. The squeeze bottle.

Another oral facilitation device is the *rubber seizure stick.* It is shaped like a tongue blade and is available from most hospital supply houses. It was designed to be placed in the mouth of a patient having a grand mal seizure to prevent him from injuring his tongue. It is useful for intraoral stimulation when the therapist cannot use his fingers in the patient's mouth.

REFERENCES

Blashy M, Fuchs RL: Am J Occup Ther 13:226, 1959.

Blashy M, Harrison HE, Fuchs EM: Orthokinetics, a preliminary report on recent experiences with a little-known rehabilitation therapy. VA Information Bull IB 10–72, 1955.

DiCarlo C, Forbis A: Chair for the child with hypertonic CNS dysfunction. Phys Ther 57:1151, 1977.

Dunkel R, Trefler E: Seating for cerebral palsied children — the sleek seat. Phys Ther 57:524–526, 1977.

Farber SD: Sensorimotor Evaluation and Treatment Procedures for Allied Health Personnel, 2nd ed. Indianapolis, Indiana University Foundation, 1974.

Fiorentino M: Reflex Testing Methods for Evaluating Central Nervous System Development, 2nd ed. Springfield, IL, Charles C Thomas Publishers, 1973.

Fuchs J: Technische Operationen in der Orthopaedie (Orthokinetics). Berlin, Julius Springer, 1927.

Fulford FE, Brown JK: Position as a cause of deformity in children with cerebral palsy. Dev Med Child Neurol 18:305–314, 1976.

Kiel JH: Basic Hand Splinting: A Pattern Designing Approach. Boston, Little, Brown and Co., Inc., in preparation.

Montgomery P, Gauger J: Dynamic trunk stabilizer for children with cerebral palsy. Phys Ther 58:447, 1978.

Neeman RL: Technique of preparing effective orthokinetic cuffs. Bulletin on Practice VI. Washington, DC, American Occupational Therapy Association, Feb. 1971.

Rider B: Study on orthokinetic cuffs. Bulletin on Practice V. Washington DC, American Occupational Therapy Association, 1970.

Ritt BJ, Belkin J: Comparative study: sling supports for subluxed hemiplegic shoulder. Presentation at the American Occupational Therapy Association national convention, Denver, Colorado, 1980.

Robinault I: Functional Aids for the Multiply Handicapped Child. Hagerstown, MD, Harper and Row, 1973.

Robins V: Should patients with hemiplegia wear a sling? Phys Ther 49:1029–1030, 1969.

Waterman M: Goals, advantages, measurements of adapted wheelchairs. Presentation at the American Occupational Therapy Association national convention, San Diego, 1978.

Zislis JM: Splinting of hand in a spastic hemiplegic patient. Archives of Physical Medicine and Rehabilitation, January 1964.

INDEX

Page numbers in *italics* indicate illustrations; those followed by (t) indicate tables.

269